Traumatology for the Emergency Doctor

Dominique Saragaglia
Ali Hassan Chamseddine

Traumatology for the Emergency Doctor

Springer

Dominique Saragaglia
Faculty of medicine
University Grenoble-Alpes
Domaine de la Merci, La Tronche, France

Ali Hassan Chamseddine
Dept. of Orthopedic Surgery
Sahel General Hospital
Beirut, Lebanon

ISBN 978-3-031-63195-5 ISBN 978-3-031-63196-2 (eBook)
https://doi.org/10.1007/978-3-031-63196-2

Translation from the French language edition: "Traumatologie à l'usage de l'urgentiste (3ème édition)" by Dominique Saragaglia and Ali Hassan Chamseddine, © Sauramps Médical 2023. Published by Sauramps Médical. All Rights Reserved.

This Springer imprint is published by the registered company Springer Nature Switzerland AG
The registered company address is: Gewerbestrasse 11, 6330 Cham, Switzerland

Preface

Traumatology has always been considered a surgical specialty. Before the 1970s, it was mainly managed by general surgeons and then gradually taken over by orthopedic surgeons. Today, with the considerable increase in the number of patients admitted to emergency departments, nonsurgical traumatology is struggling to be managed by surgeons who are often busy, either in consultation or in the operating theatre, and are barely available for traumatic emergencies requiring immediate care. Nonsurgical traumatology is difficult to learn from books because, on the one hand, the books in question are intended for more or less specialized surgeons and, on the other hand, many details do not exist in these books; these details are learned "on the job" through companionship between senior and junior surgeons.

This handbook is intended for emergency physicians and for fellows in training to become general or orthopedic surgeons. It is not an encyclopedia, nor is it a treatise compiling a large bibliography relating the opinions of various authors without always knowing what is the right thing to do or not to do. It is a compendium of the practices of a department whose head has considerable experience in orthopedic-traumatology: 41 years of experience in orthopedic surgery with more than 25,000 patients operated on and 150,000 patients in consultation and 29 years of leading and managing an academic orthopedic surgery department with an attached limb trauma emergency unit where more than 350,000 cases have been "scrutinized" during the daily morning staff meetings.

The users of this handbook will be able to find out how to make a precise diagnosis to avoid falling into the traps that are unfortunately very common in this type of traumatology, which sometimes seems benign but where ignorance and misunderstanding of certain diagnoses are sources of painful conflicts. They will also find precise guidelines, adapted to different cases, and above all indications on what is surgical, what could be, and what never is. However, they will not find information on other areas of traumatology that we no longer have experience in, such as ophthalmological, otorhinolaryngological, and maxillofacial traumatology, thoraco-abdominal, vascular, urological, and gynecological traumatology, or polytraumatology.

With this book, we aim to share our tried and tested experience, which we regularly discuss at our daily morning staff meetings attended by orthopedic surgeons, emergency physicians, orthopedic fellows, residents on duty in emergency departments, and medical students.

Domaine de la Merci,
La Tronche,
France

Dominique Saragaglia

Acknowledgments

- **Dr. Jean Jacques BANIHACHEMI**
  - Emergency doctor.
  - Grenoble-Alpes University Hospital.
- **Dr. Emmanuel BRIOT**
  - Anesthesiologist.
  - Grenoble-Alpes University Hospital.
- **Dr. Frédéric DUROURE**
  - Plastic surgeon.
  - Ex-practitioner at Grenoble-Alpes University Hospital.
- **Dr. Caroline HALLÉ**
  - Anesthesiologist.
  - Ex-practitioner at Grenoble-Alpes University Hospital.
- **Dr. Abdelhafid LEGSAIR**
  - Anesthesiologist.
  - Ex-practitioner at Grenoble-Alpes University Hospital.
- **Prof. François MOUTET**
  - Hand and plastic surgeon.
  - Ex-head of division of Hand and Plastic Surgery at Grenoble-Alpes University Hospital.
- **Prof. Jean Guy PASSAGGIA**
  - Neuro-surgeon.
  - Ex-head of Department of Neuro-Surgery at Grenoble-Alpes University Hospital.

About the Authors

Dominique Saragaglia was the Head of the Department of Orthopaedic Surgery and Traumatology at Grenoble University Medical Center—South Hospital (France) for 29 years. He has gained considerable experience in orthopedics and traumatology, having operated on over 25,000 patients and seen more than 150,000 patients in the outpatient department. He has authored more than 200 papers, as well as several books and chapters, in both French and English. He also has more than 1000 abstracts and oral presentations in national and international meetings. He is currently Professor Emeritus of Orthopedic Surgery at Grenoble-Alpes University, an honorary member of the SOFCOT (French Orthopaedic Society) and several other international societies, and a member of the French National Academy of Surgery.Every morning, as part of his daily practice as the head of the department, he would review with the residents and all staff members the trauma cases presented to the emergency department the previous day, verifying the accuracy of diagnoses and treatments. By doing so, he was able to review and analyze more than 350,000 cases, ranging from the simplest wound to the most serious trauma.

Ali Hassan Chamseddine is a member of the French College of Orthopedic surgeons, a member of the National Academy of Surgery (France), and a fellow of the American College of Surgeons. He served as President of the Lebanese Orthopedic Society, Chairman of the AO Chapter in Lebanon, and Vice-President of the Pan Arab Orthopedic Association. With 30 years of experience in surgical and academic activities in Beirut, Lebanon, he held the position of head of the Division of Orthopedic and Trauma Surgery at Sahel General Hospital-University Medical Center for 15 years and at the Faculty of Medical Sciences, Lebanese University, for 8 years. He has been responsible for the post-graduate teaching and residency program in Orthopedic and Trauma Surgery at the Lebanese University for over 15 years.Professor Chamseddine is a regular reviewer for international orthopedic peer-reviewed journals and has authored 45 papers, with more than 150 abstracts and oral presentations in national and international meetings. He has chaired and organized over ten regional and international orthopedic and trauma congresses and courses in Lebanon and the Middle East region. In addition to his orthopedic surgical practice, he has a special interest in trauma surgery and fracture treatment and has developed multiple innovative techniques in the field.

Contents

Part I

Generalities

1 Definitions

Traumatology (from Greek trauma, means injury or wound and logos: speech) is a branch of medicine dedicated to study the wounds and injuries produced by accidents or violence to the body, their mechanisms, their repair and surgical treatments, as well as their complications and sequelae. It is considered as a surgical specialty and is usually a sub-specialty of the orthopedic surgery.

Traumatism: a physical or psychological harmful action, either accidental or intentional, caused by a person or an object.

Fracture (from Latin: "fractus," past participle of "frangere," meaning rupture): the rupture of continuity or the separation of an object or a material into two or more parts in response to stress. A fracture is described with respect to:

- Affected bone and its side (i.e., right or left: humerus, radius, femur, tibia, etc.)
- Site or location in the corresponding bone: diaphyseal, metaphyseal, epiphyseal, diaphyso-metaphyseal, metaphyso-epiphyseal, etc.
- Soft tissue envelop condition: closed fracture or compound (open) fracture with or without exposed bony fragments through the open site
- Displacement: non-displaced or displaced (varus, valgus, rotation, shortening, etc.)
- Associated lesions: vascular and, or, neurologic impairment
- Cause: obstetrical, traumatic, pathologic, stress, etc.

Diaphysis (so-called shaft): the portion of a long bone located between its two extremities (so-called epiphyses). It has a tube-like shape that encloses the medullary canal.

Epiphysis: the rounded end of a long bone; its surface is covered with an articular cartilage, and its main role is to connect two adjacent bones together to make a joint.

Metaphysis: the part of a long bone located between the epiphysis and the diaphysis.

D. Saragaglia, A. Hassan Chamseddine, *Traumatology for the Emergency Doctor*, https://doi.org/10.1007/978-3-031-63196-2_1

Growth plate (so-called epiphyseal plate): a thin layer of cartilage that gives growth to the long bones, located between the epiphysis and the metaphysis.

Dislocation or Luxation (from Latin luxare): a complete displacement of one articular component (one articular surface) with respect to the other, resulting in a total loss of the normal anatomic joint configuration; it may be closed or open. A partial displacement of the articular surfaces is called sub-luxation.

Fracture-dislocation: the association of both injuries in the same joint, and at the same time (fracture and dislocation).

Sprain: an articular injury induced by a sudden distortion or a twist of the joint without permanent displacement of the articular surfaces; it involves capsulo-ligamentous lesions with different grades of severity ranging from benign (grade 1: capsulo-ligamentous simple overstretch) to intermediate (grade 2: capsulo-ligamentous partial tear) and severe (grade 3: capsulo-ligamentous complete tear).

Contusion or Bruise: typically a mechanical injury caused by a direct blow with a hard tool; it usually induces skin discoloration (Ecchymosis) without breakage. The discoloration is the result of blood leak just under the skin from adjacent disrupted blood vessels. A contusion may progress into healing or be unpredictably complicated by a skin necrosis and local infection.

Ecchymosis: as previously mentioned, an area of skin discoloration (purple and blue color) due to the effusion of blood from the ruptured capillaries into the mucosa or the sub-cutaneous tissue.

Wound: a condition where the continuity or the integrity of any living soft tissue is interrupted by a cut, a blow, or any other traumatic impact, and typically results in a skin opening or breakage.

A wound is defined according to the:

- Etiology: stab wound, gun shot, shrapnel, animal or human bite, direct blow, etc.
- Location in the body: face, eye, chest wall, arm, thigh, etc.
- Extent and importance: length, depth, etc.
- Appearance: simple, net, contused, shattered, dilacerated, etc.
- Involved tissues: skin, aponeurosis, muscle, neuro-vascular, etc.
- Septic character: clean, contaminated, infected, etc.

Hematoma: an extravasated blood in any organ, space, or tissue of the body; it may be diffuse or collected. Hematomas always develop with fractures. Small hematomas are usually absorbed unless infection arises.

Blister, Bullae, or Vesicle: a raised portion of the uppermost layer of the skin (epidermis) in the form of a closed bubble filled with fluid (serous or blood).

Skin erosion: a superficial skin lesion that induces loss of some or all of the epidermis thickness, leaving a denuded surface.

Morel-Lavallée lesion: a **closed traumatic degloving soft tissue injury** characterized by a separation of the hypodermis from the underlying fascia, with collection of lympho-hematic fluid between the tissue layers (usually in lumbar region, buttock and thigh); the fluid collection has virtually no potential for resorption. It is induced by a shearing force secondary to a high velocity trauma.

2 Bone Consolidation

Bone consolidation or bone healing is the proliferative physiological process of fracture repair; it involves complex successive stages leading to the formation of a new living bone that bridges the fracture site.

2.1 General Considerations

- *A peri-fracture hematoma*, resulting from the local bleeding from the peri-osteal vessels and the surrounding muscles, occurs after the initial trauma. It provides a rich milieu with a variety of cells that locally produce different crucial factors for the future fracture healing.
- The formation of a "*peripheral*" *peri-osteal callus* is the first step of the bone healing process; it is enhanced by the presence of controlled micro-movements at the fracture site and may be inhibited by a "too rigid" internal fixation. The periosteum itself is fundamental for the formation of the peri-osteal callus, an indispensable contributor to bone consolidation.
- In addition to the "peripheral" callus, an "internal" intra-medullary *endosteal callus* develops more slowly.
- After the formation of the two callus is complete, the *remodeling* of the newly formed bone begins. It involves a progressive resorption of the callus with a simultaneous formation of lamellar bone in adaptation to loads and according to the Wolff's law. In pediatric patients, the bone remodeling is improved by the proximity of the fracture site to the growth plate; this explains the reason why conservative orthopedic treatment is usually preferred in this age group.
- Radiodense callus is usually seen only after 3–4 weeks following the fracture; this time interval is shorter in pediatric patients and longer for metacarpal and phalangeal fractures.
- When evaluating a bone healing process, both the radiographic features and clinical assessment (especially for pain) should be considered together. For example:

D. Saragaglia, A. Hassan Chamseddine, *Traumatology for the Emergency Doctor*, https://doi.org/10.1007/978-3-031-63196-2_2

- The presence of pain on the clinical assessment should raise a red flag even if the fracture appears consolidated on the radiographs.
- In opposition, a radiographic "insufficient" callus appearance would allow weight bearing (for the lower limb) or cast removal (for the upper limb) in the absence of pain, especially in pediatric patients.

2.2 Time Frame for Bone Healing (in Days)

The following are the mean figures of time (in days) required for the consolidation of a nondisplaced or a mildly displaced fracture treated using conservative orthopedic methods, in pediatric and adult patients. Surgical treatment using internal fixation is more common in the adult group.

Fracture	Infant	Adult
Clavicle	21	45–60
Displaced humeral neck	45	60–90
Nondisplaced humeral neck	21	45
Transverse humeral shaft	60	60–90
Spiral humeral shaft	45	90
Displaced distal humerus (supra-condylar)	45	To be operated
Nondisplaced distal humerus (supra-condylar)	21	60–90
Nondisplaced lateral condyle of the elbow	21	60
Nondisplaced both forearm bones	45	60
Displaced both forearm bones	60	To be operated
Nondisplaced one forearm bone	30	60
Displaced one forearm bone	45	To be operated
Nondisplaced radial head	15	30
Nondisplaced olecranon process	21	60
Radius (buckle or torus fracture)	21	45
Distal radius	30	60
Scaphoid bone	60	90–120
Metacarpal, phalanx	21	60
Femoral shaft	60–80	To be operated
Supra-condylar femur	45	To be operated
Proximal tibia	45	60–90
Tibial shaft (isolated)	60	60–90
Both bones of the leg (tibial and fibular shafts)	60–80	90–120
Distal tibia	45	60–90
Lateral malleolus	21	45–60
Calcaneus	30	90
Metatarsals	21	45–60

- **Bone consolidation** is usually defined according to radiographic and clinical signs: callus bridging of three or more cortices on two different radiographic views with absence of pain at the fracture site on palpation and weight bearing.
- **Delayed union** is usually defined as the absence of callus formation on radiographs in the interval between the normal time of healing and 6 months post-fracture.

– **Nonunion** has been defined in various terms, such as the absence of any progressive radiographic signs of bone healing for at least 3 consecutive months after the regular time of fracture healing or the absence of fracture healing after at least 9 months from the time of the fracture. Nonunion is primarily classified into hypertrophic and atrophic types, both of which are believed to reflect different aspects of the condition's pathophysiology. Hypertrophic nonunion basically has a satisfactory biological environment and an adequate vascularity to allow bone consolidation; it is mainly caused by an inadequate stabilization of the fracture site and has a radiographic aspect of abundant nonorganized callus, the so-called elephant's foot. In opposition, atrophic nonunion usually lacks healthy biological milieu and adequate blood irrigation; it usually shows sharp margins and sclerotic fracture edges on the radiographs.

2.3 Traditional Precepts

– The younger the patient, the shorter the fracture healing time.
– In contrast with epiphyseal fractures, diaphyseal fractures in pediatric patients commonly have a smooth long term progression, as they do not involve the growth plate.
– The times required for the consolidation of diaphyseal fractures are comparable in adolescent and adult patients.
– The epiphyseal fractures have a faster healing time compared to the diaphyseal fractures.
– A persistent fracture line appearance on the radiographs is not always synonymous of nonunion: one should always consider together the radiographic and clinical presentations (i.e., pain).
– In pediatric patients, the consolidation of the diaphyseal fractures is associated with a risk of final permanent lengthening of the bone segment (more frequent with an initial anatomic or perfect reduction).
– The residual rotation deformity is not corrected by the remodeling process of bone healing.

3 Pain Control for Patients with Limb Injury in Emergency Settings

The pain control for limbs injuries involves a wide variety of scenarios related to many factors, such as the diversity of the injuries, the heterogeneous types of the patients (age, previous general condition), the context and the setting of the initial management (on the field or in the emergency department), and the qualifications and the habits of the different interveners and protagonists. This chapter discusses the outlines of the pain control methods in emergency setting; a detailed inventory of these methods is out of the purpose of this handbook.

3.1 Pain Control Using Immobilization and Fixation

The immobilization of the injured limb is the first and the simplest method to control the pain and it contributes to providing analgesia. However, the administration of an analgesic medication may be necessary prior to achieve the immobilization or the temporary fixation of the limb (undressing the patient, application of a trans-osseous traction, application of a cast or a slab).

3.2 Analgesia and Pain Control Using Systemic Drug Administration

One should distinguish hypnosis and analgesia.

3.2.1 Systemic Administration of Sedative/Hypnotic Drugs

While sedative/hypnotic drugs like benzodiazepines, antihistamines, barbiturates, ketamine, and propofol do not have analgesic effects, they can be beneficial in trauma patients due to their sedative and anxiolytic properties. These drugs can help to reduce anxiety and induce sleep, which can be particularly helpful in managing

D. Saragaglia, A. Hassan Chamseddine, *Traumatology for the Emergency Doctor*, https://doi.org/10.1007/978-3-031-63196-2_3

the psychological aspects of trauma. However, they should not be used as first line medication for pain control. On the other hand, they potentiate the effects of morphine when used together; they accordingly may improve the analgesic properties of morphine at the same time as they can exacerbate its side effects (respiratory and cardiovascular depression).

The most common used medications are as follows.

3.2.1.1 Benzodiazepines

Midazolam is a commonly used benzodiazepine in anesthesia due to its rapid onset of action (about 1 min after IV administration) and short half-life (about 1 h). However, it is important to note that the half-life can be extended in elderly and newborn patients. This is due to differences in how these individuals metabolize the drug.

- Dosage: it is typically presented in vials of 1 mg/mL. Its IV administration in adult patients is usually performed mL by mL every 5 min with the doses being titrated according to the patient's response until the desired degree of sedation is achieved. This method allows for precise control over the level of sedation, ensuring the patient's safety and comfort.
- The main side effects are excessive sedation and respiratory depression (especially in elderly patients and when associated with morphine).
- The intra-rectal route of administration is common in newborn and pediatric patients (using a cannula or a soft small catheter) generally with a delayed onset of action (10–15 min). The recommended dosage is 0.3 mg/kg (without dilution).

3.2.1.2 Anti-histaminic Drugs

Hydroxyzine (*Atarax*[R]) is the most common used anti-histamine drug. While it does have sedative and anxiolytic effects, these are generally considered to be less potent than those of benzodiazepines. It is commonly used per os (by mouth) in pediatric patients.

- Dosage is 1 mg/kg in both pediatric and adult patients. The syrup galenic form is very useful in children. Other galenic presentations are also available such as tablets and ampoules.
- The action onset of the oral form is 15–30 min; it lasts for 6–8 h and has minimal side effects.

3.2.1.3 Barbiturates, Ketamine, and Propofol

The use of these drugs is inadvisable and imprudent for non-anesthesiology specialists due to their potent effects and potential risks. These drugs require careful dosing and monitoring to ensure patient safety.

3.2.2 Analgesics Through Systemic Route of Administration

Analgesic drugs can be used according to the scheme of three levels for pain management as defined and recommended by the WHO

3.2.2.1 Level 1: Paracetamol and NSAID's

- They are used as first line analgesics for all levels of pain severity.
- They are administered according to systematic plan and doses, for expected prolonged pain, and not on a PRN basis.
- The IV route is preferred for its rapid action onset and efficacy; it is also useful in fasting patients when a surgical intervention is expected.
- NSAIDs may minimally affect the patient's hemostasis and can therefore be administered pre-operatively.

3.2.2.2 Level 2: Codeine, Tramadol, Nalbuphine

1. They are all derivatives of morphine; however, they are less potent than morphine. They are usually useful for pain level <5 (according to the Visual Analogue Scale—VAS—of 10) and when the patient is discharged (less side effects than morphine with oral route administration).
2. One should be cautious of the antagonist effect of these drugs when the use of a pure morphine agonist is anticipated, such as when morphine titration is necessary or if the patient is undergoing general anesthesia.
3. Indications and dosage:
   (a) *Codeine:*
      - can be used after the age of 15 years,
      - PO 60 mg Codeine is approximately equivalent to 10 mg morphine.

   (b) *Tramadol:*
      - available for oral route administration:
         - 50 mg in simple or double dose every 6 h,
         - 100 mg dose with a delayed or a prolonged release form allows more distanced daily administrations,
      - also available for slow IV administration in the form of 100 mg vials (maximum 600 mg daily dose).
      - Numerous generic products exist in the pharmaceutical market: Biodalgic™, Contramal™, Tradmadol™, Zamudol™, to name a few.

   (c) *Nalbuphine:*
      - can be used for IV, IM, and SC injections with doses of 10–20 mg every 3–6 h,
      - the daily dose should not exceed 160 mg,
      - the sub-cutaneous (SC) injection is painful.

3.2.2.3 Level 3: Morphine and "Morphinic" Drugs for Anesthesia (Fentanyl, Sufentanyl)

- The IV route for morphine administration is preferred in the emergency setting because of its rapid action onset and the possibility of titrating doses.
- For this category of drugs, only morphine should be used by the physicians who are not familiar with the use of the "morphinic" anesthetic drugs (major risk of respiratory depression).
- The Morphine titration for direct IV injections is performed at the dose of 1–2 mg every 5–10 min. The VAS for pain assessment, the level of sedation, and the respiratory rate should be monitored and assessed prior to each re-injection. The maintenance dose for the following hours is equivalent to the total dose that was necessary to obtain a VAS ≤3 during the initial titration; it is administered through the sub-cutaneous route every 3–4 h and always after observation and assessment of the VAS, level of sedation, and respiratory rate.
- Oxygen nasal administration (3–5 L/min) is recommended, especially for elderly patients and those with respiratory insufficiency.
- Dosage:
  - The following table shows a comparison of the doses required to obtain the same level of analgesia according to the route of administration:

Oral	Sub-cutaneous	Intra-venous	Peri-dural	Intra-thecal
1 mg	1/2 mg approximately	1/3 mg approximately	1/10 to 1/20 mg	1/50 to 1/200 mg

  - In adult, the administration of morphine is usually started as IV injection of 1 mg that is repeated every 10–15 min until complete sedation is obtained (titration). It is then relayed either with SC injections of 5–10 mg 4–6 times daily or auto-controlled perfusion (auto-controlled analgesia).
  - In patients who have previously received oral morphine, the initial starting daily dose is the half of the oral daily dose. However, it is possible to start with higher doses if the previous oral dose was insufficient for pain control.
  - In pediatric patients, morphine can also be used for pain management; however, dosage handling is more demanding in terms of precautions and team competence.
  - Classical contraindications:

    uncontrolled respiratory insufficiency (in the absence of mechanical ventilation),

    severe liver failure (with encephalopathy),

    head trauma with intracranial hypertension (in the absence of mechanical ventilation),

    uncontrolled convulsive crisis,

    associated use with other "morphinic" drugs that may potentiate respiratory distress (buprenorphine, nalbuphine, pentazocine).

3.3 Analgesia Using Inhalation of Nitrous Oxide

- Nitrous oxide is a gas that potentiate the effect of hypnotic and analgesic drugs and has poor analgesic efficacy when used alone. It is mixed to oxygen in equal parts to avoid its toxic effects (usually occurring when used alone in room air ambiance).
- The available commercialized mixtures of "Oxygen-Nitrous Oxide" (Meopa^{R}, Kalinox^{R}) can be used in association with analgesic and sedative drugs for painful interventions.
- The action onset of Nitrous Oxide is virtually immediate.
- The face mask administration of 5–10 L/min is usually sufficient.
- It is contraindicated in the presence of deep sedation or respiratory distress.

3.4 Analgesia Using Local or Loco-Regional Anesthesia

3.4.1 Local Topical Anesthesia

- **For mucosae**: Lidocaine 5% spray or Lidocaine-Prilocaine cream can be used. In order to avoid local irritation, the duration of contact of the local topical anesthetic with the mucosa should not exceed 20 min.
- **For skin**: Only Lidocaine-Prilocaine formula cream traverses the skin barrier and provides anesthesia of the whole dermis.
  - It should be applied on healthy skin and covered with occlusive dressing 1 h at least before the planned procedure.
  - It has a local vasoconstriction effect. A white local discoloration of the skin is a sign of adequate impregnation of the dermis, and hence of the usefulness and efficacy of the cream.
  - It can be used in pediatric age group patients to prepare the site of insertion of a catheter, for example
- **For eye**: Oxybuprocaine is a key reference ocular local anesthetic. Its chronic use is prohibited as it encompasses a risk of permanent corneal damage related to an induced local insensibility.
- **For sub-cutaneous tissue**:
  - Local sub-cutaneous infiltrations involve utilization of 1% Lidocaine or 1% Mepivacaine solutions. Lidocaine with Adrenaline solutions can also be used, except for digital anesthesia.
  - The infiltration should be performed either into the wound edges (when it is clean and non-contaminated) or around the wound itself.

3.4.2 Local Troncular or Nerve Block Anesthesia

- Local troncular or nerve block anesthesia is useful for the soft tissue as well as for the bony and cartilaginous anatomic structures. Good knowledge of the cutaneous sensory innervation is mandatory. However, in many situations, the innervation of the deep teguments may differ from that of superficial teguments.
- A neurostimulation device is preferably used to identify the targeted nerve; it allows a more precise and efficient local injection of the anesthetic solution with a minimal risk of needle induced nerve injury. The use of neurostimulation devices should be encouraged in the Emergency Departments. The ER physicians should be initiated and trained to use such devices.
- The use of specific utensils is highly recommended:
  - a non-traumatic needle with rounded tip (to avoid direct nerve injury),
  - a long soft extension tube to accommodate with the syringe of the local anesthetic solution,
  - and an electrical connection cable for the neurostimulation tracking.
- The use of 1% lidocaine-adrenaline solution is recommended for its minimal potential toxicity compared to other local anesthetic solutions.
- Convulsions may occur in case of an accidental intra-vascular injection of more than 100 mg of lidocaine; they usually spontaneously disappear after a few seconds. After needle introduction, the drawing back of blood into the syringe (aspiration maneuvers) and the occurrence of tachycardia (induced by intra-vascular passage of adrenaline) are early diagnostic signs of intra-vascular injection of the anesthetic solution. Injection of the solution should be slow and gradual until the occurrence of the pre-convulsive prodromal symptoms of the local anesthetic's neurologic toxicity: speech disturbance, paresthesia, tinnitus, metallic taste sensation, etc. Exceptionally, in case of significant over dosage, arrhythmias and cardiac arrest may occur (essentially with bupivacaine and ropivacaine).
- The efficacy of the nerve block on the thermo-algic sensitivity is tested by the sensibility to the cold in the area that was targeted by the injection (by application of ice or alcohol).
- Contraindications to troncular nerve block anesthesia include: infection at the site of injection, major hemostasis disorders (for deep injections), allergy to local anesthesia solutions (exceptional).
- Maximum authorized dose:
  - Lidocaine without adrenaline: 300 mg for adults, and 5 mg/kg for infants.
  - Lidocaine with adrenaline: 500 mg for adults, and 6–7 mg/kg for infants.
- The most common used nerve blocks are:
  - The femoral nerve block for femoral injuries,
  - The sciatic nerve block (or specific branch block in the ankle for wound care of the foot),
  - The brachial plexus block (or specific nerve block at the elbow or the wrist for wound care of the forearm or the hand, respectively).

3.5 Examples

3.5.1 Wounds or Burns (Mild and Moderate Surface)

- **Sedation**
  - Pediatric patient: Hydroxyzine syrup 1 mg/kg (oral) or Midazolam 0.3 mg/kg (rectal).
  - Adult patient: Hydroxyzine 1 mg/kg (oral) or Midazolam IV 1 mg titration every 5 min.
- **Analgesia**
  - Level 1: Paracetamol, NSAIDs (PO or IV).
  - Level 2:

    Pediatric patient >15 years: Codeine 1 mg/kg.

    Adult: Codeine (PO form associated to paracetamol).
- **Local anesthesia**
  - Lidocaine-Prilocaine cream applied over the wound with occlusive dressing for 20 min maximum.
  - Then injection of the wound edges with Lidocaine 1% solution with or without adrenaline (maximum 5 mg/kg).
- **Prescription on discharge**
  - Level 1: Paracetamol and NSAID's on systematic basis.
  - Level 2: Codeine or Paracetamol + Codeine if Paracetamol and NSAID's are insufficient.
  - Prescription for 4–5 days.

3.5.2 Application of Traction for a Fracture Reduction and Closed Reduction of Dislocation

- Insertion of IV line.
- Sedation: see "Wounds or burns."
- Analgesia:
  - Level 1: see "Wounds or burns."
  - Level 2: direct use of morphine (more efficient, with short half-life).
  - Level 3: Morphine in IV titration (refer to "analgesics through systemic route of administration").
- Nitrous oxide.
- Local anesthesia: Nerve block with 1% Lidocaine-Adrenaline solution (max 6–7 mg/kg) proximal to the injured area.
- Prescription on discharge:
  - See "Wounds or burns,"
  - Patient is kept on the ER until the pain is well controlled without any need for morphine.

- In case of admission:
  - Level 1: systematic administration of Paracetamol and NSAIDs.
  - Level 2: codeine or Paracetamol + Codeine if no previous morphine titration and when 3 < VAS ≤5.
  - Level 3: SC morphine every 3–4 h at the total efficient dose (as monitored during the initial titration) to obtain VAS ≤3 (associate nasal oxygen for fragile patients).
- ***All the above-mentioned analgesics can be administered from the beginning, even if surgical intervention is planned for the next few hours.***

4 Pre-anesthesia Workup for Adult Patients with Limb Injury

Many patients admitted in emergency will require anesthesia as they will undergo either a surgical intervention or a painful procedure, such as a closed reduction of a fracture or a dislocation. A pre-anesthesia consultation (by the anesthesiologist) is medico-legally mandatory; it includes a review of the medical file, the patient's history and physical examination, and the request for specific tests when needed, based on the patient's condition.

In an emergency setting, for the sake of time-saving and to avoid repetitive intravenous punctures, the ER physician usually anticipates by ordering these additional tests himself; this may be related, in some institutions, to difficult communication with the anesthesiologist (busy, not on the field, etc.).

The pre-anesthesia assessment and the explorations ordered by the ER physician should be rational and practical. However, these should be validated (and modified if needed) by the anesthesiologist, as he is the main and final assessor of the condition of patients undergoing anesthesia.

4.1 Characteristics and Particularities of Anesthesia in Traumatology

One should remember:

- The heterogeneous and wide variety of patients ranging from young athletes to elderly patients with multiple comorbidities and medications.
- The surgical treatment may be hemorrhagic and may therefore require transfusion (open treatment of femoral fracture, for example).
- The minimum pre-anesthesia fasting time may not be respected when an urgent intervention is required (open fracture, hip dislocation, knee dislocation, fracture or dislocation with neuro-vascular impairment, etc.).

D. Saragaglia, A. Hassan Chamseddine, *Traumatology for the Emergency Doctor*, https://doi.org/10.1007/973-3-031-63196-2_4

4.1.1 Pre-anesthesia Fasting

- After discussion with the surgeon, and according to the degree of emergency, the anesthesiologist is responsible for determining the required pre-anesthesia fasting time.
- However, one should know that trauma and pain modify the pH and emptying time of the stomach. Accordingly, to define the duration of fasting, it is also important to determine the time of trauma occurrence as well as the time when the patient consumed any food or beverage for the last time before the accident.

4.1.2 Pre-anesthesia Workup and Assessment

- It is recommended to limit the list of pre-operative exams based on the patient's condition.
- The pre-anesthesia workup is a complement of the initial trauma assessment; it takes into consideration:
  - The patient's age.
  - The presence of previous associated pathologies and comorbidities.
  - Any usual intake or consumption of medication.
  - The patient's history and physical exam.
  - The type and nature of the intended surgical procedure.

4.1.2.1 Electrocardiogram (ECG)

- It is recommended for:
  - males of >40 years age and females >50 years,
  - patients with cardiovascular risk factors,
  - when a clinical assessment is impossible or non-reliable,
  - patients taking drugs that can produce ECG disturbance or distortion.
- It should absolutely be done for patients with cardiovascular symptoms or antecedents.

4.1.2.2 Chest Radiography

It is recommended when a clinical cardiopulmonary assessment is impossible or not reliable.

4.1.2.3 Complete Blood Count (CBC)

- It should be requested when the surgery encompasses a potential risk of bleeding: open reduction and internal fixation of fracture of humeral shaft, femoral shaft, etc.
- It should be done when the patient presents symptoms, signs, or risk factors of anemia.

4.1.2.4 Hemostasis and Coagulation Workup

- It is not part of the routine pre-operative workup.
- The diagnosis of coagulation disorder is primarily based on the patient's past medical history and physical exam.
- It is justified when the surgery has a potential risk of bleeding; it includes PT, activated PTT, INR, and platelet count.
- It should be done when the patient is taking antivitamin K.

4.1.2.5 Blood Chemistry Workup

- It is not systematic.
- The tests include: electrolytes, creatinine, and blood sugar.
- They are requested based on the patient's condition and previous treatments (elderly patient, renal failure, diabetes, diuretic treatment, etc.).

4.1.2.6 Immunological Assessment

- It is performed in case of potential risk of surgical bleeding that may lead to transfusion.
- It includes double check of the ABO blood group and Rhesus system, the blood phenotyping, and the presence of any irregular agglutinins.
- Before the transfusion, and for medico-legal issues:
  - A patient's consent for blood transfusion should be obtained.
  - A patient's serum transaminases and serology for HIV and Hepatitis C are requested.

4.2 In Practice

The following table represents the different workups, according to the type of the procedure and the patient's characteristics

Predicted or expected intervention	Pre-anesthesia workup
Fracture of the neck of the femur	Serum electrolytes Serum creatinine, creatinine clearance CBCD PT, activated PTT, Platelets' count Blood group (ABO and Rhesus), dosage of irregular agglutinins Pre-transfusion serology for Hepatitis C and HIV ECG Chest X-ray if patient >60 years Additional tests according to patient's condition
Fracture of the femoral shaft	Serum electrolytes CBCD PT, activated PTT, Platelets count Blood group (ABO and Rhesus), dosage of irregular agglutinins Pre-transfusion serology for Hepatitis C and HIV Additional tests according to patient's condition

Predicted or expected intervention	Pre-anesthesia workup
Fracture: tibia, ankle, foot (surgery with tourniquet)	*According to patient's condition*
Closed reduction of dislocation: hip, hip prosthesis, knee, ankle Closed reduction of fracture: ankle, etc.	*According to patient's condition*
Humerus fracture: surgery without tourniquet	Serum electrolytes CBCD PT, activated PTT, Platelets count Blood group (ABO and Rhesus), dosage of irregular agglutinins Pre-transfusion serology for Hepatitis C and HIV Additional tests according to patient's condition
Humerus fracture: surgery with tourniquet	*According to patient's condition*
Fracture of the elbow, forearm bones, wrist, and hand: surgery with tourniquet	*According to patient's condition*
Closed reduction of fracture of the elbow, wrist, hand	*According to patient's condition*

Management of Wounds

5

Wound is defined as an injury that involves laceration or breaking of the soft tissues of the body; it usually implicates damage to underlying tissues. The main challenge for an ER physician is to distinguish between the types of wounds that he is able to manage alone and those he is not (requiring additional resources). The discrimination is essential to guarantee providing the most appropriate care for the patients.

5.1 Description of the Wound Is the First Fundamental Step

- *The responsible traumatic agent* can provide a primary orientation regarding the severity of the injury. Some wounds are beyond the competence of the ER physician:
  - Wounds caused by broken glass are often more jagged and extensive than they appear at first glance,
  - Wounds induced by industrial or professional tools are usually a source of extensive damage.
- *The aspect of the wound*:
  - Superficial cut wound with clear and linear edges are easy to repair,
  - Wound with contused or shredded edges or those involving multiple or deep tissues are difficult to repair by the ER physician,
  - Simple skin abrasions are often easy to manage.
- *The extent of the wound* may be a source of difficulties regarding its debridement, suture, and coverage dressing.
- *The trajectory of the wound* is a main element of its description. Is it over:
  - An area of a neuro-vascular bundle? (e.g., Scarpa's triangle, volar aspect of the wrist, etc.).
  - An important anatomic structure? (e.g., extensor tendons at the dorsal aspect of the wrist, parotid duct on the face, etc.).

D. Saragaglia, A. Hassan Chamseddine, *Traumatology for the Emergency Doctor*, https://doi.org/10.1007/978-3-031-63196-2_5

  - A “risky” or “dangerous” region? (e.g., anterior aspect of the neck, cervico-thoracic junction, near a joint, etc.).
  - … for all the above-mentioned locations, surgical exploration is mandatory.
- Finally, and above all, the *physical examination is crucial*. It must include muscular, neurologic, and vascular assessments.

Following the detailed wound examination, the ER physician must answer three questions:

- Is the wound superficial and is he able to manage it alone?
- Does the wound require exploration, after which he will seek a specialist’s opinion?
- Does the wound need to be explored and repaired by a specialist in an emergency (due to evidence or risk of injury to a neuro-vascular bundle, tendon, or other anatomic structure)?

5.2 Local Anesthesia

- Administration of local anesthetics should be performed with the patient in a comfortable supine or prone position, with surgical draping following local skin cleaning and sterilization (without shaving). The ER physician should be comfortably seated on a stable chair with a secure table and a confident working area with adequate lighting.
- Providing detailed information to the patient about the procedure is essential to ensure comfort: the first injection of the anesthetic solution is usually painful, the expected duration of the local anesthesia, etc.
- Precautions prior to the injection of local anesthetic solutions include cleansing and sterilization of the wound and surrounding area, as well as hand washing with the use of sterile surgical gloves. It is recommended for the physician to use a head cover, a face mask, and eye protection glasses.
- Injection of the local anesthetic is preferably performed at a distance from the wound; injection into the wound itself should be avoided.
- The physician should wait a few minutes after the local anesthetic injection and before starting wound exploration to allow time for the anesthetic effect to set in.
- For superficial and small wounds, the use of fine, short needle is adequate. For deep and extended wounds, a long (intramuscular) needle is more appropriate; it can be curved at 90° for easier and better infiltration around the periphery of the wound.
- Xylocaine 1% solution is preferably used at doses usually less than 5 mg/kg. It provides effective anesthesia for exploration and suture of simple superficial wounds. The association with a vasoconstrictor agent should be avoided, as it carries a risk of tissue necrosis (especially in the hands).

- After injection, the patient should be observed for signs of toxicity such as a feeling of peri-oral tingling, or an unpleasant intraoral sensation.
- True allergic reactions to local anesthetics are very rare; many reactions correspond to a vasovagal reflex secondary to anxiety and painful injection.
- In pediatric patients, anesthesia with gas inhalation can be used (refer to "Analgesia using inhalation of Nitrous Oxide").

5.3 Debridement and Exploration

- Wound debridement is a surgical procedure that should be performed very carefully with a bloodless field.
- The exsanguination of the wound can be achieved using one of the following methods according to the wound's location and nature:
  - direct compression,
  - vascular ligation (e.g., surgical ligation, electro-coagulation, or vascular clamp),
  - application of a tourniquet (i.e., blood pressure cuff) after elevating the limb and expelling venous blood by applying a special bandage (e.g., an "Esmarch" or another elastic bandage).
- The debridement consists of surgically cleansing the wound to remove foreign bodies (using high pressure lavage and direct ablation) and to excise necrotic tissues (such as skin, aponeurosis, muscle). This procedure is crucial, especially for "dirty" or contaminated wounds, and aims to prevent secondary complications (e.g., infection).
- After adequate debridement, the wound is explored to disclose any associated injuries to underlying anatomical structures (such as tendons, neuro-vascular bundles).
- For better exposure, it may be necessary to perform a surgical enlargement or extension of the wound.

Once the ER physician has completed the crucial steps of debridement-exploration, he should decide whether he is technically able to manage the wound. Accordingly:

- Wounds involving a complete tendon cut, major vessel, nerve, or articular damage are beyond the competence of the ER physician and should therefore be treated by a specialist.
- Wounds with only partial involvement of the underlying aponeurosis and muscles can be managed by the ER physician.

5.4 Suture

Wound suture should be performed using metallic surgical instruments; disposable instruments are inadequate.

After the excision of necrotic tissues, the suture of the remaining living structures is performed from deep to superficial (muscle, aponeurosis, sub-cutaneous tissue, and skin successively):

- Spontaneous muscle healing is possible without suture when the edges are close to each other. Significant muscle lesions are usually repaired with absorbable sutures (e.g., Vicryl^{R} 2.0).
- The repair of the aponeurosis is debated: while it is advised to prevent muscle herniation, it may induce compartment syndrome. It is performed with non-absorbable or slow-absorbable sutures (e.g., Vicryl^{R} 2.0).
- The sub-cutaneous tissue is sutured when it is thick, using slow-absorbable buried sutures (e.g., Vicryl^{R} 3.0).
- Interrupted stitches using nylon monofilament are preferred for skin suture; they should be performed without tension to avoid secondary wound dehiscence or skin necrosis.
- The use of sutures with fast resorption (e.g., Vicryl^{R} 3.0 or 4.0) is preferred in pediatric patients as it avoids the need for a painful experience of secondary stitch removal.
- The use of "steri-strips" is possible for small, simple wounds located in areas of low mobility.
- The use of biologic (or synthetic) glue is possible for clear and simple cut wounds, especially in children; however, its use is limited by its high cost.

Wound healing by the secondary intention method is applied when direct repair is not possible due to mild or moderate skin loss.

5.5 Use of Drain

- A drain is used when a dead space or cavity remains after wound debridement.
- It aids the healing process by removing residual oozes and necrotic material.
- Active or passive drainage can be applied according to the wound's location, extent, and depth:
  - Active drainage (e.g., Hemovac or aspiration drain) acts as a closed negative pressure system; it suctions fluid against gravity if needed and contributes to collapsing the dead space.
  - Passive drainage (e.g., Penrose drain) is usually applied for superficial wounds; it acts as open system and drains collections by capillary action, overflow, or gravity.

5.6 "Post-operative" Care

- The wound is covered with a sterile occlusive dressing.
- The dressing may be dry or "greasy" (e.g., paraffin gauze).
- The presence of associated tendon or muscle injuries may require immobilization with cast, slab, or orthotics.
- The dressing is changed after 48 h to check the condition of the wound and to disclose early signs of complications, especially infection (e.g., tension, redness, hotness, pain, oozing, etc.). The drain may be removed at the same time. If the dressing is clean, a new one is applied on day 7. In the absence of complications, suture removal is performed around day 15.
- When needed, directed secondary healing is performed using alternation every 2 days of pro-inflammatory ("greasy," vaseline-based, paraffin gauze) and anti-inflammatory dressings (cortisone-type based); it aims to control the healing process and to avoid the formation of hypertrophic proliferative granulation tissue.
- Skin erosion requires only the frequent daily application of silver sulfadiazine cream (Flamazine[R]) in thick layer, and a recommendation to avoid sun exposure.

5.7 Tetanus Prevention

Tetanus prevention is mandatory, especially for medico-legal issues, according to the following scheme:

	Moderate risk Small wound Ulcer	Important risk Large wound Wound seen with delay Gangrene
Incomplete vaccination		
– Less than 5 years	Nothing	Nothing
– Between 5 and 10 year	Nothing	1 booster
Incomplete vaccination		
Less than 10 years	1 booster	1 booster + specific Ig 250 IU
Vaccination		
– Absente – Doubtful – Less than 10 years	Complete vaccination protocol + specific Ig 250 IU	Complete vaccination protocol + specific Ig 250 IU

5.8 Antibiotics

- Infected wounds should undergo dual bacteriological sampling (swabs) for Gram stain, culture, and antibiogram.
- Antibiotic therapy does not intend to replace adequate debridement, which is always mandatory.
- Antibiotic therapy is justified in particular occasions, such as with contaminated and infected wounds, human and animal bites, and the presence of comorbidities (risk of endocarditis, immunosuppression, etc.).

6 Articular Wounds

Misdiagnosis is a major issue with articular wounds in the emergency setting; it may lead to catastrophic complications and sequelae such as septic arthritis with subsequent painful joint destruction and ankylosis.

6.1 Diagnosis

- In some occasions, the diagnosis is relatively "easy":
  - Large wounds with exposure of the articular surfaces and synovial fluid to the outside atmosphere,
  - Neglected wounds seen at a late stage of infection (fever, stabbing pain, joint swelling, local heat and redness, painful mobilization, etc.) requiring a specialists' opinion (surgery and infectious diseases).
- On other occasions, the diagnosis is more demanding; the wound is very small ("punctiform" size; induced by a bite, or the tip of a nail or knife, etc.) and located in proximity to a joint.
- The presence of *pneumarthrosis* (air in the joint) on radiographs is pathognomonic for the diagnosis of a penetrating articular wound (Fig. 6.1). Similarly, the presence of an intra-articular foreign body on simple radiographs (intra-articular radio-opaque image) is also diagnostic of an articular wound.

D. Saragaglia, A. Hassan Chamseddine, *Traumatology for the Emergency Doctor*, https://doi.org/10.1007/978-3-031-63196-2_6

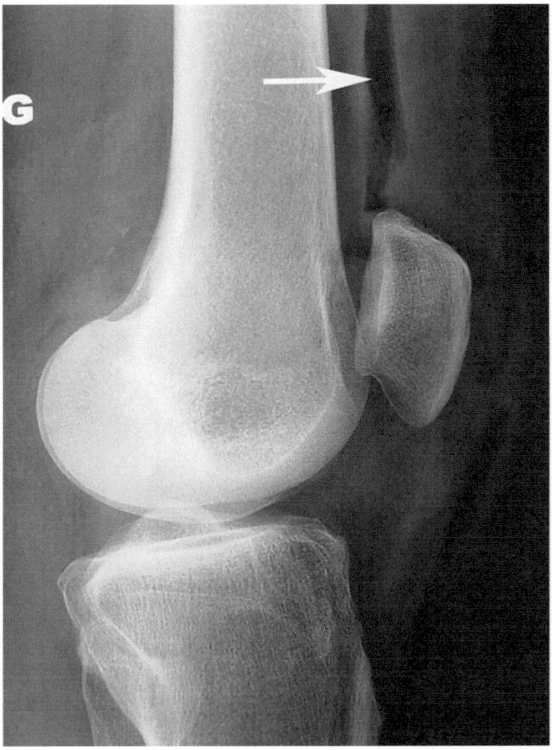

Fig. 6.1 Knee pneumarthrosis as seen on a lateral knee radiograph following a stab wound of the knee, resulting in a penetrating articular wound

6.2 Management

- *Any wound located in proximity to a joint should be meticulously explored* with optimal conditions of sterility and exposure. If the exploration reveals an articular breach, a specialized opinion is requested for further management (i.e., surgical exploration and repair in the operating room).
- Particular caution should be exercised with wounds on the dorsum of the fingers and those located around the knee (more frequent in pediatric patients).
- *Tetanus* prevention is obligatory.
- When the patient is seen in the early post-injury period, and if the wound is managed accurately (with abundant high pressure lavage and adequate debridement), the prescription of antibiotic therapy is debatable.
- If the patient is seen some time after the accident, and if the wound is contaminated or suspected to be so, treatment with antibiotics is recommended after obtaining local swabs for bacteriology.
- *Joint immobilization* using a cast or slab aids in the healing of articular structures, especially in the presence of significant capsulo-ligamentous lesions; however, it should be considered with caution and moderation as it may result in joint stiffness.
- *Post-operative rehabilitation* is crucial and should be implemented early, especially for hand injuries.
- The risk of algodystrophy is high after significant capsulo-ligamentous lesions.

7 Wounds of the Face

Facial wounds are frequent. They should be managed adequately to obtain satisfactory functional and cosmetic results. The ER physician should, first of all, check the integrity of the underlying anatomical structures: facial nerve, parotid or salivary duct, naso-lacrimal duct, eyelid muscles, etc. The management of injuries of these structures should be done by the corresponding specialist. This chapter intends to discuss only the facial "simple" wounds of the skin and mucosae.

7.1 Clinical History

- The time of the accident is important to determine, as it is recommended to repair the wound within 6 h after the injury.
- Mechanism: direct trauma, cold weapon, bite, broken glass, etc…
- History of anti-tetanus vaccine.
- Previous history and antecedents: allergy, medications intake (such as anticoagulants), comorbidities, etc.

7.2 Physical Examination

- *Characteristics of the wound*
  - Topography and location,
  - Simple, contused, loss of soft tissue (skin retraction gives a false impression of skin loss),
  - Superficial erosion, superficial wound, deep wound,
  - Dimensions (length and depth).
- *The diagnosis of injury to the facial nerve* (or its branches) is based on clinical examination, which includes a comparative assessment of the facial "sensitivity" and "motricity" on both sides.

D. Saragaglia, A. Hassan Chamseddine, *Traumatology for the Emergency Doctor*, https://doi.org/10.1007/978-3-031-63196-2_7

  - Examination of the facial motricity: primary motor assessment consists of asking the patient to whistle, blow, close his eyes, smile, frown, etc.
  - Examination of the facial sensitivity: primary sensory assessment looks for the presence sensory disturbance such as numbness, anesthesia, hyposensitivity, or even hypersensitivity, of the temporo-frontal area, tongue and palate (i.e., anterior two-thirds), cheek, jaw, nasal ala, upper lip, lower lip, etc.
  - When a facial nerve injury is suspected or confirmed, the patient should be transferred to a specialized center where microsurgical repair of the nerve can be performed, ideally without delay.
- *When a deep wound located in the jugal area* aligns with the line from the tragus to the upper lip:
  - Injury to *Wharton's duct* should be suspected.
  - The physical exam should include checking for salivary flow from the wound or blood oozing from the ostium of *Stensen's duct* at the level of the second upper molar tooth.
  - The flow of normal saline solution from the wound, following injection into the ostium, is indicative of Stensen's duct involvement.
  - The patient is transferred into a specialized department for microsurgical repair of Stensen's duct, where an intra-luminal catheter is typically inserted for at least 1 month to reduce the risk of stenosis.
- For deep wounds of the superior eyelid (palpebral):
  - The presence of *ptosis* is a sign of injury to the eyelid elevator muscle (levator palpebrae superioris) and requires specialized surgical management.
  - Wounds involving the inner (or nasal) canthus should be examined for potential lacrimal duct injury; consultation with a specialist is recommended.
- Look for other associated lesions:
  - Bony lesions: fractures of the mandible, maxillary bone, nasal bone, zygomatic bone, orbital bone, etc.
  - Ocular lesions: corneal injury, deep laceration, intra-ocular foreign body, etc.
  - Dental lesions: fractures, dislocations, etc.

It is recommended to take photographs of the initial injury.

7.3 Principles of Surgical Repair of Facial Wounds

- ***Anesthesia***
  - Local anesthesia is performed with xylocaïne^{R} 1% or 2%.
  - The use of a xylocaine-adrenaline solution can decrease local bleeding; however, it is contraindicated when the wound has poorly vascularized flaps.
  - Xylocaine spray may be used for superficial skin erosions.
- ***Brushing***: it is important to brush wounds and skin erosions that contain foreign bodies (e.g., soil, asphalt, or other particulate incrustations) as they may cause permanent tattoo-like discoloration.

- ***Washing, cleaning, and disinfection***: this process commonly uses povidone-iodine-based antiseptics (such as Betadine^R soap and solution). Cleaning and washing with a diluted hydrogen peroxide solution can facilitate recognition and removal of incrusted foreign bodies.
- ***Control of bleeding***: Active bleeding is controlled either by direct vascular ligation or selective thermo-electrical coagulation (i.e., electrocauterization).
- ***Exploration***: Meticulous exploration of the wound is crucial to identify foreign bodies (such as metal, glass, or soil) or associated injury (such as muscle, duct, neuro-vascular).
- ***Debridement of the wound edges***: debridement should be very limited, avoiding unnecessary excision of skin. All skin flaps induced by the injury should be preserved and repositioned in their initial beds, even those with seemingly precarious vascularization.
- ***Drainage***
  - It is indicated for:
    dirty and contaminated deep wounds,
    persistent oozing or bleeding after debridement,
    cavities created by the injury or during debridement.
  - It should be maintained for at least 48 h.
  - The system may be a passive-open (such as a Penrose drain) or active-closed (such as a negative pressure Hemovac drain).
- ***Closure***
  - Wound closure with sutures is preferred over Steri-strip^R.
  - Closure is performed with two-layers of sutures: sub-cutaneous (inverted stitches) and cutaneous (without tension).
  - Type of filaments and threads:
    Resorbable sutures (4.0 or 5.0) for the sub-cutaneous layer closure (Vicryl^R, PDS^R).
    Non-resorbable sutures (5.0, 6.0) for skin closure (e.g., Ethicon^R).

7.4 Post-suture Care and Instructions

- The wound should be left uncovered after suturing, with direct application of an oily or greasy pomade over the wound (e.g., Vaseline). This helps facilitate the easy removal of any crust formation.
- Antibiotic therapy is prescribed if:
  - the wound was initially contaminated,
  - the wound involves articular cartilage,
  - there was a delay in initiating wound treatment,
  - the wound is bite-induced.
- Skin stitches are typically removed on day 6 or 7.
- The use of swimming pools is prohibited for the next month.

- Sunlight exposure should be avoided for the next 6 months; it is recommended to use face protection products against sunlight to prevent permanent scar discoloration.
- Scar massage and manipulation should be performed several times daily after complete healing.
- The final plastic or cosmetic result can only be expected after 1 year.

7.5 Special Considerations Related to the Site of the Wound

- **Scalp**
  - Wounds involving the scalp are typically hemorrhagic and may involve degloving; therefore, satisfactory bleeding control, adequate drainage, and a compressive dressing for the first 48 h are essential.
  - Suture threads used for the scalp are larger than those used for the face (3.0), and stitch removal is usually delayed until day 10.
  - Hair should shaved at the edges of the wound to facilitate easier suture application.
- **Forehead**
  - The natural wrinkles of the forehead should be respected and realigned during suture.
  - The demarcation frontline between the hair and the skin of the forehead should be restored.
- **Eyebrows**
  - Care should be taken to realign the edges of the eyebrows accurately during suture.
  - A secondary specialized consultation is recommended when the injury results in partial or total loss of the eyebrows (due to abrasion).
- **Eyelids**
  - Wounds involving the eyelids can lead to significant sequelae if not adequately treated initially.
  - Specialized opinion is advised when:

    Ocular involvement is suspected,

    There is transfixiating palpebral wound,

    There is a deep wound of the upper eyelid with the presence of ptosis (suggesting involvement of the levator palpebrae superioris muscle). However, the presence of edema may mask the existence of ptosis, especially when the patient is examined after a delay.

    There is a wound in the nasal canthus area with possible involvement of the lacrimal duct.
  - For "simple" wounds involving only the eyelid's skin, with or without injury to the orbicularis oculi muscle, simple suturing with separate stitches (6.0 nylon) is adequate; sub-cutaneous stitches are not necessary as the palpebral skin is very thin.

  - Stitch removal can be performed on day 5, as the healing process is typically rapid in this area.
- **Nose**
  - An associated nasal bone fracture should not be overlooked; appropriate radiographs should be requested in any doubtful situation.
  - Repair of wounds involving the nasal ala must be very meticulous, with perfect alignment of the edges to avoid any cosmetic disturbance.
  - The temporary use of a nasal stent may be necessary to prevent scar retraction of the nasal wing.
- **Lateral facial area (jaw, cheek, parotid gland area, temple)**
- As previously mentioned, the physical examination should assess for associated injury to the facial nerve and Stensen's duct; therefore, for any suspicious or doubtful situation, a specialized consultation is essential.
- **Lips**
  - Transfixiating labial wounds should be repaired in layers, from deep to superficial, using separate stitches (resorbable 4.0 sutures for the mucosa and muscle, and non-resorbable 6.0 nylon for the skin).
  - Repair of wounds involving the muco-cutaneous junction should start at the junction landmark itself to avoid shifting the edges of the wound.
  - Suturing of the red part of the lip is performed with separate 5.0 resorbable stitches.
- **Helix of the ear**
  - The natural contours and smooth edges of the helix should be restored to avoid creating any defects or notches.
  - Transfixiating wounds of the helix are repaired with separate skin sutures after minimal excision and debridement of the cartilaginous edges.
  - Any cartilage exposed by the injury should be covered by skin during the repair process.
  - Any wound involving the cartilage requires antibiotic therapy for 8 days (e.g., Amoxicilline/Clavulanic acid).
- **Mucosae (jugal and gingival mucosae, tongue, palate)**
  - Small wounds of the tongue and palate typically do not require surgical repair; they are managed with repetitive mouthwashes for 1 week.
  - When direct repair is necessary, suturing is performed with resorbable 4.0 separate stitches.
  - Wounds of the gingival gum should be examinated for a possible associated underlying fracture.
  - Wounds of the vestibular aspect of the mandible, near the mental foramen, should be assessed for associated injury to the terminal branch of the mandibular nerve, which is clinically manifested by unilateral labio-mental anesthesia.

7.6 Special Considerations Relative to the Mechanism of Injury

- **Bites**
  - They are often caused by animals and less frequently by humans.
  - They carry a risk of infection by bacteria such as *Streptococcus pyogenes*, *Pasteurella multocida*, and *Staphylococcus aureus*.
  - Swabs for Gram stain and cultures are essential.
  - Treatment should be performed in the operating room, under general anesthesia, and includes abundant lavage, meticulous exploration, adequate debridement, and closure.
  - A high degree of caution is warranted for punctiform wounds as they may penetrate deeply and be associated with profound degloving injuries and involvement of underlying major structures (such as ducts, vessels, nerves, and muscles).
  - The steps of closure include successively: passive drainage, loose subcutaneous sutures, and separate skin stitches.
  - Initiation of antibiotic therapy with tetracycline (contraindicated for children under 8 years of age, and for pregnant and breastfeeding women), beta-lactams, or macrolides for 10 days (refer to "Bites by dogs and cats").
  - A systematic anti-rabies consultation is recommended.
- **Broken windshield**
  - Wounds induced by broken windshield are becoming less frequent.
  - They typically consist of multiple small wounds with the inclusion of foreign bodies of various sizes.
- **Skin abrasions**
  - Brushing and lavage are efficient and practical methods for the removal of embedded foreign bodies that may cause secondary permanent tattooing of the skin.
  - Small-sized abrasions can be managed under local anesthesia, with the use of a local anesthetic spray.
  - Abundant application of vaseline over the cleaned skin abrasion area can enhance healing.
- **Loss of soft tissue**
  - For superficial skin loss of small dimensions located away from any natural foramina or orifices, a controlled wound healing method is initiated. Otherwise, consultation with a specialist is required.
- **Amputations**
  - Preserve the amputated segment by placing it in a plastic bag and then putting it into an ice container.
  - The patient should be immediately transferred to a microsurgery specialized center.

8 Wounds of the Hand

Hand wounds should receive rigorous and meticulous care. Treatment is based on accurate diagnosis of the lesions which requires good knowledge of anatomy.

8.1 Diagnosis

1. **History**
   (a) Recent and past medical history: traumatic accidents, cigarette consumption, diabetes, cardiovascular events, allergies, etc.
   (b) Past vaccination history and current status,
   (c) Is the affected hand the dominant or non-dominant one?
   (d) The traumatic agent and mechanism (for example, wounds produced by broken glass are usually very deep and may reach the underlying bone).
2. **Physical examination**
   (a) The wound
   - Location with respect to any underlying important anatomical structure (such as tendons, arteries, nerves),
   - Character of the wound (simple, complex, contused, skin loss, etc.),
   - Apparent degree of contamination.

   (b) Distal to the wound
   - Vascular condition
     – Arterial assessment (capillary refill, color, local temperature),
     – The absence of external bleeding does not exclude the possibility of an arterial injury.
   - Sensitivity
     – Assessment of sensation in each individual territory of the three major nerves (median, radial, ulnar),
     – Assessment of sensation in both halves of the finger pulp to evaluate the continuity of the corresponding digital nerve,

D. Saragaglia, A. Hassan Chamseddine, *Traumatology for the Emergency Doctor*, https://doi.org/10.1007/978-3-031-63196-2_8

  - Any sensory disturbance (loss, decreased, or increased sensation) should prompt surgical exploration of the corresponding nerve.
- Finger deformity
  - Mallet finger deformity, associated with wound of the dorsal aspect of the distal interphalangeal joint, indicates an injury to the distal insertion of the extensor tendon,
  - Boutonniere deformity, associated with wound of the dorsal aspect of the proximal interphalangeal joint, suggests an injury to the central slip of the extensor tendon.
- Assessment of the active range of motion
  - The active range of motion (ROM) should be carefully examined for each joint distal to the injury.
  - A complete loss of active ROM should raise the possibility of a tendon injury (for example, loss of extension may indicate an extensor tendon injury; loss of flexion at the proximal or distal interphalangeal finger joint may suggest an injury to the flexor digitorum superficialis or profundus, respectively).
  - A wound over the course of a tendon with preserved active ROM does not completely rule out a tendon injury; it should be explored for a partial tendon lesion.

8.2 Principles of Treatment

- All simple, uncomplicated wounds, can be managed by the ER physician.
- Wounds are repaired according to their distribution in five zones for flexor tendon injuries and eight zones for extensor tendon injuries (refer to "Hand Trauma").
- Any wound located over a joint or along the trajectory of a tendon, nerve, or artery should be investigated for potential underlying injuries.
- Neurovascular and open osteoarticular injuries are considered surgical emergencies and should be treated accordingly.
- Neurovascular and complex injuries involving different structures require management by a specialized team.
- On certain occasions, tendon injuries can be managed by the ER physician (refer to "Hand Trauma").
- Open fractures of the hand generally require management by a specialized team, except for P3 open fractures without soft tissue loss.
- In case of traumatic amputation:
  - Replantation is possible if:

    the finger is well preserved and transported as previously described (the amputated segment placed in a plastic bag and kept in an ice container),

    the amputation is clean-cut (with sharp edges),

    the time since amputation is less than 6 h.
  - Contraindications for replantation include:

Multi-level amputations,
Avulsion and degloving injuries (usually with neurovascular bundle stripping),
Crush injuries,
Severe local contamination,
Patients with a severe vital prognosis,
Heavy smoker patients,
Psychiatric patients (theoretical contraindication).

Management of Wounds Induced by Dog and Cat Bites

9

In the case of a wound produced by a dog or cat bite, the ER physician should:

9.1 Clearly Define the Circumstances of the Bite

Place and circumstances of the accident, date and time of the incident, type of animal involved, animal's owner details, site and specific location of the bite on the patient's body.

9.2 Check the Patient's Anti-tetanus Vaccination Status

Refer to Chap. 5.7 in "Management of Wounds".

9.3 Disinfect and Debride the Wounds to Prevent Infection

- Consult a maxillo-facial surgeon when the wounds are located on the face for a specialized opinion.
- Thoroughly explore the wounds when they are located on the hand, due to the complex anatomy and potential for serious complications.

D. Saragaglia, A. Hassan Chamseddine, *Traumatology for the Emergency Doctor*, https://doi.org/10.1007/978-3-031-63196-2_9

9.4 Always Prescribe Preventive Antibiotic Therapy

Always prescribe preventive antibiotic therapy to prevent infections caused by common pathogens such as *Streptococcus pyogenes*, *Pasteurella multocida*, *Staphylococcus aureus*, Anaerobic germs, etc.

- ***For Adult***
- Amoxicilline/Clavulanic Acid: 1000 mg TID for 5 days.
- ***For Pediatric patients <15 years***
- Amoxicilline/Clavulanic Acid: 80 mg/kg/day divided into 3 doses for 5 days.

In case of allergy

- ***For Adult <60 kg***
  - *For superficial wound:*
  - Doxycycline 100 mg: 2 capsules in the middle of the meal as starting dose in the first day, followed by 1 capsule daily for 5 days (avoid sunlight exposure).
  - *For deep wound:*
  - Doxycycline 100 mg according to the same previous protocol + Metronidazole 500 mg, 1 capsule TID for 5 days.
- ***Adult >60 kg***
  - *For superficial wound:*
  - Doxycycline 100 mg: 2 capsules once daily in the middle of the meal for 5 days (avoid sunlight exposure).
  - *For deep wound:*
  - Doxycycline 100 mg: 2 capsules once daily in the middle of the meal for 5 days (avoid sunlight exposure) + Metronidazole 500 mg, 1 capsule TID for 5 days.
- ***Children <15 years***
  - Pristinamycine 50 mg/kg/day in 3 divided doses (can be crushed and mixed with milk, jam, or other food).

For any animal capable of scratching or biting, regardless of rabies vaccination status, and that has a known owner, the following veterinary examination schedule should be adhered to:

- First visit: within 24 h of the incident,
- Second visit: 7 days after the incident,
- Third visit: 15 days after the incident.

If the animal has escaped or cannot be identified, the patient should be directed for evaluation and follow-up at the nearest specialized center.

10 Injuries to Peripheral Nerves

Diagnosis of post-traumatic peripheral nerve injury is primarily clinical. The severity of the injury is categorized into three levels according to Seddon's classification:

- **Neurapraxia** is a condition of temporary loss of motor and sensory function induced by blockage of nerve conduction; it typically results from blunt trauma and completely recovers after a few days or weeks (6–8 weeks).
- **Axonotmesis** is a condition usually resulting from more severe blunt or crush trauma that produces serious contusion to the nerve. The axons and its myelin sheath are injured; however, the endoneurium, perineurium, and epineurium remain intact. Recovery is possible but very slow, occurring through axonal regeneration at a rate of up to 1 in per month.
- **Neurotmesis** is the most severe degree of nerve damage with complete interruption of the nerve and nerve sheath. Spontaneous recovery from this injury is not possible.

In practice:

- For blunt (close) trauma: it can be challenging to initially determine the exact degree of nerve damage severity and to predict the potential for recovery.
- For major trauma and wounds over the path of a nerve: the presence of a distal sensory deficit is highly indicative of the need for specialized surgical exploration and repair.
- EMG is not considered an "urgent" investigation. It becomes useful after 3 weeks from the trauma, coinciding with the onset of Wallerian degeneration. An initial EMG serves as a baseline study and is valuable for monitoring the progression of nerve injury.

D. Saragaglia, A. Hassan Chamseddine, *Traumatology for the Emergency Doctor*, https://doi.org/10.1007/978-3-031-63196-2_10

10.1 Upper Limb

Affected nerve	Clinical presentation	When to think about it?
Axillary	Decrease or loss of sensation of the lateral aspect of the shoulder Atrophy of the deltoid muscle (late occurrence +++) Deficient deltoid muscle on specific testing	Shoulder trauma *Before and after reduction of shoulder dislocation* (+++)
Musculo-cutaneous	Decreased power of elbow flexion Active elbow flexion maintained (brachio-radialis) Abolition of the biceps reflex	Fracture of the coracoid process Shoulder dislocation
Median	Deficit of active pronation Deficit of active flexion of the first three fingers Decrease or loss of sensation of the palmar aspect of the first three fingers Abolition of the pronator teres reflex	Elbow fracture *After reduction of elbow dislocation (+++)* *Wound of the volar aspect of the wrist*
A.I.N	Deficit of the thumb-index pinch	Forearm fracture
Ulnar	Involuntary abduction of the little finger (Wartenberg's sign) Deficit of the active adduction of the thumb Froment's sign Decrease or loss of sensation of the fifth finger	Elbow trauma Wound of the volar aspect of the wrist
Radial	Deficit of active extension of the wrist and fingers Decrease or loss of sensation of the base of the thumb and the dorsal aspect of the hand	*Fractures of the humeral shaft* (+++) Wound at the base of the thumb
P.I.O.N	Extension deficit of the metacarpo-phalangeal joint of the fingers, with preservation of the wrist extension	Fractures of the forearm

A.I.N: Anterior inter-osseous nerve, branch of the median nerve below the elbow

P.I.O.N: Posterior inter-osseous nerve, the continuation of the deep branch of the radial nerve after traversing under the pronator teres muscle

10.2 Lower Limb

Affected nerve	Clinical presentation	When to think about it?
Femoral	Decrease or loss of sensation of the medial aspect of the thigh Abolition of the patellar reflex	Hip fracture Hip dislocation
Sciatic	Motor deficit of the lower limb Loss of sensation of the lower limb	Pelvis fracture Hip dislocation Hip prosthesis dislocation
Common peroneal	Decrease or loss of sensation of the lateral aspect of the leg Deficit of dorsal flexion of the ankle and foot +++	Knee trauma (including fractures, sprains, and dislocations) Fractures of the neck of the fibula Compression by cast

Affected nerve	Clinical presentation	When to think about it?
Tibial	Decrease or loss of sensation of the posterior aspect of the leg Deficit of the calf muscles Abolition of the achilles reflex	Fractures/dislocations of the knee Direct trauma to the popliteal fossa
Superficial peroneal (musculo-cutaneous)	Decreased sensation of the first web space of the dorsal aspect of the foot	Fractures of the lower leg Compression

10.3 In Practice

- It is advocated to test the sensitivity of:
  - The pulp of the index for the median nerve injury,
  - The proximal dorsal aspect of the index for the radial nerve injury,
  - The pulp of the fifth finger for the ulnar nerve injury,
  - The lateral border of the foot for the common peroneal nerve injury,
  - The medial border of the foot for the tibial nerve injury,
  - The dorsal aspect of the foot for the superficial peroneal nerve injury.
- In the case of a fracture: it is often impossible to accurately assess the reflexes and the function of the muscular groups in the injured area due to pain, swelling, or immobilization. Therefore, a careful distal sensory examination becomes critically important to evaluate nerve function and integrity.
  - In opposition, for some fractures, a specific motor deficit distal to the fracture site can often be readily identified as a consequence of associated nerve injury (a deficit of active wrist extension associated to humeral shaft fracture suggests a radial nerve injury. A deficit of active dorsi-flexion of the ankle and foot associated to a fracture of the neck of the fibula suggests a common peroneal nerve injury.)

Stress Fractures

11

Stress fractures are fatigue-induced fractures that occur in normal bone without obvious trauma. They result from repeated stress over time and are typically seen as overuse injuries in athletes. This condition can be misleading to its clinical and radiological presentation, and it is distinct from the category of "pathologic fractures". Stress fractures have several notable characteristics:

- Recurrence: almost invariably occurs after an early return to previous activities without observing a sufficient period of rest,
- Progression: there is a possibility to progression to a complete fracture,
- Location: certain fracture locations may have significant mechanical consequences and serious repercussions on future sports activities.

11.1 Pathophysiology

Bone is normally in a perpetual remodeling process, with osteoblastic and osteoclastic activities being incessant and permanent in living bone. When unusual and repeated high stress is applied to the bone, osteoclastic activity can overwhelm the osteoblastic process. Consequently, bone resorption may exceed new bone formation, leading to a localized zone of weakness. This weakness can produce a bone "fissure" or an incomplete fracture. During the bone repair process, osteoblastic activity attempts to build up an irregular and exuberant bone at the level of the fissure. However, if a high level of stress continues to be applied, a complete fracture may occur as a consequence of the localized bone weakness.

D. Saragaglia, A. Hassan Chamseddine, *Traumatology for the Emergency Doctor*, https://doi.org/10.1007/978-3-031-63196-2_11

11.2 Radio-Clinical Aspects

11.2.1 Common Clinical Presentation

- The beginning of symptoms is rarely sudden. Patients typically report of vague pain described as "discomfort" during sports activities and physical exercises. Initially, the pain is diffuse, but gradually becomes more localized and intensifies. In a later stages, the pain may be irregularly alleviated by rest but eventually becomes constant, interfering with sports practice.
- Occasionally, localized swelling and tenderness are noted.
- The pain may exhibit pseudo-inflammatory characteristics, despite normal biological markers.
- A detailed patient history often reveals the underlying cause:
  - Unusual physical sustained and repeated overactivity: For example, a long military march or excessive training.
  - Sports practice at higher level without adequate preparation or training.
  - Participation in successive competitions without proper physical rest or preparation or too soon after recovering from illness or injury.
  - Engagement in sports activities with different or new habits or environmental changes (such as training on hard or inclined training surfaces or using new types of shoes).

11.2.2 Roentgenographic Assessment

- In the early stage (i.e., the first 3 weeks after pain onset), radiographs are typically normal, as stress fractures may not be visible on X-rays immediately following the onset of symptoms.
- In the later stage (i.e., 1 month after pain onset), radiographs usually reveal an image of a "hairline fracture," which indicates a thin fracture line that has become visible as the bone starts to respond to the injury.
- In the more advanced stage, a periosteal reaction, such as exuberant callus formation can be observed surrounding the fracture line area.

11.2.3 Bone Scintigraphy (Bone Scan)

- It has high sensitivity,
- It has no specificity,
- The results should be interpreted in light of the clinical context and presentation for better diagnostic confirmation
- It is performed using Technetium-99m,
- It typically shows a positive image of a localized "hyper-fixation" ("hot spot") in the very early stage (as early as 48 h) (Fig. 11.1),

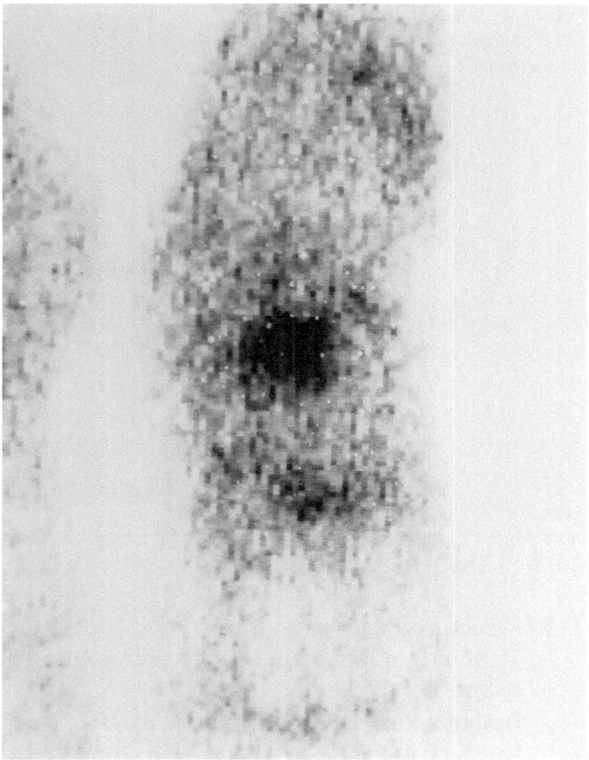

Fig. 11.1 Scintigraphy image of a stress fracture of the tarsal navicular bone

- The isotope fixation is positive in both early and late stages of the exam, on both periosteal and endosteal sides.

11.2.4 CT Scan (Guided by Bone Scintigraphy)

- CT scan cuts are oriented by the area of "hot spot" identified in the bone scan, when it has been previously performed.
- It can reveal an image of "hairline" fracture or minimal sub-periosteal ossification as early as 10 days after the onset of pain (Fig. 11.2).

11.2.5 MRI

- MRI can show a positive image of a stress fracture from the first 24 h after the onset of symptoms.
- MRI is particularly useful in doubtful situations, especially when there is an absence of suggestive clinical history or circumstances.

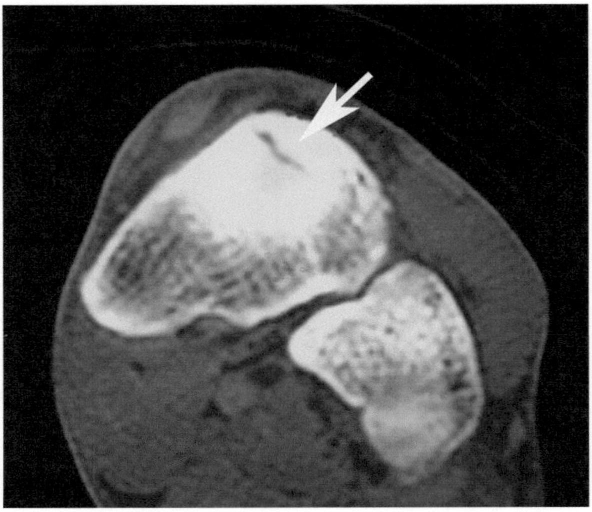

Fig. 11.2 Image of a tarsal navicular bone stress fracture on CT scan

11.3 Treatment

- **Pre-fracture stage**
  - Treatment, primarily involves a strict rest and non-weight bearing period of 6–8 weeks.
  - Resuming activity is permitted only after the pain has disappeared. If pain reoccurs, rest and non-weight bearing must recommence.
- **Stage of confirmed fracture**
  - Orthopedic conservative treatment is the initial treatment of choice in most cases.
  - Persistence of the radio-clinical features and symptoms after 5 months suggests non-union, warranting surgical management, including bone graft and internal fixation.
  - Surgical treatment is mandatory for any displaced fracture regardless of the stage of progression.
  - There is an elevated risk of algodystrophy.
- **Preventive or prophylactic measures**
  - Ensure the observance of rational and balanced measures in terms of gradual training, intensity, and frequency of activities, as well as participation in competitions.
  - Maintain well-adjusted behaviors and habits, and ensure the use of secure accessories and a safe environment for training and practice, including appropriate footwear and playing fields.

11.4 Topographic Forms with Respect to the Affected Bone

11.4.1 Tibia

- It represents the most frequent site of stress fractures.
- The most common location is the mid third of the shaft.
- The primary differential diagnosis includes medial tibial stress syndrome (MTSS) or shin-splint syndrome, also known as "aponeurositis" of the posterior tibialis muscle. This condition shares similar clinical symptoms and presentation with stress fractures, but may recur. In contrast, "hot spot" images on scintigraphic examination typically appear only in the late phase and may also affect the fibula.

11.4.2 Calcaneus

- It represents the 2nd most common site of stress fractures.
- Radiographic image is positive only in late stage.
- The clinical presentation frequently mimics Achilles tendinitis.

11.4.3 Femur

- The femoral neck (intra-capsular) corresponds to the most common site of stress fractures in the femur, and this location carries a potential for severe prognosis.
- A misdiagnosis can lead to the development of a complete femoral neck fracture, which is a very serious complication in young patients as it may progress to avascular necrosis of the femoral head.
- Bilateral femoral neck involvement is not uncommon; it requires a long period of complete rest.
- Diaphyseal and distal femoral involvements are rare.

11.4.4 Metatarsals

- Metatarsals are a classically well-known site of stress fractures.
- Diagnosis is often made retrospectively, when the radiographs reveal exuberant callus formation.
- The necks of the metatarsals are frequently involved.
- Multiple and bilateral involvements are not exceptional presentations.

11.4.5 Tarsal Navicular Bone

- For track race runners, the "outside foot" is more frequently involved than the other foot.
- Despite adequate initial treatment, pseudarthrosis is frequent and typically requires surgical management, including internal fixation and bone grafting.

11.4.6 Pelvis

- The ilio-pubic and ischio-pubic rami are the primary pelvic sites of stress fractures.
- In adolescent patients, the differential diagnosis primarily includes bony avulsions of the ischiatic tuberosity, iliac spines, and symphysis pubis.

11.4.7 Spine

- Low back pain in young patients who practice horse riding and gymnastics should prompt consideration of an isthmic stress fracture (isthmic spondylolysis). The risk of progression to spondylolisthesis is not uncommon in these cases.
- Sacral involvement in athletes with low back pain is not rare.

11.4.8 Upper Limb

Particular sites of stress fractures of the upper limb are associated with specific activities:

- Fractures of the hook process of the hamatum are commonly associated with racket sports due to the repetitive forces exerted on the wrist and hand.
- Both bones of the forearm are at risk in throwing sports, where repetitive stress can lead to fractures.
- Fractures of the clavicle are frequently seen in patients who carry heavy loads, as the clavicle is subjected to increased stress.

11.5 In Conclusion

The diagnosis of stress fracture should be considered in patients presenting with localized bone pain that intensifies progressively, especially after unusual overuse or overexertion, and without obvious trauma.

Initial radiographs may be normal despite the presence of symptoms.

Bone Scintigraphy usually confirms the diagnosis, showing increased uptake in the affected area.

More elaborate investigations, such as MRI, may be requested in cases of diagnostic uncertainty to rule out other conditions like tumors or osteomyelitis.

Preventive measures include the careful observance and adaptation of the patient's physical and sports activities, taking into account their age, level of practice, and physical and musculo-skeletal conditions.

Acute Muscular Injuries

12

Acute muscle injuries refer to muscular damage that occurs secondary to a distinct traumatic event. A precise history and meticulous clinical examination are usually sufficient to orient the diagnostic regarding the injury and its potential severity.

Initial mismanagement in the early post-traumatic period may lead to severe muscular sequelae with serious repercussion on future sports activities.

It is important to distinguish between injuries occurring during the activity itself (subject of the current chapter) and those occurring after the activity which are mainly related to physical overuse (such as cramps, contractures, etc.).

12.1 History

Patient's history and questionnaire should look for:

- Whether the patient had an inadequate worm-up before starting the activity,
- Any excessive, erroneous or overly hard training techniques that were used,
- The level of fatigue and overuse from training and competition sessions,
- Whether there was insufficient recovery from a previous injury,
- Mechanism of accident:
  - Sudden acceleration or deceleration,
  - Sudden forceful contraction of an over elongated muscle that crosses two joints,
  - Unexpected simultaneous contraction of two antagonist muscles,
- Intensity and type of initial pain:
  - The initial pain is not always directly related to the degree of severity of the trauma,
  - A sudden onset of severe pain usually indicates a serious muscle injury, as opposed to a progressive onset,
  - An audible "snap" or "pop" accompanied by a feeling of a "mass" can signify a serious injury,

D. Saragaglia, A. Hassan Chamseddine, *Traumatology for the Emergency Doctor*, https://doi.org/10.1007/978-3-031-63196-2_12

- An Immediate stop of the ongoing activity usually corresponds to a severe injury.

12.2 Clinical assessment

- Inspection: look for ecchymosis, deformity, notching, etc.
- Palpation: feel for a gap, mass (hematoma), localized tenderness, etc.
- Assessment of muscular passive stretching and elongation:
  - Adductor muscles: perform passive hip abduction with the patient in a supine position.
  - Hamstring muscles: perform passive hip flexion with the knee in an extension position.
  - Quadriceps muscle: perform passive knee flexion, with the patient in a prone position.
  - Sural triceps muscle: evaluate passive dorsal foot flexion with the knee in both extension and flexion position successively (to separately assess the gastrocnemius and soleus muscles).
- Assessment of muscle's contraction power against resistance.

12.3 Clinical Grading of Muscle Injury Severity

12.3.1 Grade 1 (Mild)

Only a small number of muscle fibers are involved.

- The pain and tenderness may have started during the activity or been delayed ~~to~~ until the next day,
- The pain is alleviated by rest and reawakened by mobilization against resistance,
- The functional disturbance is mild,
- The palpation of the affected muscle area is tender,
- There is no hematoma or ecchymosis present,
- The progression is smooth with recovery expected after a rest period of 7–14 days.

12.3.2 Grade II (Moderate)

A significant number of fibers are torn.

- The pain has occurred during the activity,
- The pain is sudden, intense, and persists at rest,
- The patient had to immediately stop the sports activity; he could barely walk, with limping, on the affected limb,
- The pain is exacerbated by muscle contraction and active motion of the limb.
- Palpation:

  - A gap is palpable in the belly of the superficial muscle,
  - There is a localized tenderness surrounded by an area of muscle guarding reactive muscle defense.
- There is a delayed occurrence of ecchymosis.

12.3.3 Grade III (Severe)

Complete tear or rupture of the muscle belly.

- There is a very severe and sudden pain with audible pop,
- There is an immediate and complete functional disability,
- Swelling occurs very early after the injury,
- There is a tender and palpable gap surrounded by an area of ecchymosis.

12.4 Progression

- For minor and simple injuries, the progression is usually satisfactory after appropriate and early treatment.
- Severe injuries may have a complicated progression resulting in secondary sequelae that can lead to functional repercussions and impair the ability to resume sports activities at the same previous level. This may be due to:
  - A healing process that results in the formation of granulomatous and fibrous scar tissue,
  - Cystic formation due to the encapsulation of a local collection, such as a hematoma or serous fluid,
  - The formation of local calcifications and ossifications.

12.5 Diagnosis

While the diagnosis of muscular injuries is usually evident, evaluating the degree of severity can be misleading and a source of confusion.

- ***Radiographic assessment*** is helpful for differential diagnosis (anterior superior iliac spine avulsion, ischial tuberosity avulsion, etc.).
- ***Ultrasound assessment***
  - is a quick and easy examination
  - It helps:
    confirming the diagnosis,
    visualizing the size and location of the injury,
    measuring the size of intra-muscular or musculo-tendinous gaps or retractions,

measuring the dimensions of any existing hematoma (large hematoma may require surgical drainage),
excluding other differential diagnoses, such as phlebitis.

- **MRI**
  - Is not a routine examination,
  - However, it is very helpful for making an accurate diagnosis and defining the injury in the early post-trauma period. This is particularly true for high level athletes and when discussing surgical indications,
  - It is of primary importance in demonstrating the muscle's actual anatomic condition during the sequela stage.

12.6 Management

- *For benign or mild injuries* (grade I), confirmed by ultrasound, a short period of rest (10–15 days) combined with physiotherapy is usually sufficient to promote healing and **allow for a gradual return to** sports activities.
- *For more severe injuries* (grade II and III):
  - Initial measures include applying ice, a compressive elastic bandage, elevation (when appropriate), and rest, with the aim of limiting local bleeding and preventing hematoma formation.
  - An ultrasound is performed a few days after the trauma, preferably on day 7, when the hematoma is well-defined.
  - Healing time is relatively long, ranging from 6 to 12 weeks. Physiotherapy and rehabilitation aim to ensure uneventful and smooth healing of the injury, minimizing the incidence of complications such as fibrotic scar tissue, cystic formation, encapsulation of a well-defined hematoma, calcification, and so on.
  - Surgery may be indicated for:

    drainage of large hematoma if ultrasound-guided needle aspiration fails,
    Surgical repair for tendon avulsions and avulsion-fractures such as those of the ischial tuberosity or anterior superior iliac spine is crucial. Early diagnosis is key to performing timely and adequate surgical repair, allowing for complete recovery, or "restitutio ad integrum."

Methods of Limbs Traction 13

Traction is usually a temporary treatment for certain fractures, used while waiting for the final management strategy to be implemented. However, it may occasionally correspond to the final treatment (patients with absolute surgical contraindications, some pediatric fractures, etc.). The general aim is to align the fracture fragments and reduce inert-fragmentary motion in order to:

- Relieve pain,
- Reduce bleeding at the fracture site,
- Decrease incidence of neuro-vascular complications.

The installation of a fracture's traction system follows strict precautions and rules with respect to the technique and the accessories to use.

13.1 Types of Tractions and Material to Use

13.1.1 Skeletal Traction

Skeletal traction requires absolute surgical aseptic precautions. It is usually performed using local anesthesia with additional sedation if needed. It involves the trans-osseous insertion of a wire or pin distal to the fracture site. A special metallic stirrup or bow is then connected to the pin (or wire), allowing a string with weights to be attached to pull the limb and align the fracture site. Skeletal traction can be achieved with either a Kirschner wire or Steinmann pin.

1. **Kirschner wire (1.8–2.0 mm)**
   (a) Insertion can use either a power drill or a hand drill,
   (b) Special stirrup or traction bow is needed.

D. Saragaglia, A. Hassan Chamseddine, *Traumatology for the Emergency Doctor*, https://doi.org/10.1007/978-3-031-63196-2_13

   (c) Advantages:
      - Easy insertion,
      - "Small" trans-osseous tunnel.
   (d) Disadvantages
      - Cannot be used for:
         - substantial weight,
         - prolonged time.
      - Risk of:
         - Pin cutting through the bone, especially in osteoporotic bone,
         - Local infection, especially when left in place for long time.
2. **Steinmann pin (4–5 mm)**
   (a) Should never be inserted using a hammer, to avoid the risk of inducing a fracture,
   (b) Pin insertion uses a Jacobs chuck with a T-handle attachment, a hand drill, or a slow speed power drill,
   (c) A special stirrup or traction bow is used.
   (d) Advantages:
      - Allows the application of greater weight, over a longer period of time,
      - Less risk of pin cut-out through the bone.
   (e) Disadvantages:
      - Technically demanding (e.g., femoral trans-condylar),
      - More risk of local infection.

13.1.2 Skin Traction

- Applied directly to the skin,
- Quick application and less invasive than skeletal traction,
- Uses special adhesive bandages and tapes.
- Disadvantages:
   - Suitable only for light weight (less than 5 kg) and short durations of traction,
   - May cause constriction and subsequent vascular impairment due to an over-tightened bandage,
   - May lead to skin necrosis and avulsion, particularly in elderly individuals with fragile and thin skin,
   - May result in insufficient fracture reduction and pain relief,
   - Traction may frequently become untied and loosened.

13.2 Different Sites of Tractions

13.2.1 Upper Limb

Trans-olecranon traction is the only type of skeletal traction that can be applied in the upper limb (Fig. 13.1).

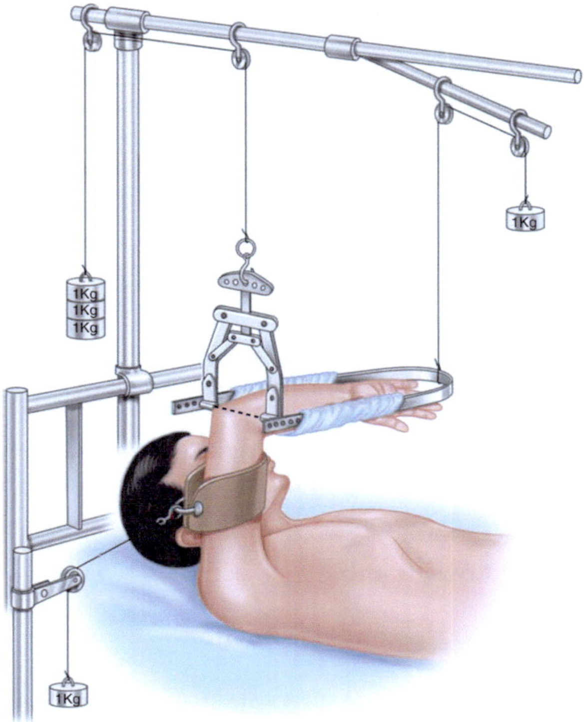

Fig. 13.1 Schematic illustration of a trans-olecranon skeletal traction

- It may be indicated for displaced humeral fractures (whether proximal, shaft, or distal) in particular situations:
  - For patients whose final treatment is delayed due to polytrauma or other reasons,
  - Following debridement and closure of an open fracture, while awaiting final treatment via open reduction and internal fixation,
  - In small or emerging facilities where specialized surgical care is unavailable or when a transfer to more specialized healthcare center is anticipated.
- The traction system is applied under local anesthesia with sedation.
- Traction involves the use of either a Kirschner wire or a special olecranon screw inserted perpendicular to the long axis of the ulna.
  - The Kirschner wire is 1.8–2.0 mm
  - The olecranon screw corresponds to:

    special "olecranon wing screw,"

    or bent Schanz screw (3.0–4.0 mm),

    or cancellous screw (4.0 mm) with a metallic loop fashioned around its neck for attachment of the string.
- Insertion of the Kirschner wire:
  - 3 cm distal to the tip of the olecranon,
  - Just deep to the sub-cutaneous posterior edge of the ulna,

- The wire is inserted from medial to lateral in the frontal plan (to avoid injuring the ulnar nerve), and perpendicular to the long axis of the ulna.
- Insertion of the screw:
  - 3 cm distal to the tip of the olecranon,
  - The screw is inserted from the posterior border of the ulna, perpendicular to its long axis, in the sagittal plan (postero-anterior direction), directed toward the coronoid process.
- Positioning of the patient on traction :
  - Patient in supine position,
  - Shoulder at 90° anterior flexion,
  - Elbow at 90° flexion,
  - A stockinette dressing is applied to the forearm for comfort reasons and to suspend the forearm in a horizontal position in front of the patient's face and upper chest.
  - Traction begins with a 3 kg weight, and is increased until the patient's ipsilateral scapula lifts off the bed, typically reaching to 6–7 kg.

13.2.2 Lower Limb

13.2.2.1 Trans-condylar Traction

- Technique
  - Administer local anesthesia (±sedation) at the suggested sites of pin entry and exit, injecting deep to the periosteum. A femoral block is an alternative option.
  - Make a stab incision at the medial side of the distal femur, just 2–3 cm proximal to the upper border of the patella,
  - *Insert* a Steinmann pin manually from medial to lateral, parallel to the joint line, using a Jacobs chuck with a T-handle, to avoid the femoral artery.
  - *Make* another stab incision on the opposite side where the pin emerges under the skin.
  - *Mount* a special stirrup with an attached string on the pin.
- Setup and positioning
  - Use a standard bed, with or without a special mobile frame, or a special orthopedic bed equipped with traction-suspension accessories (Figs. 13.2 and 13.3)
  - The weight used to apply traction can be up to 20% of the patient's body weight, ranging from 10 to 20 kg, depending to the fracture displacement.
- Indications
  - Displaced fractures of the pelvic ring,
  - Displaced fractures of the acetabulum.
- Complications of prolonged period of traction:
  - Knee stiffness,
  - Osteitis of the femur at the pin entry and exit sites.

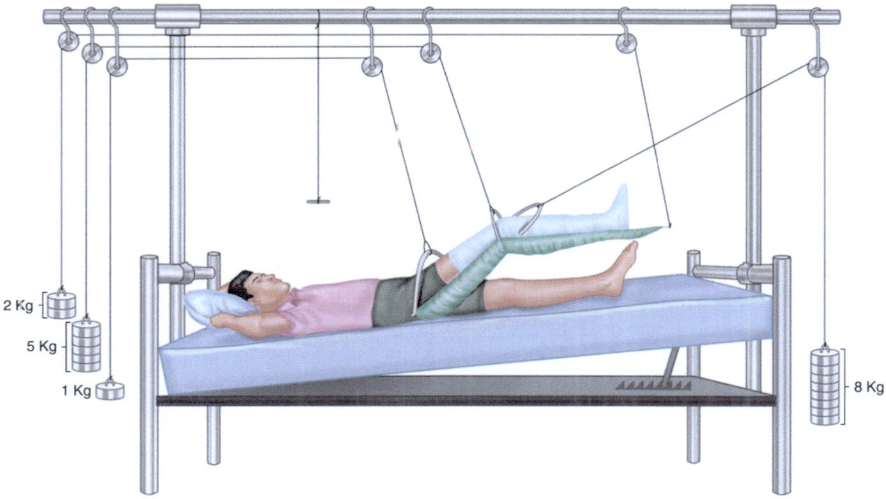

Fig. 13.2 Schematic illustration of a special orthopedic bed with the traction-suspension accessories

Fig. 13.3 Photo of a patient treated with a traction-suspension method for an undisplaced fracture of the acetabulum

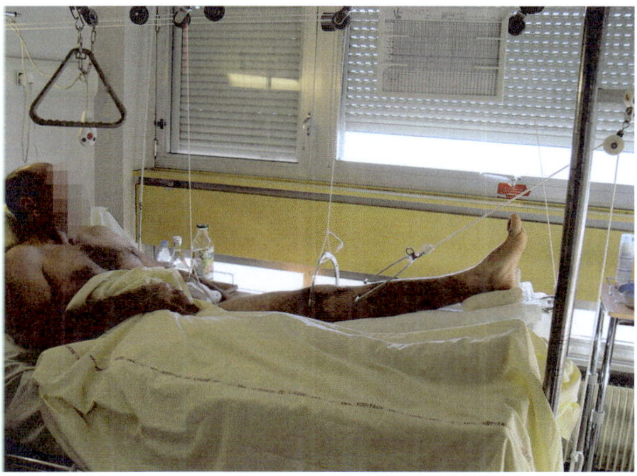

13.2.2.2 Trans-Tibial Traction (Fig. 13.4)

1. Technique
   (a) Administer local anesthesia (±sedation) at the suggested sites of pin entry and exit, injecting deep to the periosteum.
   (b) Insert a Steinmann pin manually, from lateral to medial, parallel to the joint line, to avoid the fibular nerve, using a Jacobs chuck with a T-handle or a hand drill. Alternatively, insert a Kirschner wire using a power drill.
   (c) For adults, the pin's entry point is 1–2 cm posterior to the anterior tibial tuberosity. For pediatric patients, the pin's entry point is distal to the anterior

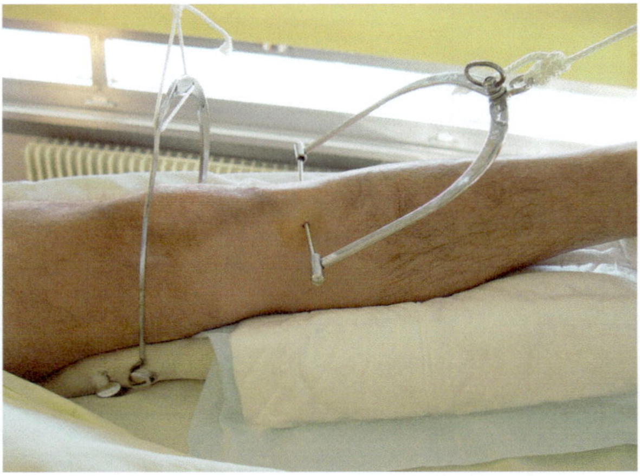

Fig. 13.4 Photo of a patient with a trans-tibial skeletal traction using a Steinmann pin

tibial tuberosity to prevent injury to the center of ossification and avoid iatrogenic secondary epiphysiodesis.

(d) Mount a special stirrup or bow with a string on the pin.

2. Indications: trans-tibial traction is typically used as a provisional treatment for displaced femoral fractures pending final treatment. This includes fractures of the proximal femur (neck, pertrochanteric) shaft, and distal end, whether or not there is articular involvement.
3. Setup and positioning
   (a) Proximal femur fractures
   - Displaced femoral neck
     - Young adult (<65 years)
       Apply 8–10 kg of traction for fracture reduction if surgery (internal fixation) is delayed or postponed,
       Orthopedic bed with special traction-suspension accessories.
     - Old patients (>65 years)
       Traction with 8–10 kg,
       Skin traction is another option (5 kg maximum),
       Orthopedic bed with traction-suspension accessories.
   - Displaced pertrochanteric fractures
     - Traction with 10–12 kg,
     - Orthopedic bed with traction-suspension accessories.

   (b) Femoral shaft fractures
   - Apply traction with 10–15 kg which may be up to 20% of body weight,
   - Orthopedic bed with traction-suspension accessories.

   (c) Distal femur
   - Traction with 10–12 kg,
   - Use an orthopedic bed with traction-suspension accessories, positioning the knee at a 45° flexion.

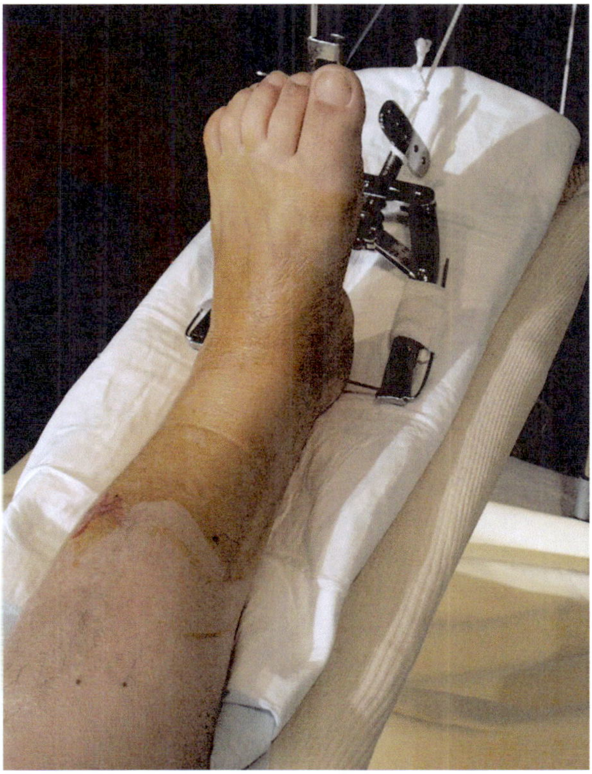

Fig. 13.5 Photo of a temporary trans-calcaneal skeletal traction using a Kirschner wire while awaiting for the final treatment of a tibial fracture

13.2.2.3 Trans-Calcaneal Traction (Fig. 13.5)

- Technique
  - Administer local anesthesia deep to the bone at the suggested entry and exit points for the pin or wire,
  - Insert the Steinmann pin using Jacobs chuck with T-handle, or hand drill, or the Kirschner wire using a power drill, from medial to lateral across the posterior part of the calcaneus to avoid the posterior tibial neuro-vascular bundle,
  - The entry point is located 2 cm posterior and distal to the tip of the medial malleolus,
  - Insert the pin horizontally and perpendicular to the limb's longitudinal axis, ensuring it exits on the heel's opposite side, distal, and posterior to the tip of the lateral malleolus.
- Indications
  - Tibial plateau fractures,
  - Tibial shaft fractures,
  - Tibial pilon (plafond) fractures (not bimalleolar fractures).

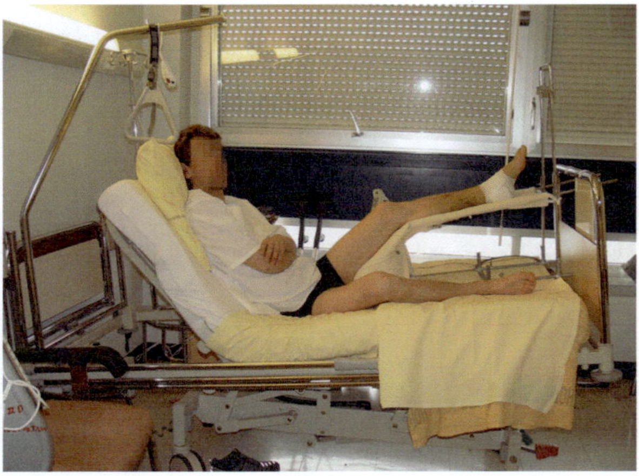

Fig. 13.6 Photo of a movable articulated beam frame used for positioning of the lower limb in the bed

- Setup and positioning
  - Traction weight 6–8 kg according to fracture's location,
  - Movable beam frame for leg positioning (Fig. 13.6),
  - Position in 45° knee flexion for tibial shaft and pilon fractures,
  - Position in knee extension for tibial plateau fractures.

13.2.3 Multiple Tractions

Usual indications for multiple tractions include the presence of ipsilateral or bilateral lower limb multiple fractures in patients with major contraindications for early surgical repair. A trans-condylar or trans-tibial traction (e.g., for a pelvic or femoral fracture) can be simultaneously applied with a trans-calcaneal traction (e.g., for a tibial fracture) on the same lower limb. An orthopedic bed with traction-suspension accessories is required for this setup.

13.2.4 Conclusion

- Skeletal traction is not without risk, particularly when over a long period, as it may lead to complications such as local infection,
- The weight used in traction should be adjusted based on the reduction of fracture displacement as determined by successive radiographic evaluations,
- Patient positioning in the bed is a meticulous task that should avoid unnecessary equipment and installations, as comfort is crucial (Fig. 13.7),
- Use of specific setup (orthopedic bed with traction-suspension accessories) is important for the patient's comfort and nursing care,

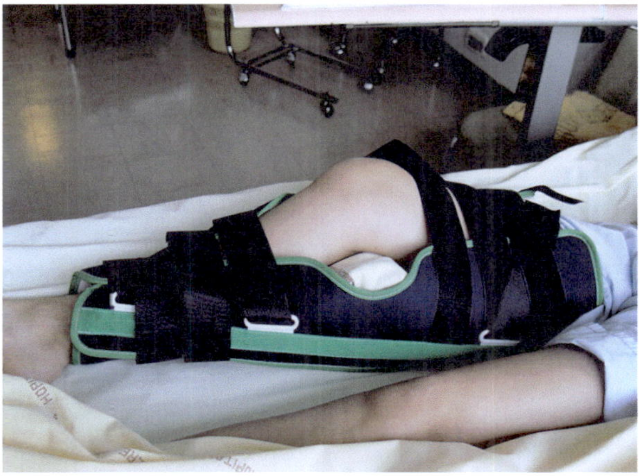

Fig. 13.7 Bad example of an immobilization system applied for a tibial plateau fracture

- Skeletal traction is a rigorous procedure that may serve as the final treatment or be maintained for an extended period in specific cases, such as polytrauma, acetabular fractures, and pelvic ring fractures,
- Skin traction should be used with caution and is generally reserved for exceptional cases, such as small children.

Part II

Traumatic Injuries of the Upper Limb

14 Clinical Assessment of Chronic Painful Shoulder

A comprehensive physical examination of the shoulder in the early post-traumatic period is often difficult and hazardous, as it may lead to dislocation or displacement of an underlying non-displaced fracture. However, it can be performed later, away from the initial trauma, and when there is no fracture or dislocation present.

For osteo-articular injuries, both physical examination and history are important to guide the para-clinical investigations and diagnosis.

The first step in the assessment is to obtain the patient's history and details of the trauma, including the circumstances of occurrence (such as road traffic accident, sports, or domestic incidents), the type of trauma (direct or indirect), the character and severity of pain, and the degree of functional disability. The second step involves inspection, followed by the evaluation of active and passive shoulder mobility. Finally, provocative and dynamic maneuvers are performed to assess shoulder stability and the condition of the rotator cuff.

14.1 Inspection

The patient should be undressed for inspection, comparing both sides. The inspection looks for:

- Muscle atrophy (deltoid, supra-spinatous fossa, infra-spinatous fossa, trapezius),
- Scapular winging, which may be due to paralysis of the serratus anterior muscle caused by injury to the long thoracic nerve (Fig. 14.1),
- Any modification or deformity of the acromio-clavicular joint or sterno-clavicular joint,
- Any modification or deformity of the shoulder, such as obliteration of the delto-pectoral sulcus, flattening of the antero-lateral aspect of the deltoid muscle, or bulging of the posterior aspect of the deltoid.

D. Saragaglia, A. Hassan Chamseddine, *Traumatology for the Emergency Doctor*, https://doi.org/10.1007/978-3-031-63196-2_14

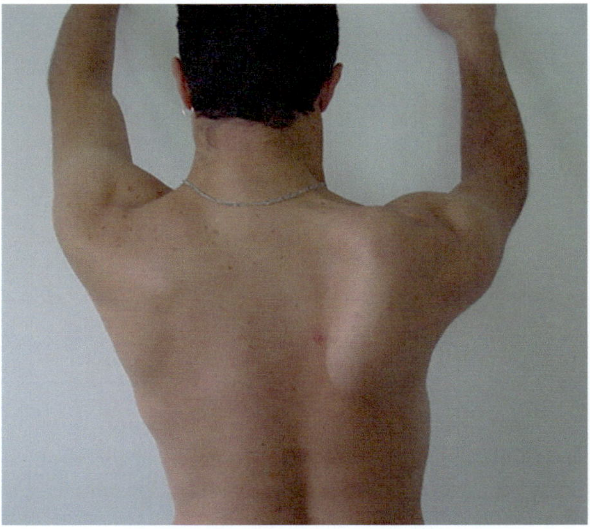

Fig. 14.1 Photo of a patient with a scapular winging seen from behind

14.2 Evaluation of Active and Passive Shoulder Motion

Among the six elementary shoulder movements, three are fundamental for diagnostic orientation:

- Anterior elevation or flexion is measured using goniometer, with the normal value being 180°.
- Internal rotation (Fig. 14.2) is measured by having the patient place their hand behind their back and to push it as high as possible. The internal rotation is evaluated by measuring the distance between the thumb and the spinous process of C7, or by noting the vertebra reached by the hand, typically T4–T8, or the lower pole of the scapula.
- External rotation (Fig. 14.3) is measured with the elbow flexed at 90° the elbow at the side, and the arm abducted at 90° successively. The normal value for external rotation is considered to be between 70 and 80°.

Simultaneous concomitant decrease of passive and active range of motion (ROM) for the above three movements is usually sign of *adhesive capsulitis*, and less frequently omarthrosis (especially in the elderly).

For patient with normal passive ROM and decreased active ROM, rotator cuff disease should be considered and particularly *pseudoparalytic shoulder* (Fig. 14.4).

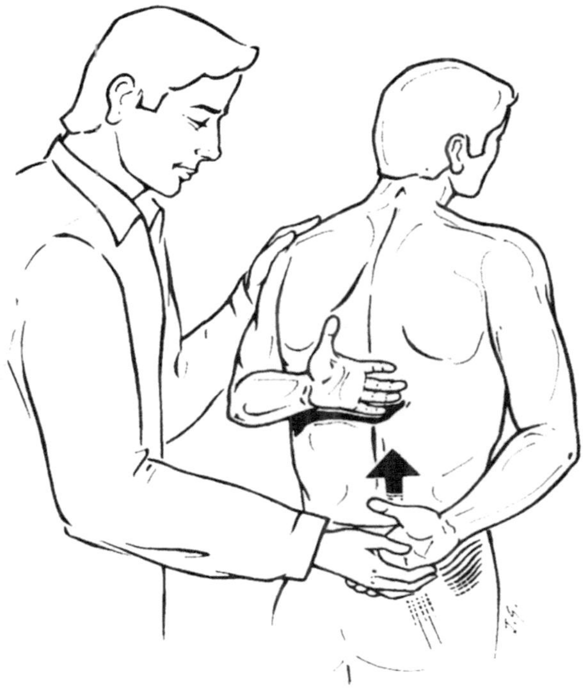

Fig. 14.2 Illustration of the evaluation of the shoulder internal rotation

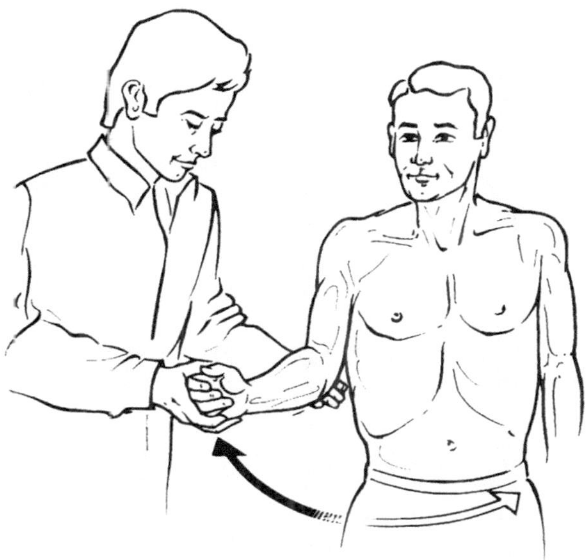

Fig. 14.3 Illustration of the evaluation of the shoulder external rotation with the elbow at side

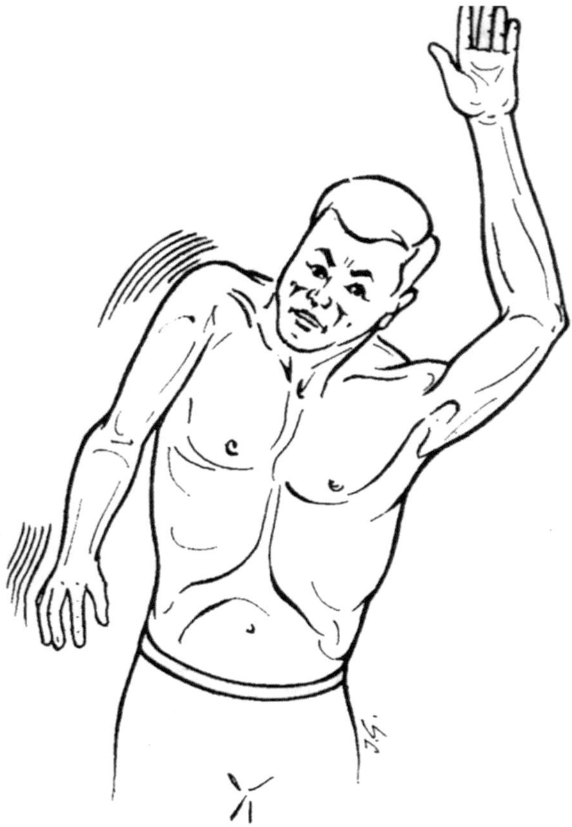

Fig. 14.4 Illustration of a patient with absence of active shoulder elevation

14.3 Provocative and Dynamic Maneuvers

14.3.1 Sub-acromial Impingement

Sub-acromial impingement classically corresponds to degenerative changes of the rotator cuff tendons secondary to chronic and repetitive conflict with the antero-inferior acromial edge-spur and the antero-lateral border of the coraco-acromial ligament.

- *Neer's maneuver*: the examiner (placed behind the patient's shoulder) locks the scapula with one hand (to prevent scapular movement) and raises, with the other hand, the patient's upper limb in passive elevation with the elbow extended (in a position between anterior flexion and abduction, usually in the scapular plane); the upper limb is placed in internal rotation during the maneuver. Positive maneuver corresponds to pain at 60–120° of elevation as the greater tuberosity impinges against the sub-acromial arch. In addition, pain disappears when the examiner brings the upper limb in external rotation.

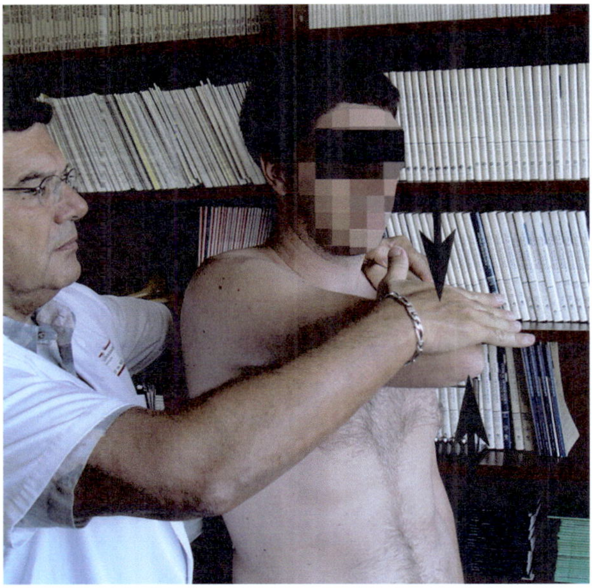

Fig. 14.5 Illustration of the Yocum maneuver

- *Yocum's maneuver* (Fig. 14.5): the patient's hand of the affected side is placed over the opposite shoulder, with the arm at 90° anterior elevation and elbow flexion. The patient is then asked to push their elbow upwards against resistance by the examiner's hand; the maneuver is positive for impingement if the patient feels pain.
- *Hawkins' maneuver* (Fig. 14.6): the scapula of the affected side is locked by the examiner; the patient's arm is passively brought at 90° anterior shoulder elevation with 90° elbow flexion, followed by forced passive internal rotation of the shoulder. The maneuver is positive for impingement if the patient feels pain.

14.3.2 Assessment of the Rotator Cuff Muscles

The rotator cuff is basically composed of four muscles: supra-spinatus, infra-spinatus, teres minor, and sub-scapularis. Although the intra-articular portion of the long biceps tendon is not structurally part of the rotator cuff tendons, it participates in rotator cuff pathology and should be considered alongside it. Each one of the rotator cuff muscles should be individually assessed with a specific test.

1. *Supra-spinatus: Jobe's test* (Fig. 14.7)
   (a) The arm is abducted at 90° and brought 30° forward into the scapular plane with internal rotation (thumb directed to the floor).
   (b) The examiner applies downward pressure on the patient's arm while the patient attempts to maintain the initial position.
   (c) The test is positive:

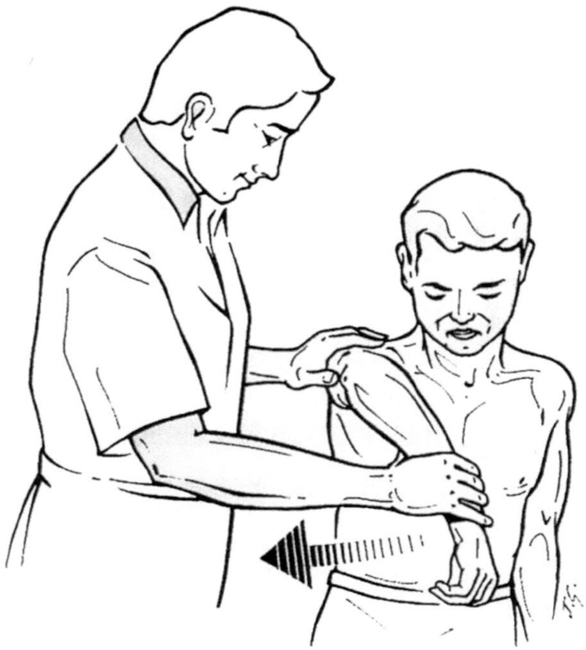

Fig. 14.6 Illustration of the Hawkins maneuver

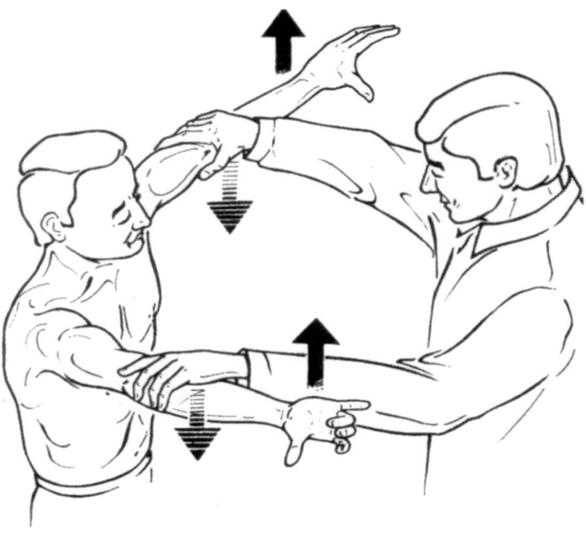

Fig. 14.7 Illustration of the Jobe maneuver

- for supra-spinatus weakness if the patient is unable to maintain the position,
- or for supra-spinatus impingement if the patient feels pain during the test.

2. *Infra-spinatus and teres minor:*

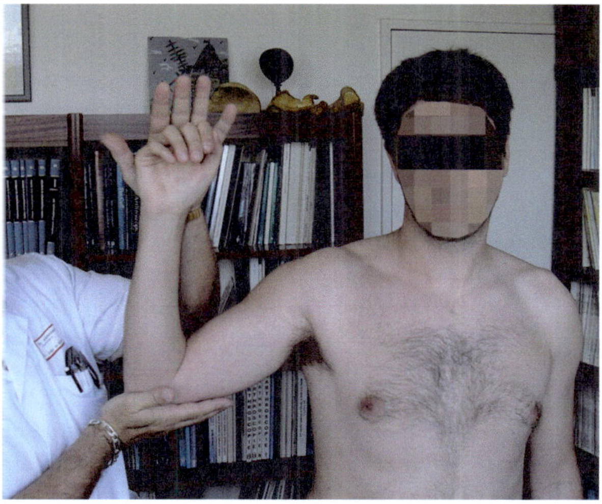

Fig. 14.8 Photo of the Patte maneuver

(a) *Patte's maneuver* (Fig. 14.8)
- The examiner is positioned behind the patient's back,
- The patient positions their shoulder in 90° of external rotation position with the elbow 90° flexed and the arm 90° abducted,
- The patient is then asked to push into further external rotation of the shoulder against the examiner's resistance,
- Muscular force is evaluated according to the following scale:
  - 5: symmetrical normal muscular power,
  - 4: decreased muscular power,
  - 3: shoulder positioning in external rotation is only possible against gravity (failure to maintain external rotation against resistance),
  - 2: absence of active external rotation (with arm 90° abduction and elbow 90° flexion),
  - 1: only muscular contraction is possible,
  - 0: absence of muscular contraction.

(b) Two additional signs can also be used for evaluation of the function of the supra-spinatus and teres minor muscles:
- *The Hornblower's sign*: the examiner brings the patient's shoulder into 90° external rotation position with the elbow 90° flexed and the arm 90° abducted. The patient is then asked to maintain this position. The hornblower's sign is positive if the patient fails to hold the position: the arm spontaneously falls in internal rotation with the hand dropping below the level of the elbow. In daily life activities, this sign is seen when the patient wants to eat: as they try to bring their hand to the level of their mouth, they should elevate their elbow above the horizontal line with internal rotation of the arm, miming the hornblower's position.
- *The "swing gate" sign*: the examiner holds the patient's hand and brings their shoulder in external rotation with the arm at side and the elbow 90°

flexed; when the examiner releases the hand of the patient, it swings back and hits his their abdomen. In addition, the so-called *drop sign* has the same significance; however it is explored with the arm passively abducted at 90° in the scapular plane and the shoulder brought in external rotation: the sign is positive when the patient is asked to slowly lower the arm causing them to drop the arm to their side.

3. *Sub-scapularis:*
   (a) *Lift-off test or Gerber's maneuver* (Fig. 14.9): the patient makes a fist with their hand and brings it around their back to the lumbar spine region; he is then asked to lift the hand away from the back and to maintain the position. The test is positive when the patient is unable to lift the hand off the back, and it is more specific for the distal part of the sub-scapularis.
   (b) *Belly-press test or Napoleon sign* (Fig. 14.10a, b): the patient is asked to press their abdomen with their hand palm, while the elbow is passively brought in front of the trunk (shoulder internal rotation). The test is positive when the elbow swings back to the trunk, and it is more specific for the proximal part of the sub-scapularis.
4. *Long head of Biceps*: Multiple tests have been described; however none of them is specific for the pathology of the long head of the biceps.

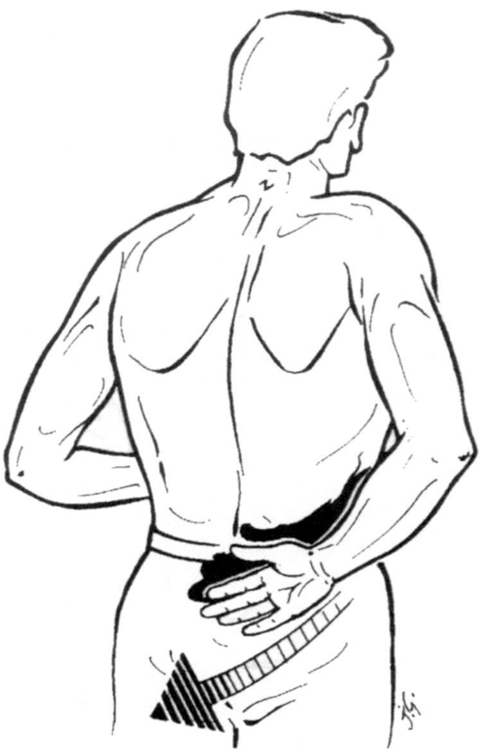

Fig. 14.9 Illustration of the lift-off test of Gerber

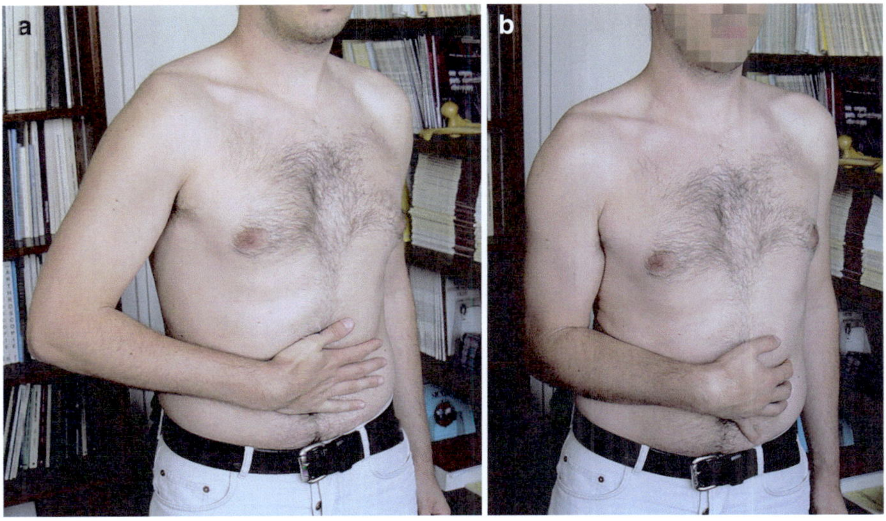

Fig. 14.10 (**a**) Negative belly-press test: the elbow remains distant from the trunk. (**b**) Positive belly-press test: the elbow swings back to the trunk and the patient is unable to press their abdomen with their hand palm

(a) *Palm-up test (Speed's test)*: the test is considered positive if the patient feels pain in the bicipital groove during active forward elevation of their shoulder against resistance with the elbow in extension and forearm in supination.
(b) *Yergason's test*: the patient's elbow is 90° flexed with the forearm fully pronated. The patient is then asked to actively bring their forearm in supination while the examiner makes contra-resistance by holding their wrist in pronated position. The test is considered positive if the patient feels pain in the bicipital groove.
(c) *Popeye Sign*: the patient is asked to make elbow flexion to 90° while the examiner performs contra-resistance. The test is positive for proximal rupture of the long head of the biceps tendon when a bump appears in the middle of the arm at the level of the muscle belly.

14.3.3 Assessment of Shoulder Instability

14.3.3.1 Anterior Instability

Testing of anterior instability is better achieved with the patient in supine position. Two tests are usually performed:

– *Apprehension test* (Fig. 14.11): with the elbow 90° flexed and the arm 90° abducted, the examiner progressively brings the shoulder into a position of extreme external rotation. The test is positive if the patient feels a sensation of

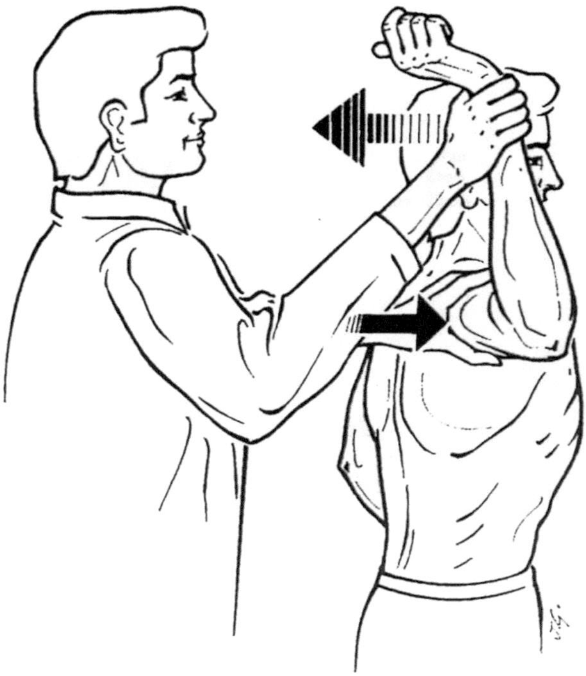

Fig. 14.11 Illustration of the apprehension test

instability and resists against the examiner's maneuver because they fear their shoulder is going to dislocate.

- *Relocation test*: when the patient feels apprehension of dislocation during the previous maneuver, the examiner applies an antero-posterior directed force to the anterior aspect of the shoulder to relocate the humeral head into the glenohumeral joint; the patient consequently feels reassured with the immediate disappearance of the instability sensation.

14.3.3.2 Posterior Instability

Apprehension to posterior stress test: the patient's elbow is 90° flexed with the arm placed at 90° forward elevation with mild adduction and shoulder internal rotation. One of the examiner's hands stabilizes the scapula of the patient, and the other hand applies an antero-posterior force to the patient's elbow.

The test is considered positive if the patient apprehends or fears a posterior subluxation, or if the examiner feels a posterior displacement of the humeral head.

14.3.4 Assessment of Laxity

- Passive external rotation of the shoulder of more than 80–85°, with the elbow at side, can indicate laxity.

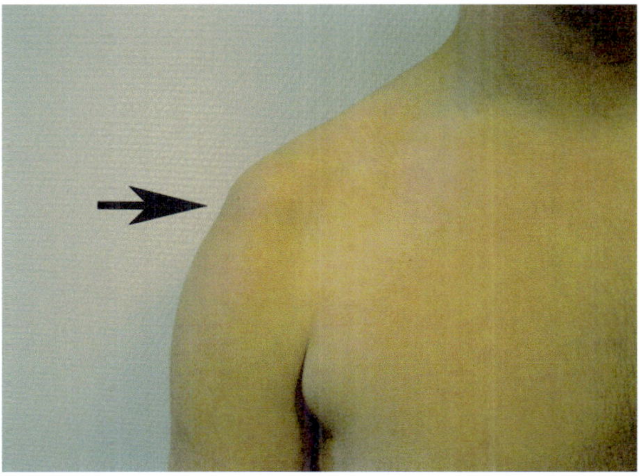

Fig. 14.12 The sulcus sign

- *Anterior drawer test*: the patient's scapula is stabilized by one of the examiner's hands; the other hand seizes the humeral head and applies an anteriorly directed force. An excessive anterior translation of the humeral head is considered positive for anterior laxity.
- *Posterior drawer test*: the patient's scapula is stabilized by one of the examiner's hands; the other hand seizes the humeral head and applies a posteriorly directed force. An excessive posterior translation of the humeral head is considered positive for posterior laxity.
- *Sulcus sign* (Fig. 14.12): the patient in standing position facing the examiner, with their arms at their side. The examiner seizes the patient's arms and pulls them inferiorly in an attempt to induce gleno-humeral "de-coaptation." The test is considered positive when a sulcus appears at the supero-lateral edge of the humeral head, below the latero-inferior border of the acromion.

Fractures of the Clavicle

15

Fractures of the clavicle are very common traumatic injuries in sports practice as well as in road traffic and domestic accidents. They usually occur in young adults and are typically induced by a direct traumatic impact to the lateral aspect of the shoulder or to the clavicle itself.

15.1 Patho-anatomy

Fractures of the clavicle can be schematically categorized into three types based on their location: medial third, middle third, and lateral third.

15.1.1 Fractures of the Medial Third

- They represent the least common location (5%),
- They are usually non-displaced,
- They may be either simple or comminuted.

15.1.2 Fractures of the Middle Third

- They represent the most common location (70–85% of cases).
- They may be simple (two parts), segmental, or comminuted (three or more fragments), or with an intercalated displaced fragment producing skin tenting.
- The lateral main fragment is usually displaced infero-medially (by the effect of gravity: weight of the arm), and the medial main fragment is commonly displaced postero-superiorly (traction induced by the sterno-cleido-mastoid muscle).

D. Saragaglia, A. Hassan Chamseddine, *Traumatology for the Emergency Doctor*, https://doi.org/10.1007/978-3-031-63196-2_15

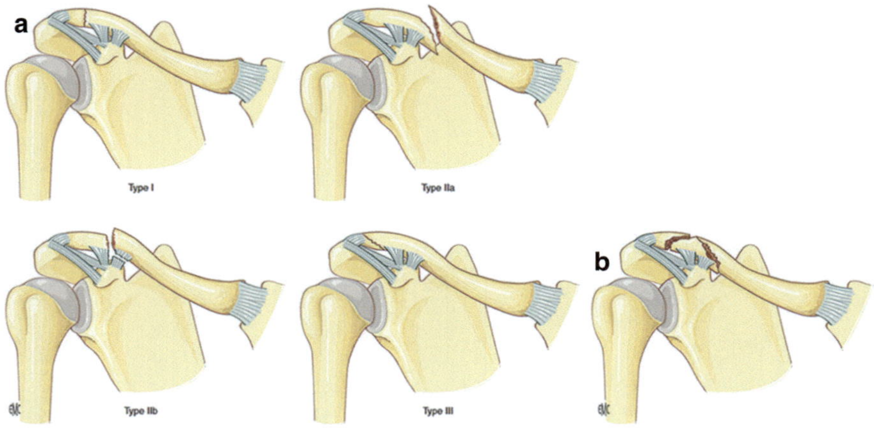

Fig. 15.1 Neer fracture classification (type I, type IIa, type IIb, type III fractures) and Latarajet fracture (Reproduced with permission of Elsevier Masson from Saragaglia D, Chirurgie et traumatismes de la clavicule, articulations acromioclaviculaire et sternoclaviculaire incluses. EMC -techniques chirurgicales - Orthopédie-Traumatologie 2019;14(1):1-16 [Article 44-230])

15.1.3 Fractures of the Lateral Third

- They represent the second least common location (10–15%).
- The fracture pattern may affect the acromioclavicular joint.
- Neer's classification is commonly used for their description: three types of fractures are distinguished according to their location with respect to the coracoclavicular ligaments:
  - Type I: the fracture is located lateral to the coracoclavicular ligaments (Fig. 15.1).
    If the ligaments are intact, the fracture is stable.
    If the ligaments are disrupted, the fracture is unstable and is considered equivalent to an acromioclavicular dislocation.
  - Type II: the fracture is located at the level of the coracoclavicular ligaments, with two sub-types:
    Type IIa: medial to the coracoclavicular ligaments (Fig. 15.1),
    Type IIb: through the coracoclavicular ligaments (Fig. 15.1). A particular variety of type IIb fracture is distinguished: the so-called Latarjet fracture which corresponds to an inferior bone fragment that remains attached to the coracoclavicular ligaments (Figs. 15.1 and 15.2).
  - Type III: the fracture involves the acromioclavicular joint (Fig. 15.1).

15.2 Management

1. ***Physical evaluation*** to identify potential complications which are very rare:

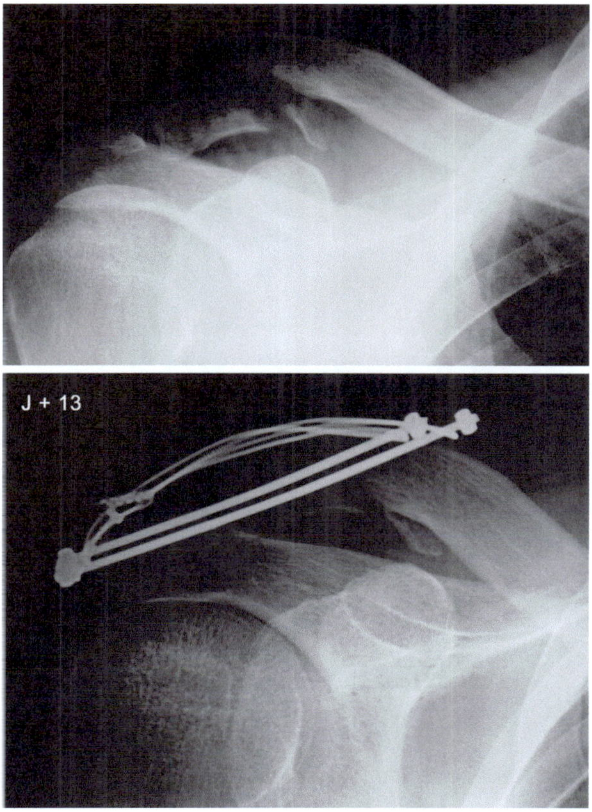

Fig. 15.2 "Figure of 8" fixation using metallic pins and wire for the treatment of a Latarjet fracture

   (a) Neurovascular (brachial plexus, subclavian vessels),
   (b) Pulmonary (lung and pleura: pneumothorax, lung injury, etc.),
   (c) Cutaneous (skin tenting or opening).
2. ***Radiographic assessment***
   (a) Antero-posterior view, preferably in a standing position if the patient's condition permits.
   (b) Antero-posterior view with a 15–30° cephalic tilt.
   (c) Shoulder radiographs to evaluate associated injuries (e.g., proximal humerus fracture).
   (d) Chest X-rays if there is suspicion of pneumothorax or lung injury.
   (e) CT scan which is useful to assess fractures of both extremities of the clavicle (i.e., fractures of the lateral-acromial extremity and medial-sternal extremity).
3. ***Treatment*** is commonly debated: conservative versus operative.
   (a) *Conservative treatment*:
      - Attempting to reduce the fracture is generally considered useless.
      - Ideal or complete immobilization is neither available nor realistic.
      - The "Figure of 8" brace or strap (Fig. 15.3) is commonly used:

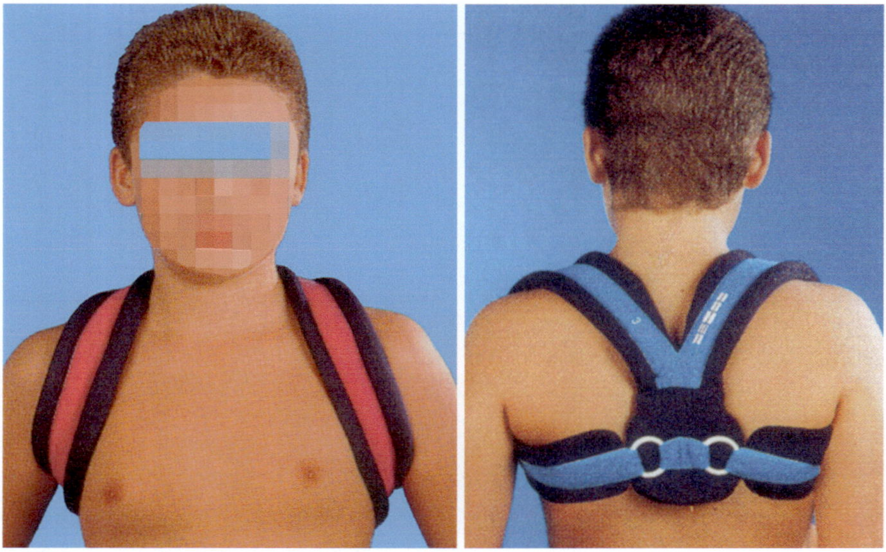

Fig. 15.3 "Figure of 8" brace for clavicular fracture

- Until pain completely disappears (4–6 weeks),
- It requires continuous readjustment,
- It can be uncomfortable for the patient as it may induce skin friction-irritation and neurovascular compression, especially in the axillary region (upper limb edema, numbness, etc.).

• Arm sling:
- There is no difference in functional and cosmetic results compared to the "Figure of 8" brace,
- It is less painful and more comfortable than the "Figure of 8" brace,
- It has better patient's compliance than the "Figure of 8" brace.

(b) *Surgical treatment:*

• Principally corresponds to open reduction and internal fixation with plate and screws.

• Indications:
- Absolute indications:
  Vascular injury,
  Skin tenting,
  Vertically displaced intercalated fragment, impinging with the skin,
  Open fractures,
  Fracture pattern equivalent to acromioclavicular dislocation.
- Relative indications:
  Bilateral clavicle fracture,
  >2 cm shortening,
  Polytrauma.

16 Sternoclavicular Dislocations

Sternoclavicular dislocations are rare injuries. They usually occur after high-energy trauma and are more frequent in road traffic than in sports accidents.

16.1 Patho-anatomy

- The direction of displacement of the medial end of the clavicle defines two types of dislocations:
  - ***Anterior dislocations***: they only cause cosmetic disturbance, usually with no or minimal functional disability. The clavicle is usually displaced in an antero-superior direction.
  - ***Posterior dislocations***: they are less common than anterior dislocations. They may produce compression to the trachea and esophagus, causing dyspnea and dysphagia, respectively. The clavicle is usually displaced in a postero-inferior direction.
- A lesser degree of injury corresponds to sprain without incongruence of the sternoclavicular joint.

16.2 Clinical Presentation and Assessment

- A painful bump at the corresponding sternoclavicular joint.
- Palpation:
  - Tender prominence,
  - Abnormal vertical or horizontal mobility of the joint, induced by the examiner.
- Neurovascular assessment of the affected upper limb (compared to the opposite side):
  - Pulse asymmetry or lessening,
  - Venous congestion,
  - Tingling and paresthesia.

D. Saragaglia, A. Hassan Chamseddine, *Traumatology for the Emergency Doctor*, https://doi.org/10.1007/978-3-031-63196-2_16

  - Neurovascular disturbances typically occur in posterior dislocations.
- Dysphagia and dyspnea are typically present in posterior dislocations.

16.3 Imaging Assessment

- ***Radiographic diagnosis*** is challenging due to the difficult visualization of the sternoclavicular joint on simple radiographs.
  - Recommended view: Antero-posterior view including both sternoclavicular joints in one field with a 40–50° cephalic tilt of the beam (for comparison).
  - it shows superior displacement (in anterior dislocations) or inferior displacement (in posterior dislocations) of the medial end of the clavicle compared to the opposite side.
- ***CT scan***
  - is the most accurate diagnostic tool,
  - useful to differentiate very medial clavicle fractures from dislocations,
  - axial cuts are useful to visualize the direction of displacement and the presence of compression of the mediastinal elements (trachea, esophagus, aorta, etc.).

16.4 Management

- There is no adequate orthopedic treatment that allows stabilization of the sternoclavicular joint with any type of external brace or bandage.
- Sprains with congruent joints are treated conservatively: pain control, arm sling for analgesic purposes and comfort, and restoration of range of motion. However, residual pain and discomfort may persist for 3–12 months.
- Displaced acute dislocations may benefit from attempt at closed reduction under anesthesia. However, post-reduction immobilization is not reliable.
- Surgical treatment using open reduction and stabilization is suggested for anterior dislocations with significant displacement and for posterior dislocations, especially when associated with complication (dysphagia, dyspnea, vascular impairment, etc.).
- Surgical excision of the medial end of the clavicle is suggested for persistent painful dislocations. This usually leads to satisfactory results.

Acromioclavicular Dislocations 17

Acromioclavicular joint (ACJ) dislocations are common sports-related injuries (bicycle, rugby, combat sports, etc.) and also occur due to road traffic and domestic accidents.

17.1 Patho-anatomy and Clinical Correlation

Several classifications have been described. Rockwood's classification, which includes six types, is the most commonly used in the English-language literature. In France, many authors prefer the simpler three-type Julliard's classification, which is widely popular for its simplicity.

17.1.1 Grade I of Julliard (Type I and II of Rockwood) (Fig. 17.1)

- This grade involves an injury only to the *acromioclavicular ligaments*.
- Clinically, it manifests as pain and tenderness over the acromioclavicular joint without deformity or abnormal movement under stress.

17.1.2 Grade II of Julliard (Type III of Rockwood) (Fig. 17.2)

- This grade involves two associated injuries: tears of the *acromioclavicular* (AC) and *coracoclavicular (CC) ligaments*.
- Clinical findings include pain and tenderness over the acromioclavicular joint, along with an abnormal antero-posterior "drawer" under stress, tested by the examiner seizing the acromial end of the clavicle with a thumb-index pinch and applying antero-posterior drawer movement.
- ACJ *incongruence is tpyically intermittent* and often becomes apparent under axial longitudinal loading stress.

D. Saragaglia, A. Hassan Chamseddine, *Traumatology for the Emergency Doctor*, https://doi.org/10.1007/978-3-031-63196-2_17

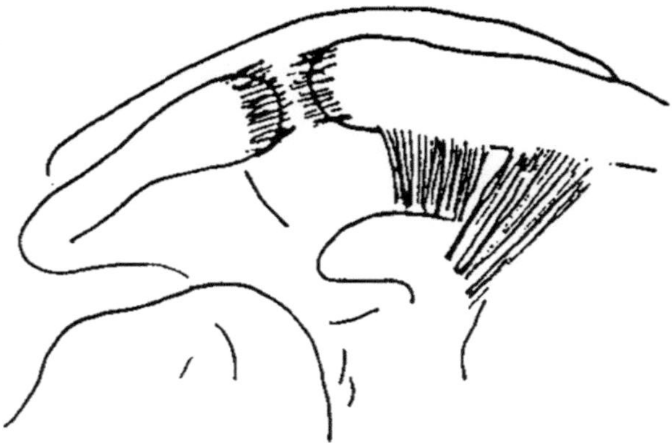

Fig. 17.1 Acromioclavicular dislocation of grade I of Julliard (type I and II of Rockwood)

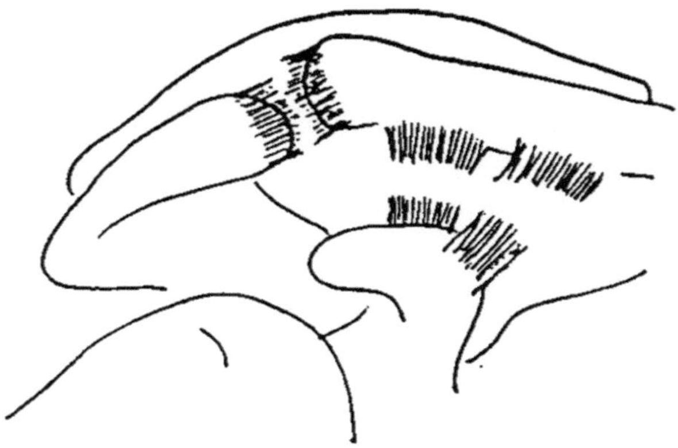

Fig. 17.2 Acromioclavicular dislocation of grade II of Julliard (type III of Rockwood)

17.1.3 Grade III of Julliard (Type V of Rockwood) (Fig. 17.3)

- This grade involves three associated injuries: tears of the *AC and the CC ligaments*, with a rupture of the *delto-trapezius periosteal envelope* or attachment.
- ACJ incongruence is typically permanent, with a deformity and an abnormal shoulder contour compared to the opposite side, often described as a "*stair step-like*" appearance (Fig. 17.4). The shoulder may hang limply downward when standing.
- The lateral extremity of the clavicle is displaced upward.
- Examination reveals abnormal excessive vertical and horizontal instability of the acromial end of the clavicle, characterized by "*piano key-like*" vertical mobility and horizontal antero-posterior "drawer" movement).

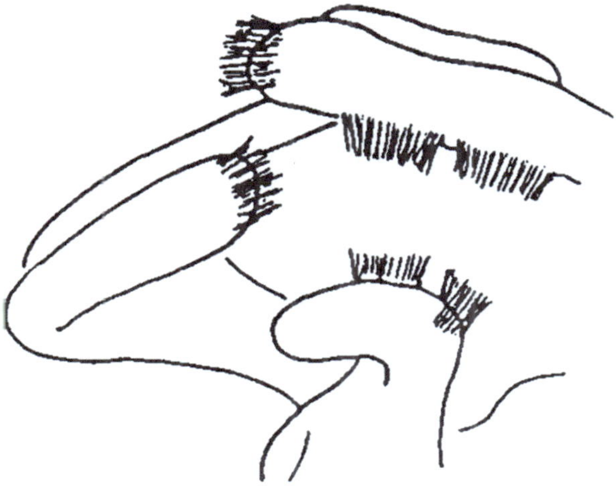

Fig. 17.3 Acromioclavicular dislocation of grade III of Julliard (type V of Rockwood)

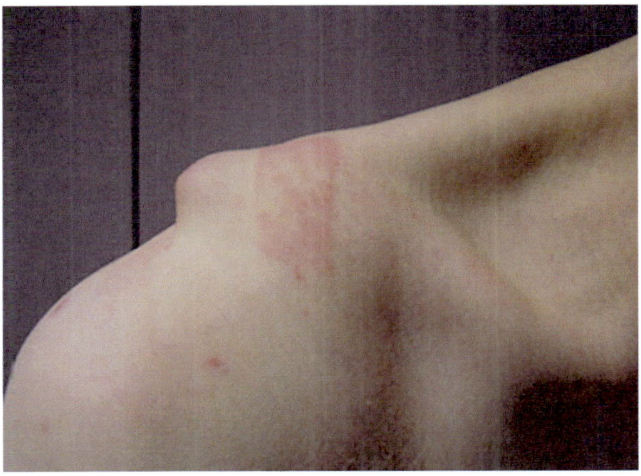

Fig. 17.4 "Stair step-like" appearance of an acromioclavicular dislocation of grade III of Julliard (type V of Rockwood)

17.1.4 Particular Presentations

- ***Type IV of Rockwood*** involves the same patho-anatomic injuries as type V (or III of Julliard) with the addition of posterior dislocation of the lateral extremity of the clavicle.
- ***Type VI of Rockwood*** involves the same patho-anatomic injuries as type V (or III of Julliard) with the addition of inferior dislocation of the lateral extremity of the clavicle.
- ***Equivalent of ACJ dislocation***
  - Fractures involving the "acromial" end of the clavicle, located lateral to the CC ligaments or through it, are associated with rupture of the ligaments.
  - Latarjet's fracture, which is an avulsion-fracture of the clavicular insertion of the CC, the so-called Latarjet's fracture.

- ***Fracture of the base of the coracoid process***
  - A displaced fracture may coincide with a displaced ACJ dislocation, without rupture of the CC ligaments (the coracoclavicular space remains normal, without enlargement).
  - Red flag: A displaced ACJ dislocation with a preserved coracoclavicular radiographic space should prompt consideration of displaced fracture of the base of the coracoid process (Fig. 17.5). Delayed treatment of a coracoid fracture can lead to complications, such as nonunion.

17.1.5 Radiographic Assessment

1. Radiographic assessment is indispensable for an accurate appreciation of the injury grade and to disclose any possible associated lesions.
2. The displacement of the dislocated ACJ is assessed by measuring the coracoclavicular distance, which is the space between the apex of the coracoid and the inferior border of the clavicle.
3. Recommended views:
   (a) Antero-posterior radiographs of both ACJs are used to compare the displacement of the affected side with the normal appearance of the opposite side.
   (b) Antero-posterior radiograph with 15–25° cephalad tilting of the beam (Zanca view).
   (c) Stress view (Fig. 17.6):
   - Performed when there is clinical suspicion of ACJ dislocation with a "normal" radiographic presentation ("congruent" ACJ).
   - Technique:
     - Patient in a standing position,
     - Comparative AP views of both shoulders,

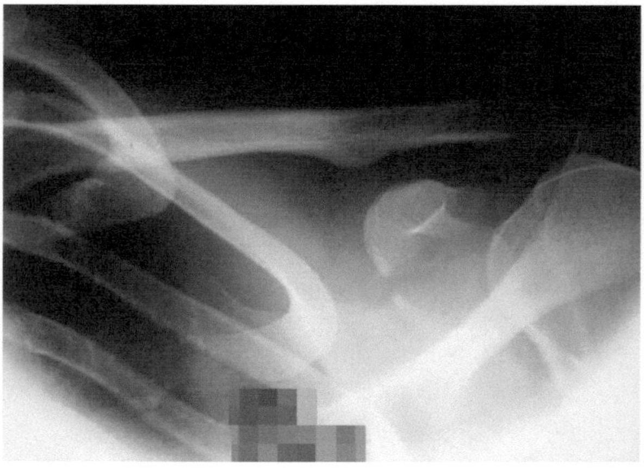

Fig. 17.5 Acromioclavicular dislocation with fracture of the base of the coracoid process: note the preservation of the coracoclavicular space distance

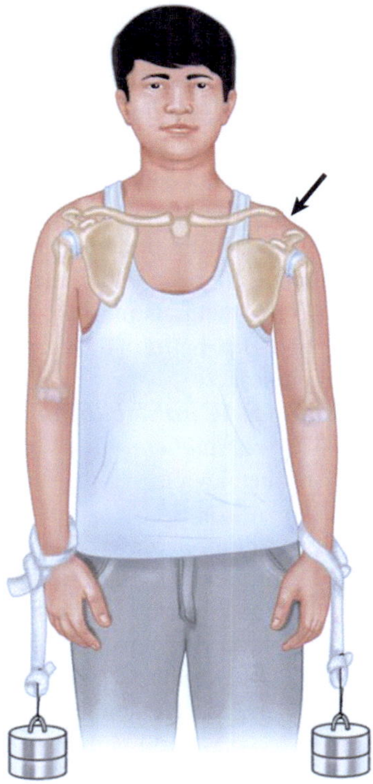

Fig. 17.6 Illustration of the radiographic stress view using weight attached to the wrists

- And a weight is attached to the patient's wrists (hanging the upper limb in elbow extension): 10 kg for males and 5 kg for females.
- Useful for differentiating between Grade I and II. An increased coracoclavicular and acromioclavicular space on the affected side indicates Grade II injury.

17.1.6 Management

Treatment remains controversial.

- ***For Grade I and II of Julliard (type I, II, and III of Rockwood):*** Conservative treatment is recommended.
  - Apply ice to the ACJ,
  - Rest,
  - Strapping (typically no beneficial),
  - Use an arm sling for a short period (10–20 days),
  - Control pain with Paracetamol and NSAID's,
  - Begin early rehabilitation to restore the range of motion,

- Pain may persist for up to 3 months (consider corticosteroid infiltration if needed),
- Resume sports activity 4–6 months after the injury.

- ***Grade III of Julliard (type V of Rockwood):*** Surgical treatment is indicated**.**
  - Early consideration of surgical treatment (within 7 days post-injury) is recommended.
  - The treatment aims to reduce and stabilize both the ACJ and the CC space.
  - The authors' preferred method involves open reduction and stabilization with a tension band using one Kirschner wire, which is removed after 2 months.
  - Other methods include: arthroscopic assisted repair (using artificial ligament and flip button), hook plate fixation, CC screw fixation (Bosworth technique), etc.
- ***Residual ACJ instability and pain***
  - *For residual chronic pain* with stable ACJ: Simple excision of the lateral end of the clavicle.
  - *For residual ACJ instability*:

    Authors' preferred method: Modified Cadenat procedure (French technique): open reduction and temporary stabilization of the ACJ (tension band fixation for 2 months) with reconstruction of the CC ligaments (using the coracoacromial ligament).

    Other method: Modified Weaver-Dunn procedure: excision of the lateral end of the clavicle with reconstruction of the CC ligaments (using the coracoacromial ligament).

Fractures of the Scapula 18

Fractures of the scapula are rare injuries, as this bone is normally well wrapped and protected by an important muscular envelop. They are rarely isolated injuries and are usually associated with other injuries in polytrauma patients.

18.1 Patho-anatomy

Scapula fractures can be categorized as extra-articular or articular. However, some extra-articular fractures that are displaced may functionally be considered intra-articular due to their impact on shoulder function. This is due to architectural disorientation or misalignment of the gleno-humeral joint or the coracoacromial arch, such as in the case of fracture-rupture of the coracoacromial arch or floating shoulder.

18.1.1 Extra-Articular Fractures

- Most frequent (50%),
- Location
  - Scapular body,
  - Scapular spine,
  - Scapular distal tip or angle.

18.1.2 Articular Fractures (Figs. 18.1, 18.2, and 18.3)

- Glenoid fossa and glenoid rim fractures (10%),
- Displaced scapular neck fractures (25%),
- Displaced coracoacromial arch fractures (acromion: 8%, coracoid process 7%). (Displacement is defined as 10 mm or 40° angulation compared to the opposite side)

D. Saragaglia, A. Hassan Chamseddine, *Traumatology for the Emergency Doctor*, https://doi.org/10.1007/978-3-031-63196-2_18

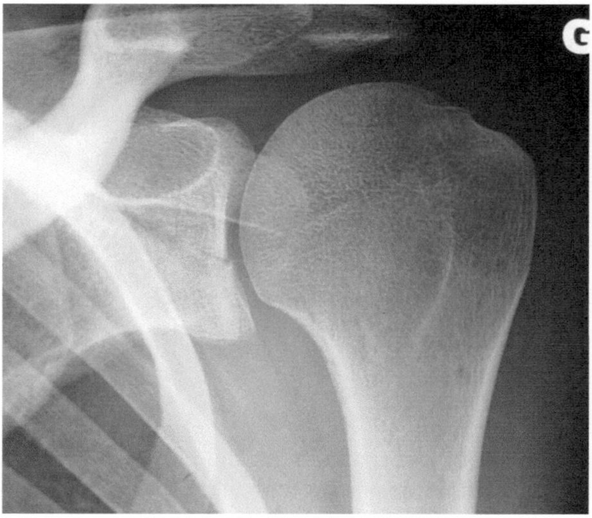

Fig. 18.1 Subtle transverse fracture of the glenoid fossa

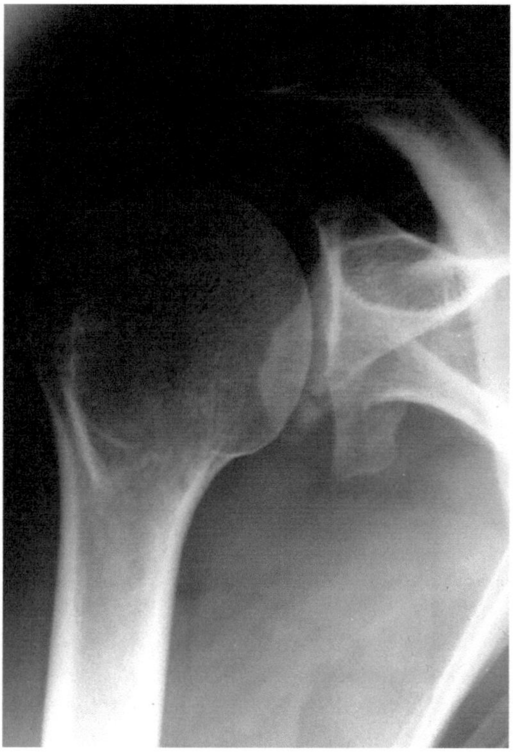

Fig. 18.2 Garth view showing a fracture of the antero-inferior glenoid rim

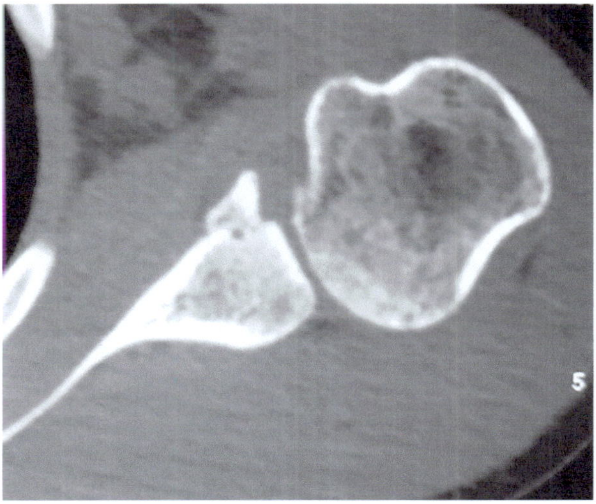

Fig. 18.3 Axial CT scan cut showing a fracture of the antero-inferior glenoid rim

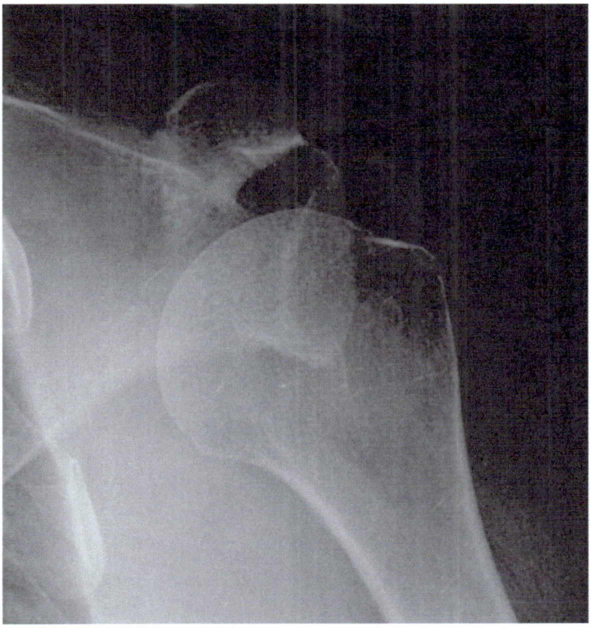

Fig. 18.4 Antero-medial gleno-humeral dislocation with coracoid process fracture

18.1.3 Other Fractures

- Fractures of the *coracoid process:*
  - Fractures of the tip and the horizontal part of the coracoid (Figs. 18.4 and 18.5) can be associated with anterior dislocation of the shoulder.
  - Fractures of the base of the coracoid (Fig. 18.6): can be associated with acromioclavicular joint dislocation.

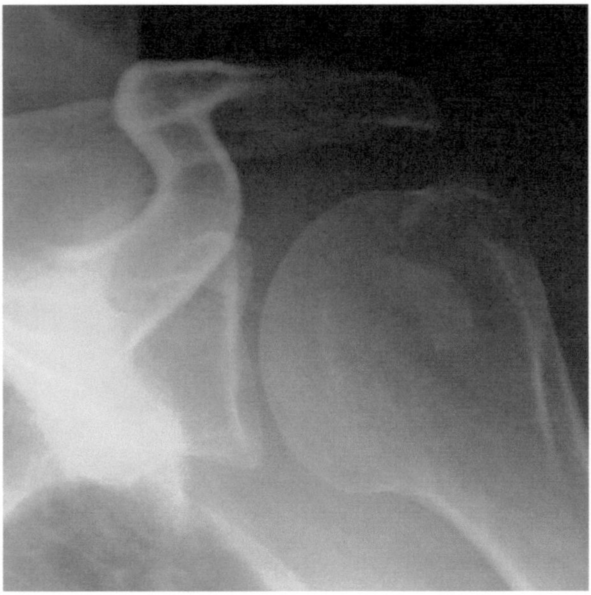

Fig. 18.5 Radiograph of the same shoulder as shown in Fig. 18.4 after reduction of the dislocation

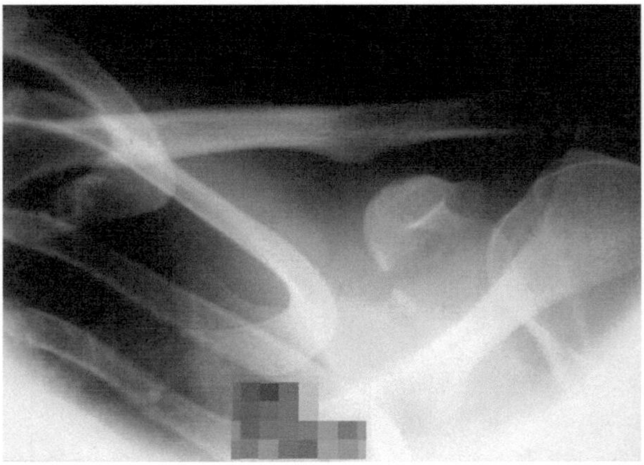

Fig. 18.6 Fracture of the base of the coracoid process with acromioclavicular dislocation

- *Complex fractures of the Glenoid fossa and Glenoid neck:* these fractures are commonly associated with an impaction of the humeral head into the scapula.
- *Floating shoulder:* this injury pattern is characterized by a double rupture of the Superior Shoulder Suspensory Complex (SSSC) which is a bone-soft tissue ring composed of five elements: the Glenoid, CC ligaments, lateral part of the clavicle, ACJ, acromion.

18.2 Clinical Presentation

- The common clinical presentation usually includes shoulder pain, disability, ecchymosis, bruises, etc.
- Fractures of the Glenoid rim may be associated with shoulder dislocation (anterior rim with anterior dislocation, and posterior rim with posterior dislocation).
- Scapular fractures typically occur as part of a more complex traumatic presentation in polytrauma patients with other associated injuries caused by the same event:
  - Pulmonary injury (lung contusion, hemothorax, pneumothorax, etc.),
  - Vascular injury to the ipsilateral upper limb,
  - Ipsilateral brachial plexus injury,
  - Rib fractures,
  - Clavicle fracture,
  - Humerus fracture,
  - Head trauma,
  - Intra-abdominal injury (e.g., spleen injury).

18.3 Radiographic Assessment

- Antero-posterior, scapular, and axillary shoulder views are typically helpful in demonstrating scapular fractures; however, CT scans provide a better analysis of the fracture pattern.
- Radiographs of the ribs are suitable for revealing associated fractures.
- Chest radiographs are useful for detecting hemo-pneumothorax.
- ***CT scan with 2D and 3D reconstruction*** is essential for documenting and analyzing the fracture pattern, which is crucial for guiding therapeutic decision.

18.4 Management

- *Extra-articular fractures with preservation* of the architectural orientation and alignment of the gleno-humeral joint and the coracoacromial arch: the treatment is usually conservative, and involves the following:
  - Arm sling,
  - Pain control: Paracetamol, NSAID's, Codeine if needed,
  - Early rehabilitation to restore the range of motion,
  - A satisfactory outcome is commonly expected after 2 months.

- *Articular fractures*:
  - Conservative treatment (as above) for undisplaced fractures.
  - Surgical treatment (open reduction and internal fixation) is indicated for:
    Displaced fractures,
    Fractures involving shoulder impaction,
    Fractures involving destabilization of the coracoacromial arch.
- *Fractures of the coracoid process*:
  - Fractures involving the tip of the coracoid: simple observation and conservative treatment (after reduction of associated shoulder dislocation, when present).
  - Fractures involving the base of the coracoid: treatment of the associated ACJ dislocation by reduction and stabilization (see corresponding chapter).

Traumatic Shoulder Dislocations 19

Three types of shoulder dislocations (glenohumeral) are distinguished according to the direction of displacement of the humeral head: anterior, posterior, and inferior dislocations (Figs. 19.1 and 19.2).

Particular note is made for recurrent anterior dislocations.

19.1 Acute Anterior Dislocations

Traumatic anterior shoulder dislocation typically occurs in young active males and accounts for more than 95% of all shoulder dislocations. It is very common in sports-related injuries and domestic accidents.

19.1.1 Clinical Findings (Undressed Patient)

- Obliteration of the delto-pectoral sulcus,
- Flattening of the antero-lateral aspect of the deltoid muscle with sharp prominence of the lateral border of the acromion,
- Lateral sub-acromial void (on palpation).
- The arm is spontaneously positioned in irreducible abduction and external rotation,

19.1.2 Radiographic Findings

- An antero-posterior radiograph is usually sufficient for diagnosis.
- In cases of doubt, additional views such as axillary and scapular views can be taken.
- On the AP view, the humeral head is located lateral, inferior, or medial to the coracoid process.

D. Saragaglia, A. Hassan Chamseddine, *Traumatology for the Emergency Doctor*, https://doi.org/10.1007/978-3-031-63196-2_19

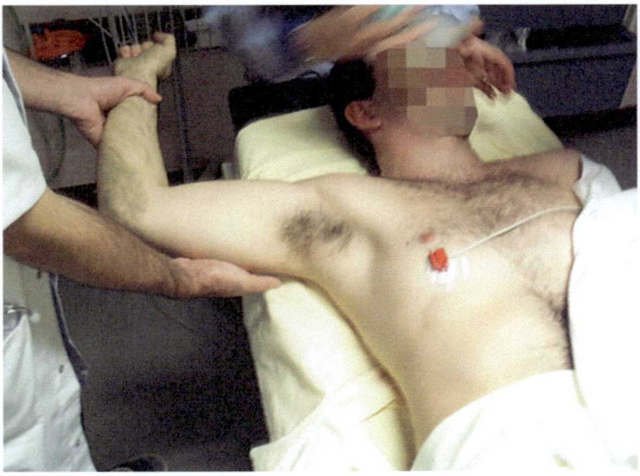

Fig. 19.1 Photo of clinical presentation of a patient with "luxatio erecta" or inferior dislocation

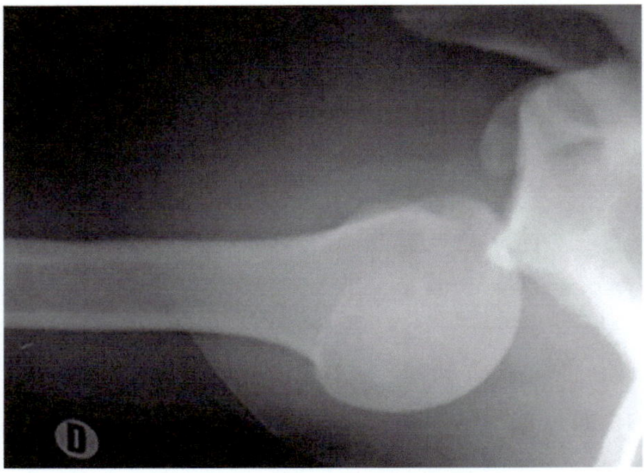

Fig. 19.2 Radiographic presentation of a luxatio erecta

- It is important to always check for *associated bony lesions*:
  - Fracture of the glenoid rim (antero-inferior): Bony Bankart lesion (Fig. 19.3).
  - Impaction of the humeral head (postero-superior): Hill-Sachs lesion (Fig. 19.4).
- A CT scan is indicated for the evaluation and assessment of associated bony injuries (glenoid rim fracture, Hill-Sachs lesion, tubercle major fracture, etc.).
- An MRI is indicated for the assessment of the rotator cuff condition (when needed).

19.1.3 Patho-Anatomy of Associated Lesions

- ***Bony lesions***
  - Fractures of the coracoid process (Fig. 18.4):
    Rare, usually overlooked,
    Secondary to direct impact with the humeral head.

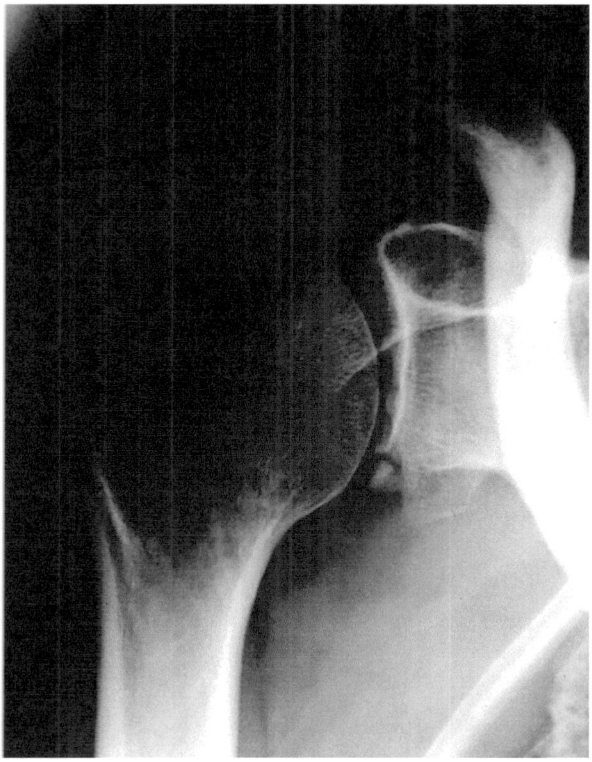

Fig. 19.3 Fracture of the antero-inferior glenoid rim seen after reduction of the dislocation

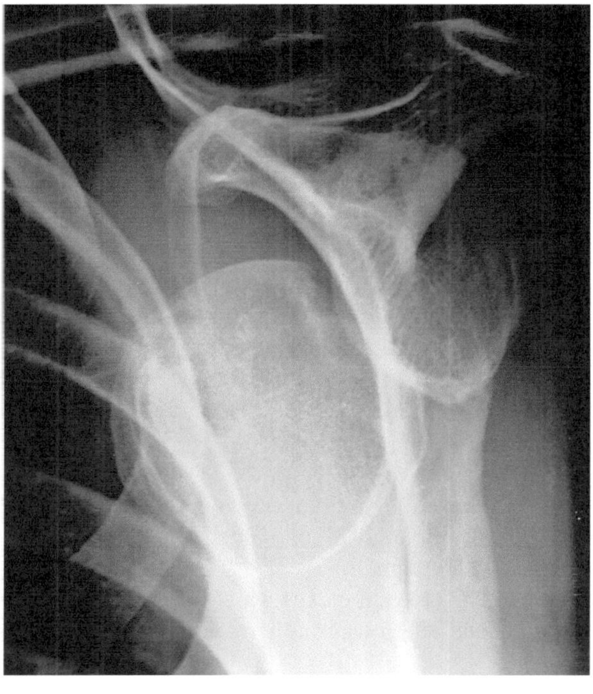

Fig. 19.4 Impaction of the humeral head seen on the "Y scapular view" with the humeral head riding over the antero-inferior glenoid rim

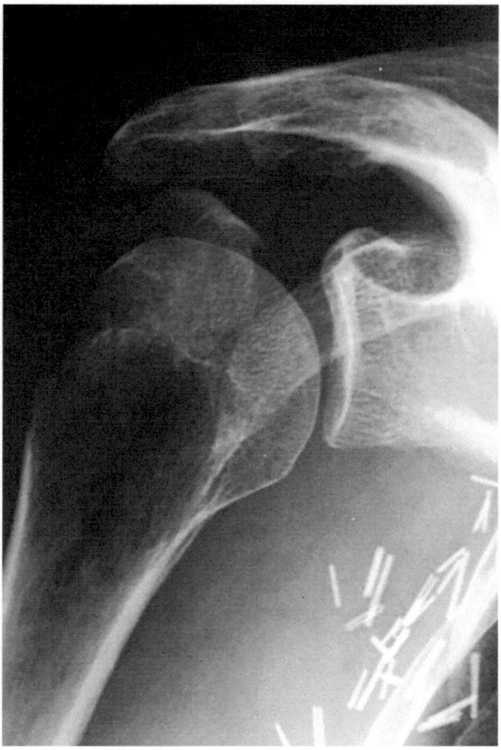

Fig. 19.5 Fracture-avulsion of the tubercle major (greater tuberosity) remaining displaced after reduction of a shoulder dislocation (indication for surgical treatment)

- Fracture of the tubercle major: common injury (20–40% of cases) (Fig. 19.5).
- Undisplaced fracture of the humeral neck

  May be missed on initial radiographs,

  Red flag: Risk of complete fracture displacement during closed reduction.

- ***Rotator cuff lesion***
  - Usually seen after the age of 40 years (Figs. 19.6 and 19.7).
  - 5–10% of cases, possibly even more.
  - These lesions are commonly missed in the initial post-traumatic period.

    They should be differentiated from brachial plexus lesion in cases of pseudoparalytic shoulder,

    An early MRI assessment is recommended if there is any doubt.
- ***Neurologic lesions***
  - Seen 5–10% of cases.
  - They involve:

    The axillary nerve, which may cause loss of sensation of the lateral aspect of the shoulder and humeral head "ptosis" on post-reduction AP shoulder radiograph).

    The brachial plexus which may be incompletely affected.

    These lesions usually regress within a few weeks.

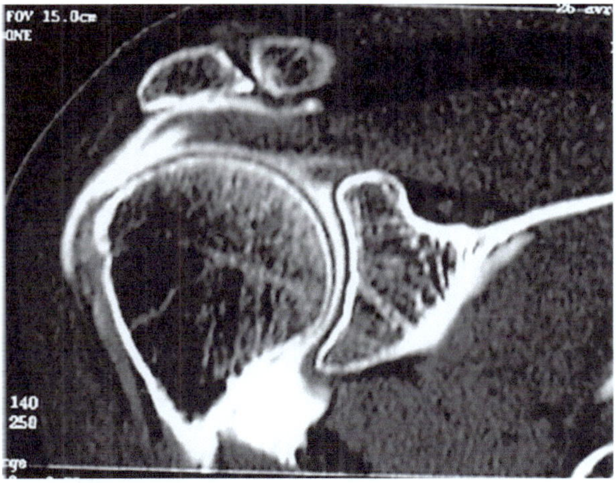

Fig. 19.6 Rotator cuff rupture seen on arthro-CT after reduction of an anterior shoulder dislocation in a 55 years old female patient

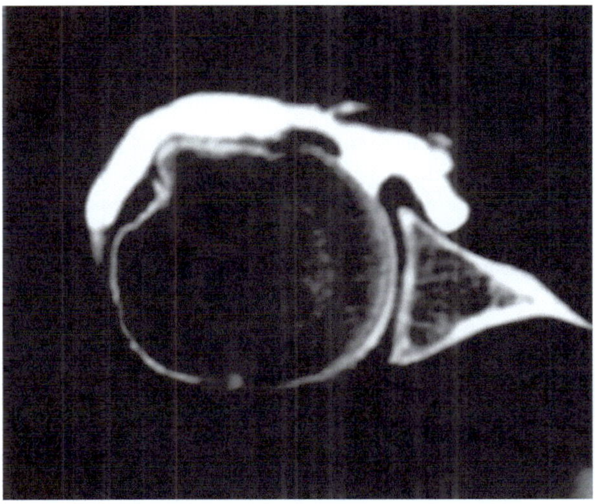

Fig. 19.7 Dislocation of the tendon of the long biceps with rupture of the sub-scapularis tendon seen on arthro-CT after reduction of an anterior shoulder dislocation in a 50 years old male patient

- ***Vascular lesions***
  - They are exceptional,
  - They usually involve arterial contusion with intimal injury, rather than rupture,
  - There is a common association with brachial plexus injury.

19.1.4 Treatment

- ***The treatment begins with an urgent closed reduction*** followed by:
  - Sling immobilization with elbow at side (Fig. 19.8) which has better patient compliance than immobilization in external rotation.
  - Rehabilitation with sub-scapularis reinforcement after the arm sling is removed (the duration of immobilization is detailed below).

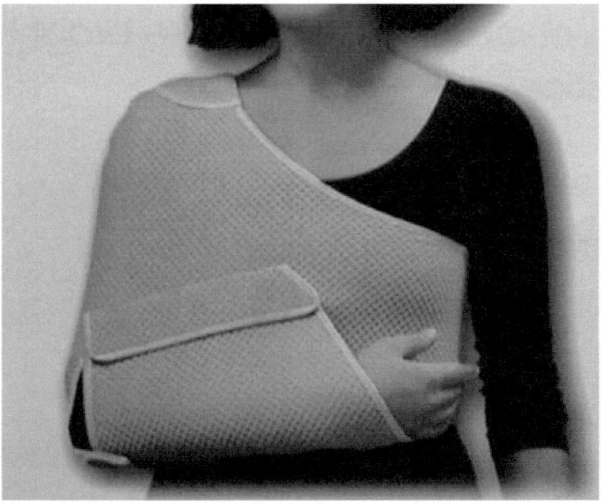

Fig. 19.8 Photo of a patient with a sling immobilization (elbow at side)

- ***Method of reduction***
  - Red Flag: Closed reduction should not be attempted in the ER when the dislocation is associated with a fracture of the humeral neck.
  - All reduction methods require the patient to be completely relaxed and confident.
  - The administration of IV or IM analgesics and muscle relaxants may be necessary if the patient is anxious or uncooperative.
  - General anesthesia is reserved for cases where closed reduction attempts have failed despite the use of systemic analgesia and muscle relaxation.
  - The best method of reduction is the one that the practitioner is most proficient in.
  - Authors' preferred methods:

    1st method: *Milch maneuver*: the patient is positioned supine with the elbow flexed at 90°. The operator applies longitudinal traction to the upper limb while simultaneously exaggerating the shoulder's abduction and external rotation. Following the feeling of a reduction "click," the practitioner then brings the arm into adduction and internal rotation.

    2nd method: *FARES method or "handshaking" technique*: the patient lies in a supine position. The operator firmly grasps the patient's hand and wrist with both hands, as if shaking hands, ensuring the patient's elbow is extended and the forearm is in neutral rotation. The operator then applies gentle longitudinal traction to the upper limb while progressively abducting it. Simultaneously, the practitioner applies continuous rapid vertical oscillations (2–3/s) to the patient's upper limb through their wrist. These oscillations are cycled approximately 5 cm above and below the horizontal level. When abduction exceeds 90°, the upper limb is gently brought into external rotation while the oscillating movements and gradual abduction. As soon as the reduction is perceived, typically at

approximately 120° of abduction, the upper limb is smoothly brought into internal rotation with the elbow flexed and the forearm crossing the chest.
3rd method: the patient is seated, with the affected upper limb hanging at the side of the chair. A counter-support is placed into the axilla (chair back), and the elbow is flexed at 90°. Longitudinal traction is applied to the arm, accompanied by external rotation.

- ***Duration of immobilization*** (as preferred by the authors)
  - Patients under 35 years:
    6 weeks of sling immobilization,
    Rehabilitation for an additional 6 weeks,
    Resumption of sports activities at 3 months.
  - Patients over 35 years:
    Only 3 weeks of sling immobilization to avoid shoulder stiffness (adhesive capsulitis),
    Rehabilitation after sling removal to restore the range of motion.
- ***Surgical treatment***
  - Some authors advocate for arthroscopic early repair in high-level professional players under 25 years of age, although the authors' opinion supports conservative management as first-line treatment.
  - Open surgical reduction is rarely indicated and is usually reserved for dislocations that are irreducible by external maneuvers.
  - Delayed early surgical treatment is indicated for:
    Fractures of the anterior glenoid rim greater than 25%,
    Fractures of the tubercle major that remain displaced after closed reduction, as assessed by CT scan,
    Rotator cuff lesion, as assessed by MRI.

19.2 Recurrent Anterior Dislocations

- Recurrent anterior dislocation is a frequent injury in young athletes under 25 years of age, with 40–80% of recurrent dislocations reported in the literature.
- Treatment for an episode of recurrent dislocation includes closed reduction followed by 8 days of sling immobilization. Rehabilitation is usually not effective in restoring long-term shoulder stability.
- Surgical treatment for shoulder stabilization is often suggested after the second episode of dislocation in young athlete patients.

19.3 Acute Posterior Dislocation

- Acute traumatic posterior shoulder dislocation is a rare condition, accounting for 2–4% of all shoulder dislocations.
- It exceptionally occurs during sports practice.

- It is usually secondary to conditions such as epilepsy (30–40% of cases) and electrocution.
- The diagnosis can be challenging and may be missed in 50–80% of cases. This is often due to a lack of awareness or knowledge about the condition and ignorance and poor-quality radiographs in emergency settings.

19.3.1 Clinical Presentation

- Patient presentation
  - Spontaneous presentation with the arm at side and the shoulder held in irreducible internal rotation,
  - Prominence of the coracoid process,
  - Flattening of the anterior aspect of the deltoid,
  - Obliteration of the posterior sub-acromial space.
- Physical examination
  - Absence of any external rotation of the shoulder when the elbow is flexed at 90° (Fig. 19.9),
  - Possible external rotation of the forearm (supination) when the elbow is flexed at 90°,
  - Limited external rotation of the forearm when the elbow is extended.

19.3.2 Radiographic Assessment

1. *Standard Radiographs*
   (a) True AP view of the gleno-humeral joint (Figs. 19.11 and 19.12):
   - The radiographic view and quality are frequently inadequate in emergency settings.
   - The following radiographic signs are usually subtle and commonly overlooked due to lack of awareness:
     - Overlap between the humeral head and the glenoid rim,
     - Double contour sign or "trough line sign" (Fig. 19.12),
     - "Light bulb sign,"
     - "Rim sign": a widened joint space, with more than 6 mm between the glenoid rim and the humeral head.

   (b) Lateral views:
   - When the radiographic findings of the AP view are doubtful, one or more of the following lateral views is requested:
     - Axillary view which is usually difficult to achieve due to pain and patient discomfort, as it requires shoulder abduction,
     - Bloom and Obata view (angle up view) (Fig. 19.10),
     - Lateral scapular Y view (Fig. 19.14),
     - Garth view (apical oblique view).
   - Lateral views show (Figs. 19.13 and 19.14):

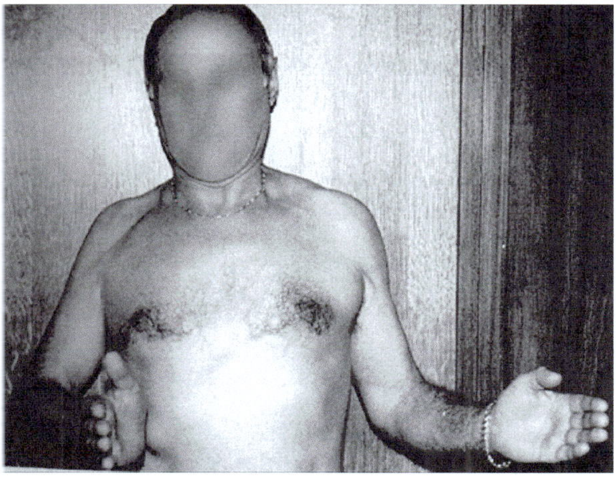

Fig. 19.9 Photo of a patient with a posterior dislocation of the right shoulder. Note the position in irreducible internal rotation with the elbow 90° flexed, and the flattening of the anterior deltoid

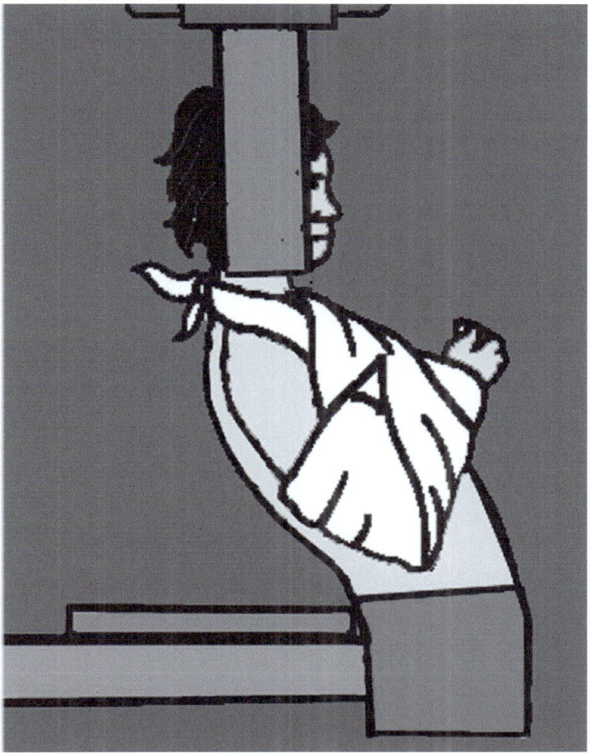

Fig. 19.10 Illustration of the bloom and obata view

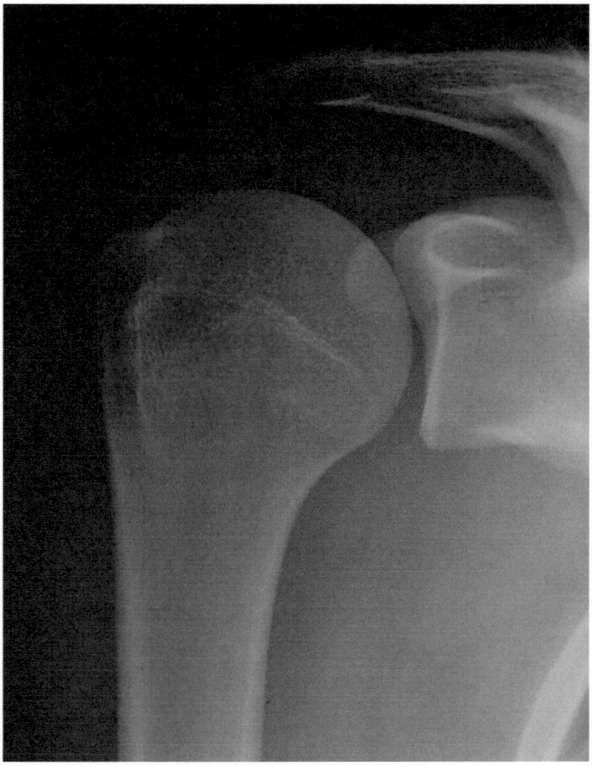

Fig. 19.11 True AP radiograph of a normal right shoulder. Note the perfect visualization of the glenohumeral joint line

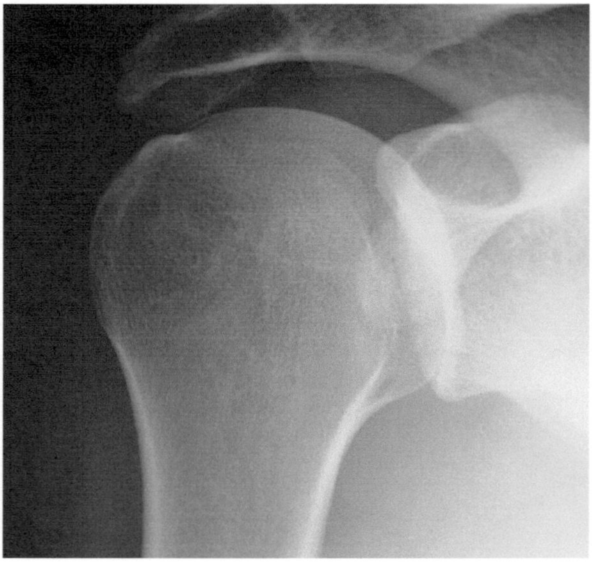

Fig. 19.12 True AP radiograph of a right shoulder with posterior dislocation. Note the double contour aspect of the humeral head

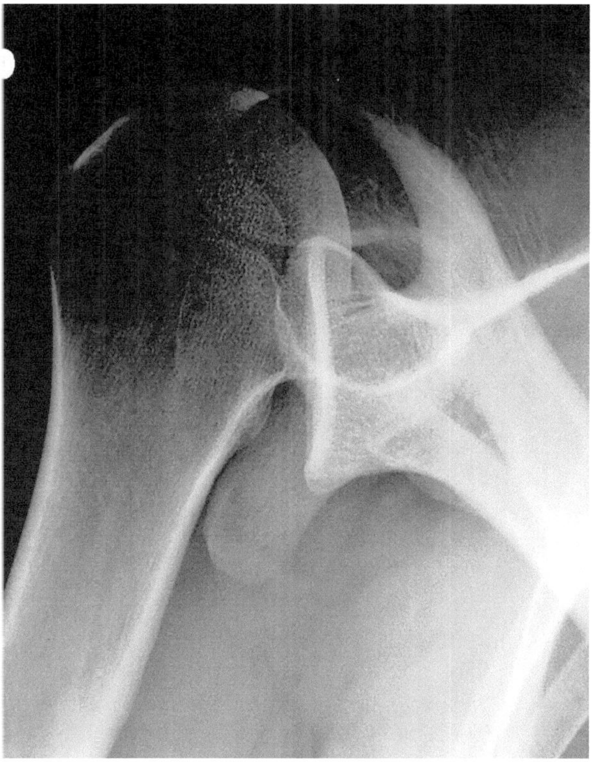

Fig. 19.13 Posterior shoulder dislocation seen on Bloom and Obata view

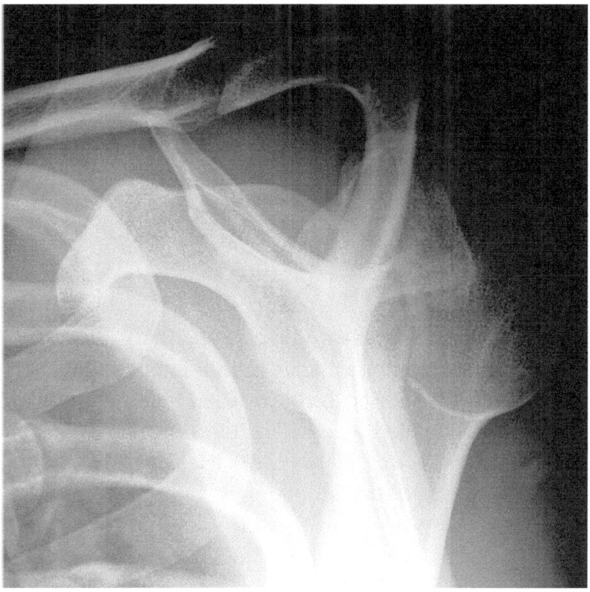

Fig. 19.14 Posterior shoulder dislocation seen on the Y scapular view. Note the widened distance between the humeral head and the tip of the coracoid process

- Posterior displacement of the humeral head (the anterior aspect of the humeral head is locked over the posterior glenoid rim: a part of the humeral head is located behind the glenoid fossa while the other part remains in contact with it).
- Impaction of the anterior aspect of the humeral head: McLaughlin or Reverse Hill-Sachs lesion (the anterior aspect of the humeral head is impacted over the posterior glenoid rim).

2. ***CT Scan with 2-D or 3-D reconstruction***
   (a) It is not requested in emergency.
   (b) It is useful to:
   - Confirm the diagnosis in doubtful situations,
   - Visualize the McLaughlin lesion and assess its size (percentage of the impacted humeral head surface),
   - Disclose presence of tubercle minor fracture,
   - Disclose presence of humeral head split.

19.3.3 Treatment

- *Orthopedic treatment*
  - Closed reduction

    Should be done in emergency, by orthopedic surgeon, under general anesthesia: gentle traction with internal rotation (to disengage the humeral head from the posterior glenoid rim), followed by external rotation with adduction.

    Red Flag: risk of complete humeral head split during reduction (starting from a pre-existing large McLaughlin lesion).
  - Immobilization

    Internal rotation of the shoulder is prohibited in order to avoid redeslocation.

    Use of shoulder brace with 60° Abduction and 30° external rotation (Figs. 19.15 and 19.16).

    Or immobilization with the elbow at the side and the shoulder in 30° of external rotation.

    Duration: 45 days.
- *Surgical treatment*
  - Indications

    Unstable closed reduction (usually with McLaughlin lesion >25%),

    Irreducible dislocation with gentle maneuver,

    Dislocation with concomitant fracture susceptible to iatrogenic displacement,

    Associated glenoid fracture.
  - The aim is ideally to fill the McLaughlin lesion (defect between 25 and 50%) using one of the following techniques:

    Transposition of the sub-scapularis tendon into the humeral head defect,

    Transposition of the lesser tuberosity with the sub-scapularis into the humeral head defect,

    Bone autograft underneath the humeral head cartilage,

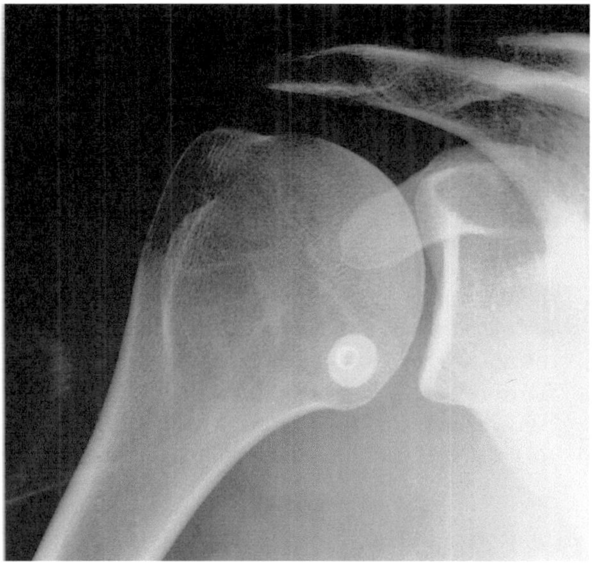

Fig. 19.15 Shoulder AP radiograph for the same patient as shown in Fig. 19.12 after reduction and immobilization with an abduction-external rotation shoulder brace

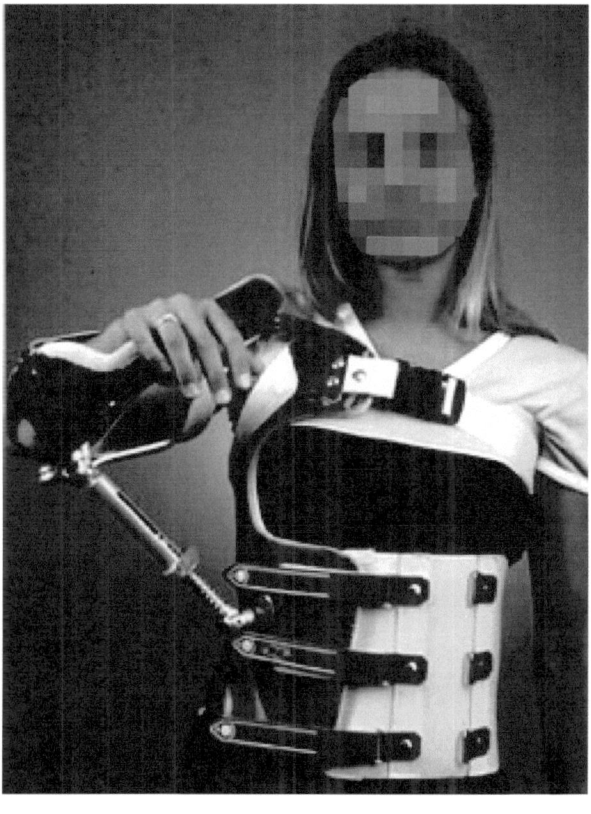

Fig. 19.16 Photo of an abduction shoulder brace in position

Segmental bone allograft into the humeral head defect.
 - Shoulder prosthesis is suggested for:
 Associated comminuted humeral head fracture,
 Unreconstructible large defects of the humeral head (>50%).

19.4 Acute Inferior Dislocation (Luxatio Erecta)

- Acute traumatic inferior shoulder dislocation is an extremely rare condition: 1% of all shoulder dislocations.
- It typically occurs with forced hyperabduction mechanism to the upper limb, often associated with high velocity trauma.
- It involves the inferior displacement of the humeral head, which becomes lodged below the glenoid fossa (Figs. 19.1 and 19.2).
- It is associated with neurovascular complication in 40–60% of cases.

19.4.1 Clinical Presentation

- The patient presents with the upper limb in an overhead position and extreme abduction-elevation (Fig. 19.1).
- The physical examination should assess the distal pulses and the brachial plexus.

19.4.2 Radiographic Assessment

- Antero-posterior shoulder radiographs demonstrate complete displacement of the humeral head beneath the inferior pole of the glenoid fossa, with the arm in extreme abduction (Fig. 19.2).
- An MRI of the shoulder is useful after reduction to assess the rotator cuff, which is a common site of associated injury.

19.4.3 Treatment

- Closed reduction performed by an orthopedic surgeon under general anesthesia:
  - Gentle traction is applied with external rotation followed by internal rotation and adduction when reduction click is perceived (countertraction is applied during the maneuver),
  - Neurovascular assessment is conducted after reduction.
  - Immobilization is recommended for short period (3 weeks).
- Rehabilitation after sling removal.

20 Fractures of the Proximal Humerus

Fractures of the proximal humerus are common in the elderly. They rarely occur in sports practice, except for skiing, where they happen in younger patients. The use of CT scan plays a major place in identifying the injury pattern, especially for displaced 3- and 4-part fractures.

20.1 Patho-anatomy

- There are two main classifications commonly used for these fractures: Neer's classification and the AC classification.
- Neer's classification is very popular; it is based on the number of fragments: 2, 3, or 4 fragments.
  - the basic fragments are:
    The humeral head,
    The lesser tuberosity,
    the greater tuberosity,
    the humeral shaft.
  - Fracture–dislocations are included into the classification, encompassing both anterior and posterior dislocations

D. Saragaglia, A. Hassan Chamseddine, *Traumatology for the Emergency Doctor*, https://doi.org/10.1007/978-3-031-63196-2_20

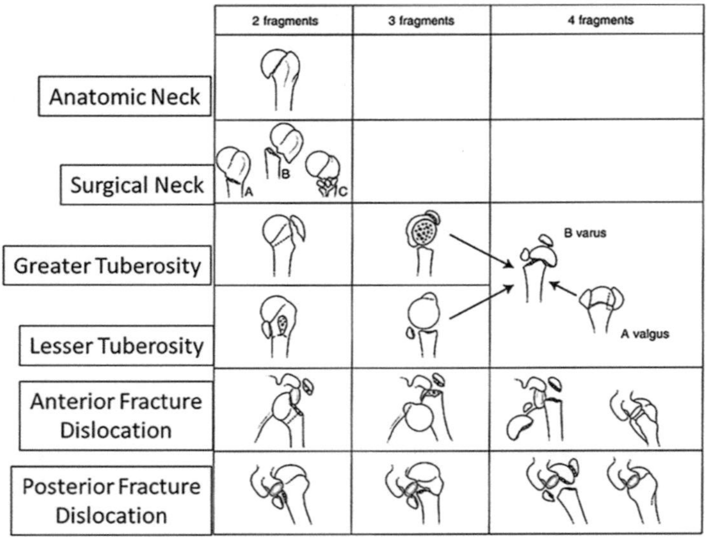

Neer's classification:

- AO classification includes 27 sub-types of fractures and is not used in the daily practice.
- Several types of fractures are usually seen in the daily practice, from the simplest one to the most complex:
  - ***Fracture of the greater tuberosity*** (Fig. 20.1)
    It may be either isolated or associated with anterior shoulder dislocation (20–40%);
    It may be overlooked in emergency when the fracture is not displaced,
    The bone fragment may have variable size (as a bone chip indicating a rotator cuff avulsion-fracture).
  - ***Fracture of the lesser tuberosity*** (Fig. 20.2)
    Exceptional,
    Often overlooked,
    The bone fragment is usually displaced medially pulled by the subscapularis.
  - ***Fracture of the surgical neck*** (Fig. 20.3)
    It involves a variable degree or amount of displacement,
    It is usually not at risk for osteonecrosis of the humeral head.
  - ***Fracture of the anatomic neck***
    Exceptional,
    It encompasses a variable major risk of osteonecrosis of the humeral head.
  - ***3 and 4 part fractures*** (Fig. 20.4)
    The most frequent types of articular fractures,

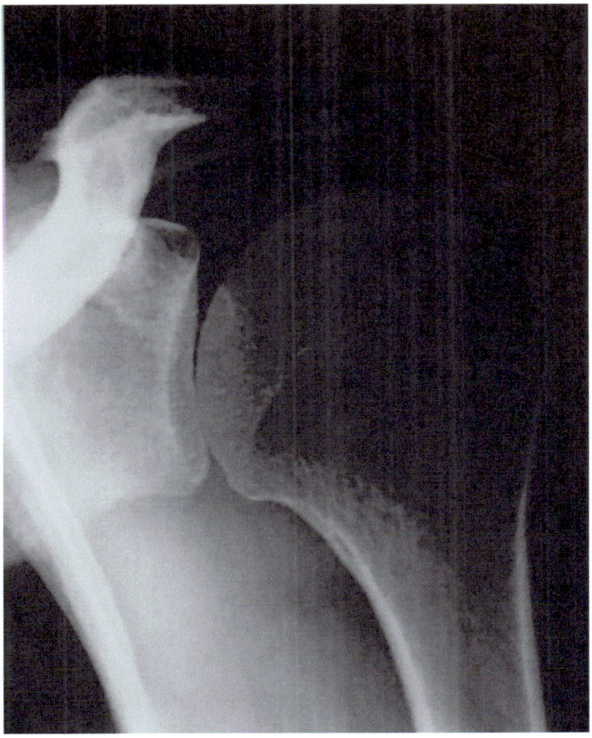

Fig. 20.1 AP shoulder radiograph showing a very minimally displaced fracture of the tubercle major (greater tuberosity)

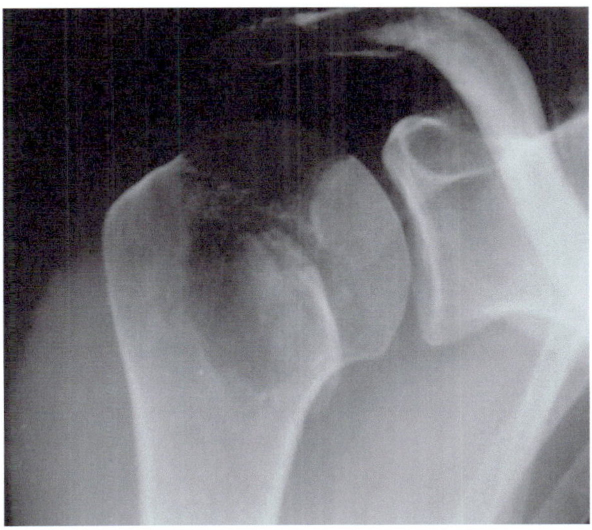

Fig. 20.2 AP shoulder radiograph showing a fracture of the tubercle minor (lesser tuberosity)

It involves a variable degree or amount of displacement,

It encompasses a variable major risk of osteonecrosis of the humeral head (>30%).

– ***Anterior and posterior fracture–dislocations*** (Figs. 20.5 and 20.6).

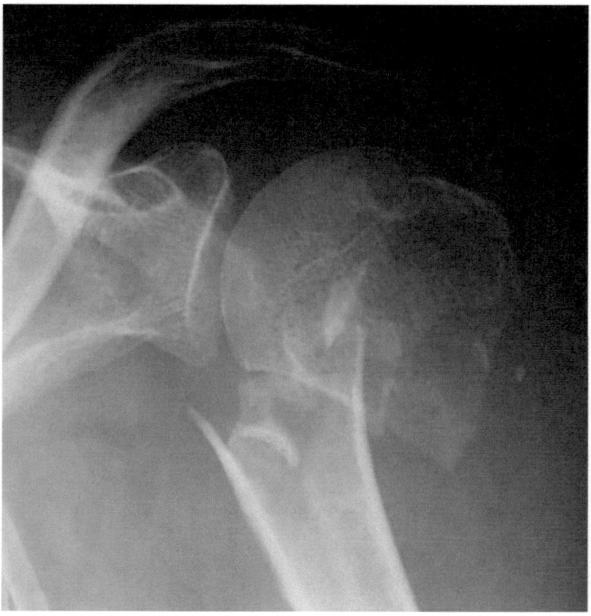

Fig. 20.3 Displaced fracture of the surgical neck of the humerus seen on AP shoulder view

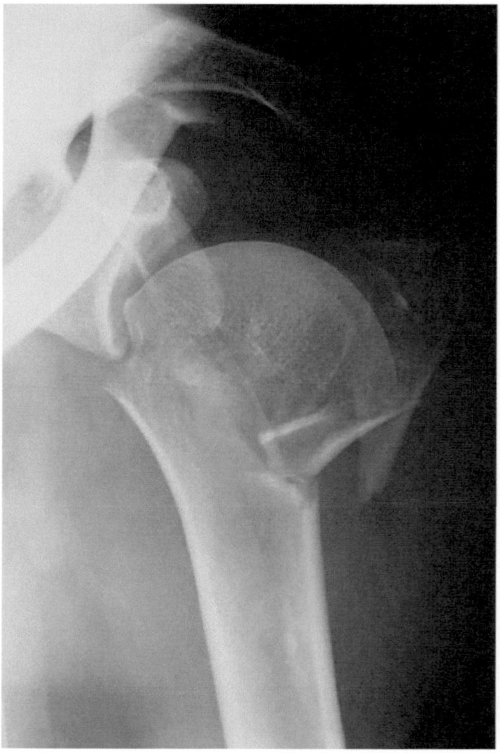

Fig. 20.4 Associated displaced fractures of the humeral neck and the tubercle major on AP shoulder view

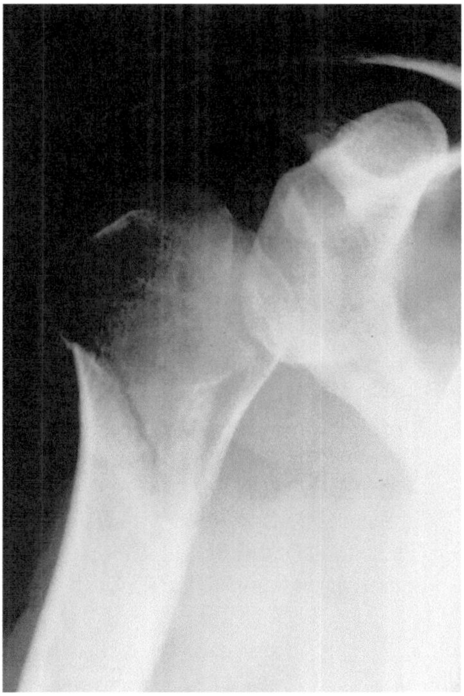

Fig. 20.5 Suboptimal AP shoulder view revealing an ill-defined fracture–dislocation, suggestive of a posterior dislocation characterized by a “light bulb” appearance

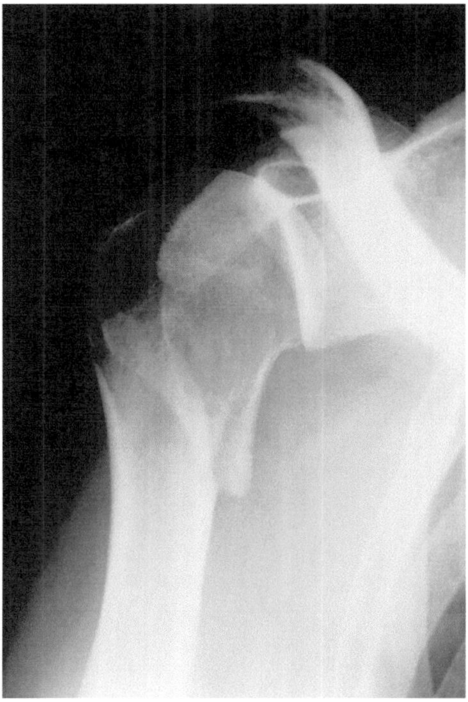

Fig. 20.6 True AP shoulder view for the same patient as shown in Fig. 20.5. The diagnosis of posterior dislocation is now evident with an image of humeral head-glenoid rim overlap

20.2 Traps and Pitfalls

- Undisplaced fractures of the greater tuberosity, as well as fractures of the lesser tuberosity, can be easily overlooked in an emergency setting.
- Adequate radiographic views are necessary to make the right diagnosis.
- ***A CT scan with 3D reconstruction*** is usually required to determine the appropriate therapeutic approach, particularly in cases of uncertainty.

20.3 Management

- **Physical examination** should always assess the neuro-vascular condition of the upper limb.
- **Radiographic shoulder views include:**
  - True AP view (Grashey view),
  - Lateral Y scapular view,
  - Lateral trans-thoracic view (Fig. 20.7).
- **CT scan (2D and 3D)** is mandatory for therapeutic decision (especially for pre-operative planning) (Fig. 20.8).

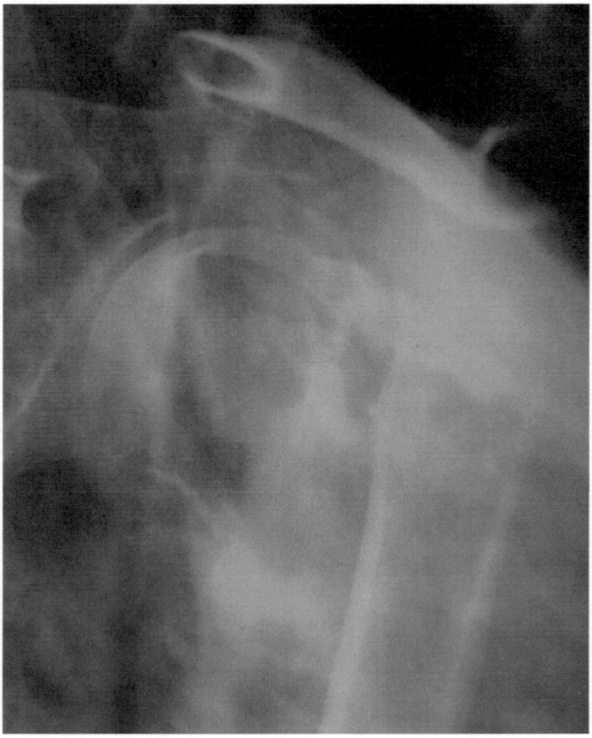

Fig. 20.7 Lateral trans-thoracic view of the shoulder showing a fracture–dislocation with significant displacement. Note the important anterior displacement of the humerus with potential impalement of the deltoid muscle

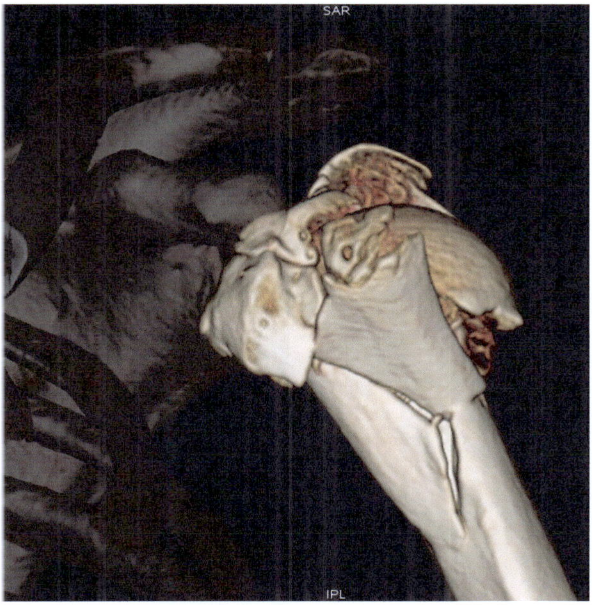

Fig. 20.8 3D CT scan of a four-part fracture of the proximal humerus

20.4 Treatment

- ER physicians can initiate the treatment for the majority of proximal humerus fractures, as only 15–20% of cases typically require surgical intervention.
- Based on Neer's classification, surgical treatment (Fig. 20.9) in young active patients is indicated for the following displacements of the basic fragments (previously defined):
  - Humeral head in varus or valgus angulation >20–30°, compared to the opposite side,
  - Head-Shaft displacement >50% of the humeral shaft diameter,
  - Fracture–dislocations
  - Greater tuberosity displacement >2–5 mm,
  - Lesser tuberosity fracture in most of the cases.
  - Other factors should also be considered for the decision-making (of operative versus non-operative) and for the type of the surgical treatment (open reduction with internal fixation versus shoulder prosthetic replacement):
    Patient's age and comorbidities,
    Patient's functional demands,
    Patient's expectations,
    Fracture's complexity,
    Fracture's initial displacement,
    Presence of osteoporosis.

In the ER, the initiation of conservative non-operative treatment typically involves the use of a special brace for shoulder immobilization, such as a sling and swathe or an arm sling shoulder immobilizer. This is usually followed by an early clinical and radiographic follow-up with an orthopedic-trauma surgeon 5–7 days post-trauma.

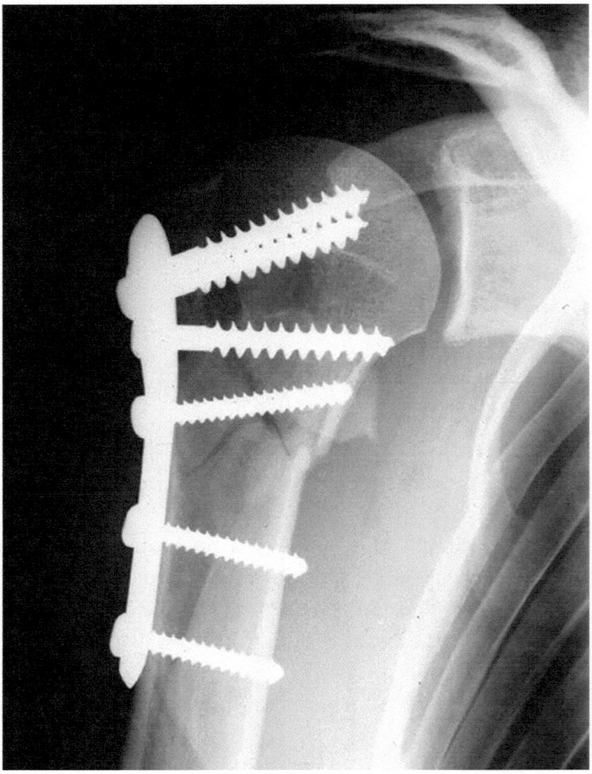

Fig. 20.9 AP shoulder X-ray showing an internal fixation of a proximal humerus fracture using plate and screws

21 Management of Shoulder Trauma with "Normal" Radiographs

This chapter focuses on patients who arrive to the ER for post-traumatic shoulder pain and or disability but without any evident pathological conditions or abnormalities in radiographic images.

21.1 Clinical Presentation

21.1.1 History and Patient's Interrogation

- Circumstances of the accident and mechanism of the injury,
  - Description of any abnormal feeling,
  - Presence of post-traumatic disability.

21.1.2 Physical Examination

- Undress the patient's upper body,
- Inspection for any apparent deformities,
- Palpation: clavicle, acromioclavicular joint, coracoid, acromion, humeral head.
- Range of motion (ROM):
  - Active ROM: flexion, extension, abduction, adduction, internal rotation, external rotation, circumduction.
  - Passive ROM
- Testing of the power of the different muscle groups.

D. Saragaglia, A. Hassan Chamseddine, *Traumatology for the Emergency Doctor*, https://doi.org/10.1007/978-3-031-63196-2_21

21.1.3 Radiographic Assessment

- Attentive reexamination of the initial radiographs,
- Look for any subtle or suspicious images,
- Repeat the radiographs if the initial views are inappropriate or the quality is inadequate:
  - True AP "Grashey" view with "neutral rotation," "internal rotation," and "external rotation" of the shoulder,
  - Oblique apical view ("Garth" view) (Fig. 21.1),
  - Lateral scapular "Y" view,
  - Lateral glenoid view (when feasible),
  - Comparative views are helpful in doubtful cases.

21.1.4 Diagnosis of Injury

21.1.4.1 Acromioclavicular Dislocation

- Is usually grade 1 or 2: absence of deformation and "normal" radiographs,
- Focal pain and tenderness at the acromioclavicular joint,

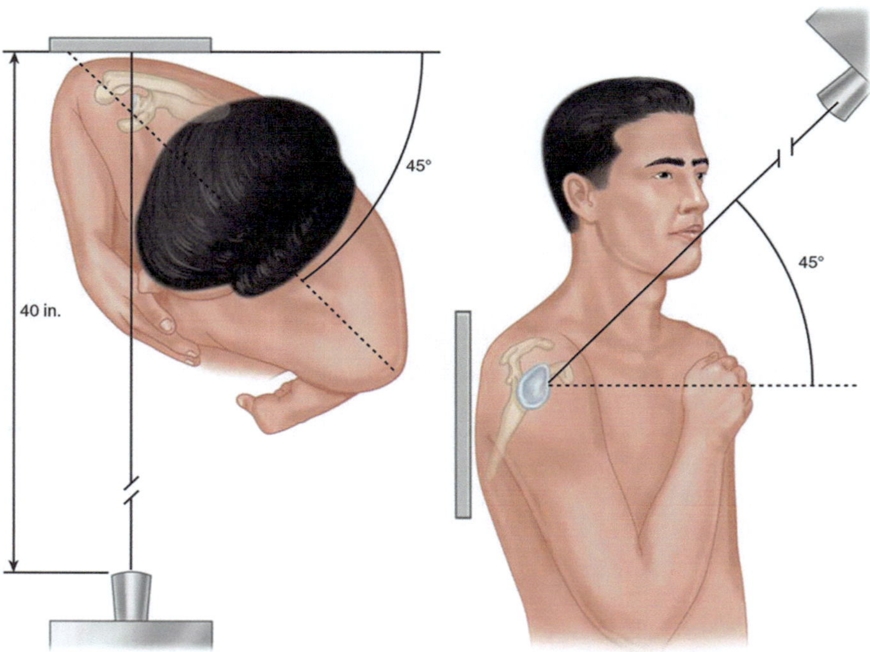

Fig. 21.1 Illustration of the "Garth" oblique apical view

– Stress radiographs are beneficial in differentiating grade 1 from grade 2 (refer to chapter acromioclavicular dislocations).

21.1.4.2 Undisplaced Fracture of the Tubercle Major (Greater Tuberosity) (Figs. 21.2 and 21.3)

– Lateral sub-acromial tenderness (at the level of the greater tuberosity),
– Painful normal active ROM,
– If the initial radiographs are not clear, a repeat series of shoulder radiographs (as previously detailed) should be performed after an interval of 8 days.
– A shoulder MRI is beneficial for revealing fractures that are undetectable on simple radiographs.

21.1.4.3 Anterior Shoulder Instability

- Mainly in young adult.
- It may manifest in different forms:
  – Episode of evident dislocation spontaneously reduced,
  – Episode of transient subluxation,
  – Painful shoulder due to unknown episode of dislocation.
- The patient may report a subtle feeling of their shoulder "moving in and out."

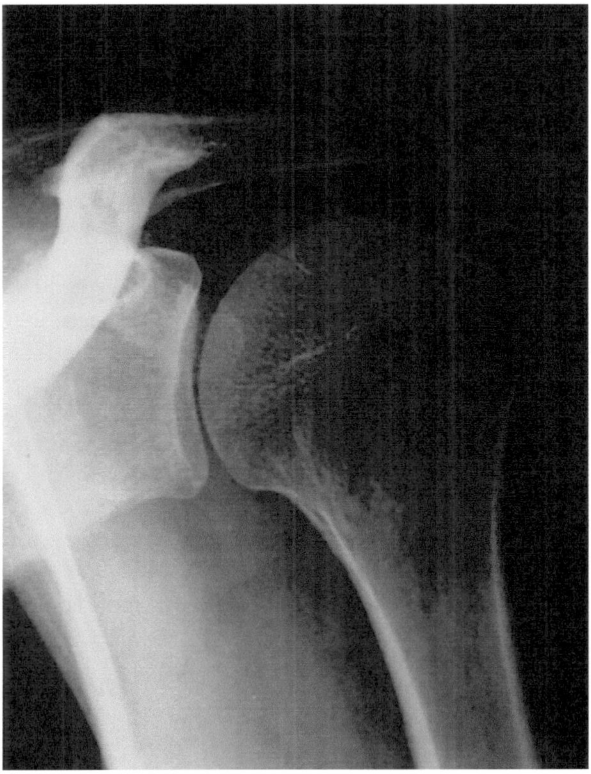

Fig. 21.2 AP shoulder view showing an undisplaced fracture of the tubercle major

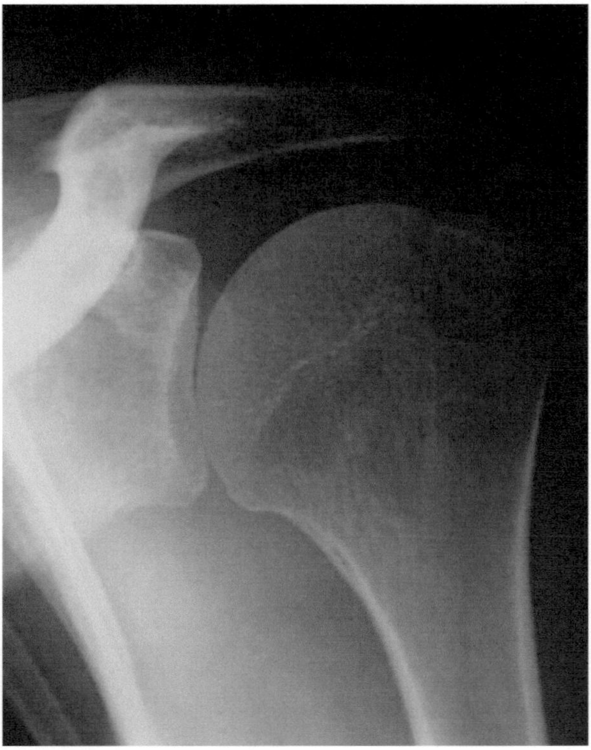

Fig. 21.3 Radiograph of the same patient as shown in Fig. 21.2 after 8 days with a better visualization of the tubercle major fracture

- Shoulder exam usually reveals:
  - Anterior shoulder pain in Abduction-External Rotation,
  - Apprehension to dislocation or subluxation in extreme abduction-external rotation.
- Fine and attentive analysis of the radiographs may reveal the following radiographic signs (on the "Garth" oblique apical view, lateral glenoid view, and "Grashey" true AP view with different rotations) (Figs. 21.4, 21.5, and 21.6):
  - Hill-Sachs lesion (impaction of the postero-superior aspect of the humeral head),
  - Fracture-avulsion of the antero-inferior bony glenoid rim, the so-called bony Bankart lesion.
- Shoulder MRI shows:
  - lesion of the antero-inferior glenoid capsulo-ligamento-labral complex (Bankart lesion),
  - lesions previously suspected on the radiographs (Hill-Sachs and bony Bankart).

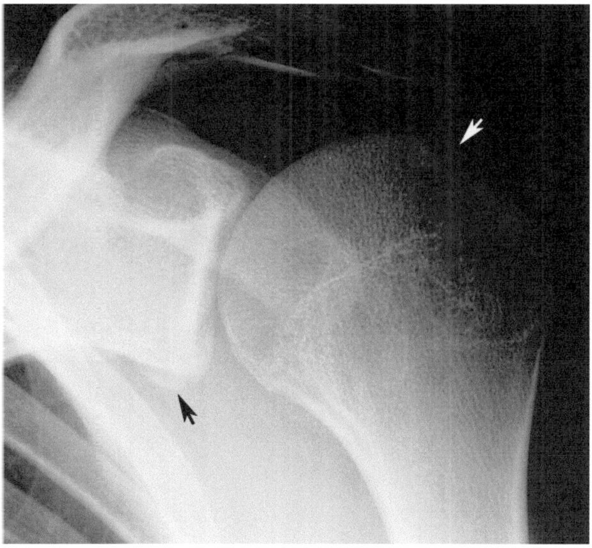

Fig. 21.4 AP shoulder view of a patient with an anterior shoulder instability showing a Hill-Sachs lesion of the humeral head and a bony Bankart lesion of the antero-inferior glenoid rim

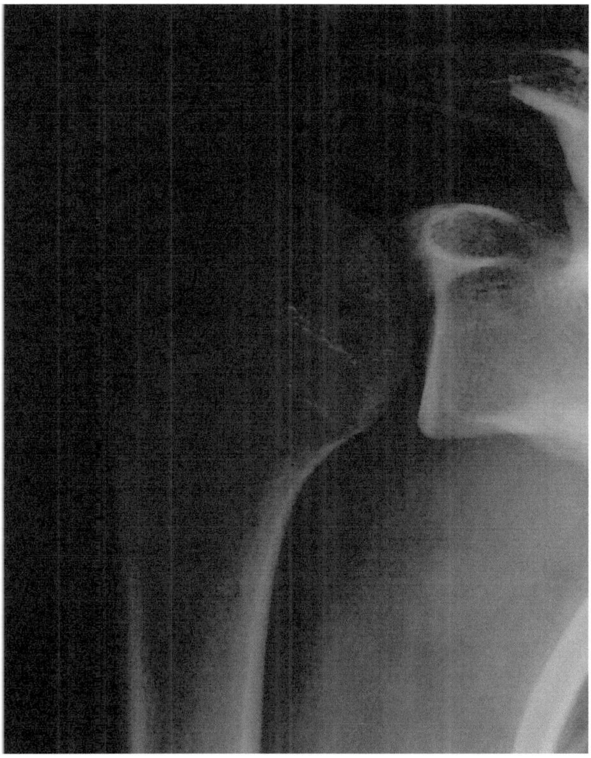

Fig. 21.5 AP radiographic view in external shoulder rotation interpreted as "normal"

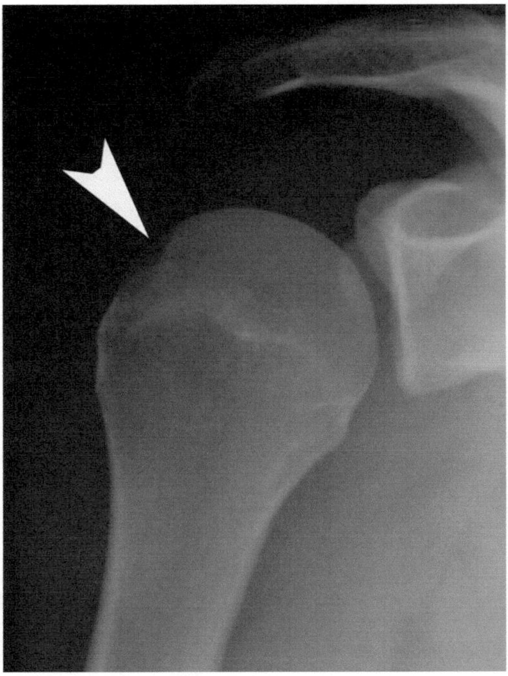

Fig. 21.6 AP radiographic view in internal rotation of the shoulder for the patient from Fig. 21.5, revealing a Hill-Sachs lesion indicative of anterior instability

21.1.4.4 Tear of the Rotator Cuff Tendons

- Patient presentation for post-traumatic shoulder pseudo-paralysis is highly suggestive of acute rotator cuff tear: *arthro-scanner* or *arthro-MRI* is recommended for prompt diagnosis and early repair.
- In some cases, the physical exam may reveal:
  - Shoulder pain that is triggered by passive antero-lateral elevation, which could suggest an impingement of the rotator cuff with the coraco-acromial arch,
  - Positive Jobe's test (weakness is suggestive of supra-spinatus tear).
- Initial radiographic assessment may reveal signs of chronic rotator cuff disease:
  - Decrease of the sub-acromial space (Fig. 21.7),
  - Indirect signs of chronic impingement at the superior border of the tubercle major and, or the inferior border of the acromion: sclerotic changes with or without intra-osseous cysts.
- If any doubt persists following the initial evaluation, the patient should be reassessed after a period of 1 week:
  - If the patient's condition has improved: send for rehabilitation and reassess after 1 month,
  - If there is no improvement in the patient's condition, it may be beneficial to seek a specialized orthopedic opinion for further assessment. This could involve a shoulder ultrasound, complemented by an arthro-scanner or arthro-MRI, particularly for young patients where a traumatic rotator cuff rupture is very uncommon (Fig. 21.8).

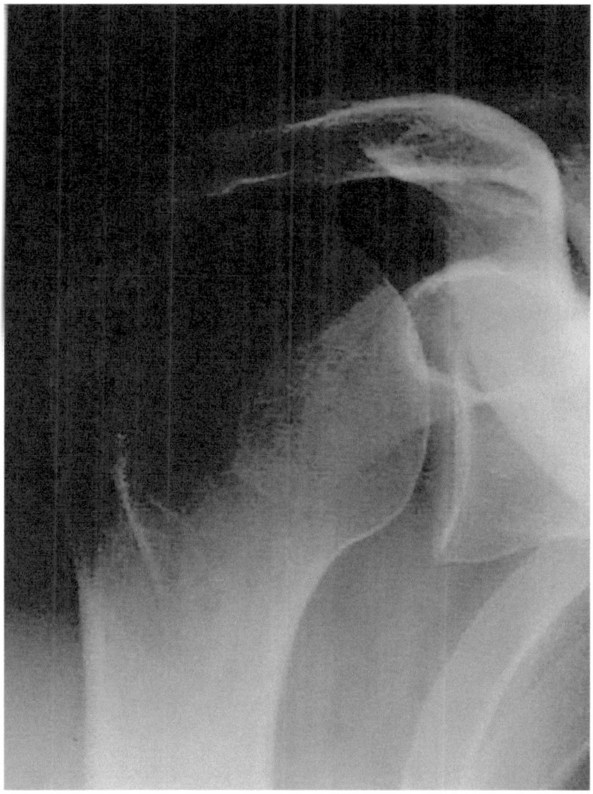

Fig. 21.7 AP shoulder X-ray revealing a severe narrowing of the acromiohumeral space in a 60-years-old patient, suggestive of chronic rotator cuff rupture ("incidental finding" after shoulder trauma)

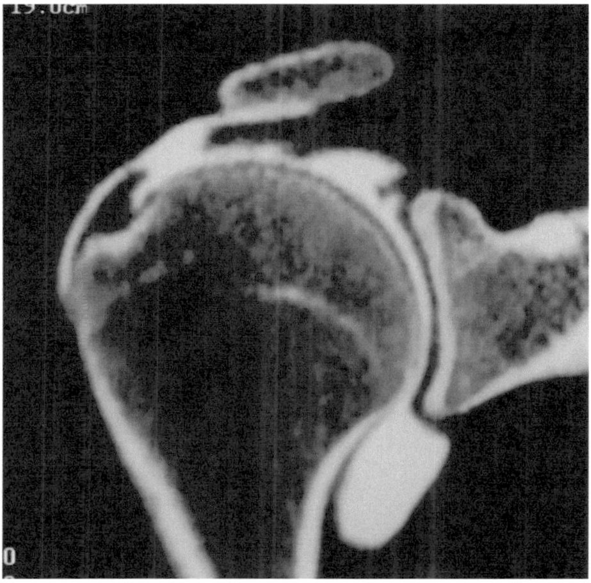

Fig. 21.8 Coronal cut of a right shoulder arthro-CT in a 22-years-old patient revealing a post-traumatic rotator cuff rupture (snow-board accident)

21.1.4.5 Posterior Shoulder Dislocation

- The diagnosis is often overlooked during the initial presentation to the ER.
- The causes of misdiagnosis are usually the following: inadequate radiographic views, inappropriate quality of the initial radiographs, poor physical exam findings with radiographic assessment concluded as "normal."
  - Clinical examination
    Anterior prominence of the coracoid process (especially in thin patients),
    Bulging of the posterior aspect of the deltoid (humeral head prominence),
    Flattening of the anterior deltoid muscle,
    Shoulder presentation in irreducible internal rotation,
    Loss of both passive and active shoulder external rotation (with elbow flexed).
  - Radiographic assessment (refer to Chap. 19)
    Plain radiographs are fundamental for the diagnosis.
    A CT scan is crucial for confirming the diagnosis and planning the treatment.
  - Reduction under GA is mandatory as soon as possible.
- Diagnosis is much more difficult in cases of *posterior subluxation* or *spontaneously reduced dislocation*.
  - The clinical examination provides a little guidance for the diagnosis.
  - The radiographs may, in some occasions, show a double contour image of the humeral head (Fig. 21.9).
  - The MRI is essential to disclose the type of injury in such situations.

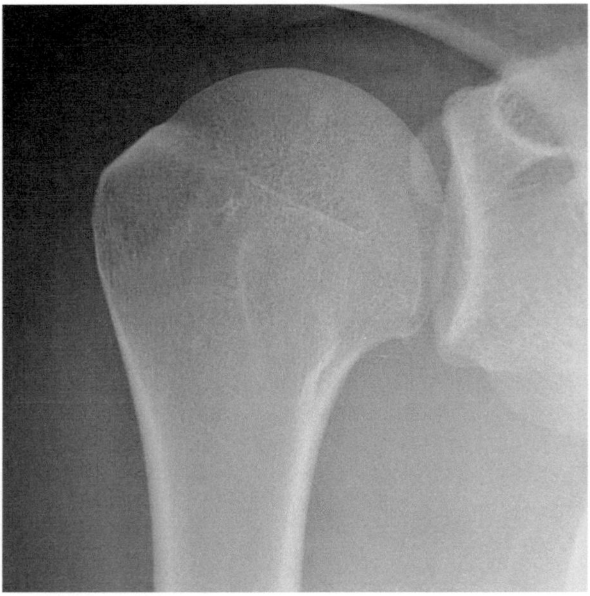

Fig. 21.9 True AP shoulder X-ray revealing a double contour image of the humeral head after spontaneous reduction of a posterior shoulder dislocation (McLaughlin or reverse Hill-Sachs lesion)

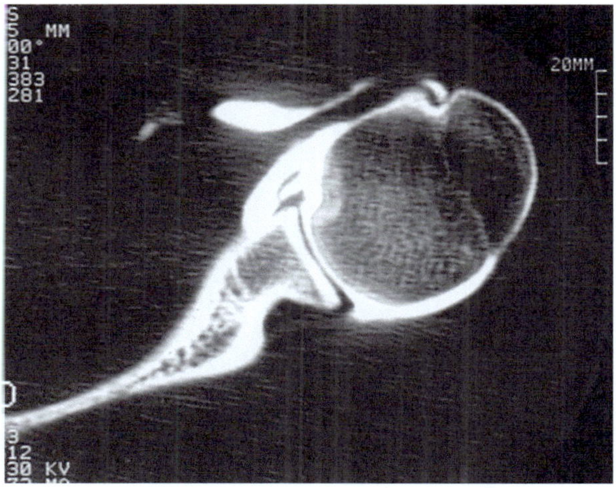

Fig. 21.10 Axial cut of shoulder arthro-CT showing a McLaughlin lesion located at the anterior aspect of the humeral head

  - In many cases, an arthro-scanner, which is prescribed in response to persistent shoulder pain, will allow for a diagnosis to be made (Fig. 21.10).

21.1.4.6 Fracture of the Tubercle Minor (Lesser Tuberosity) (Fig. 21.11)

- It is frequently disregarded or undiagnosed at initial presentation to the ER because of misinterpretation of the initial radiographs.
- The clinical examination reveals painful internal and external shoulder rotation, with significant decrease of the power of active internal rotation.
- A complete radiographic shoulder series assessment is crucial for the diagnosis (true AP "Grashey view," lateral scapular "Y view," Oblique apical "Garth view"): the ER physician should not rely on the interpretation of the only AP view (frequently of inadequate quality).
- A *CT scan with 2-D and 3-D reconstruction* should be requested in case of doubt.
- The treatment is commonly surgical.

21.1.4.7 Shoulder Contusion

- Final diagnosis of "shoulder contusion" should not be made unless the ER physician has ruled out any possible traumatic injuries, and the diagnosis does not correspond to any of the previous entities.
- Management:
  - Shoulder rest (arm sling or sling and swathe),
  - Analgesics and NSAID's,
  - Reassessment 1 week later.

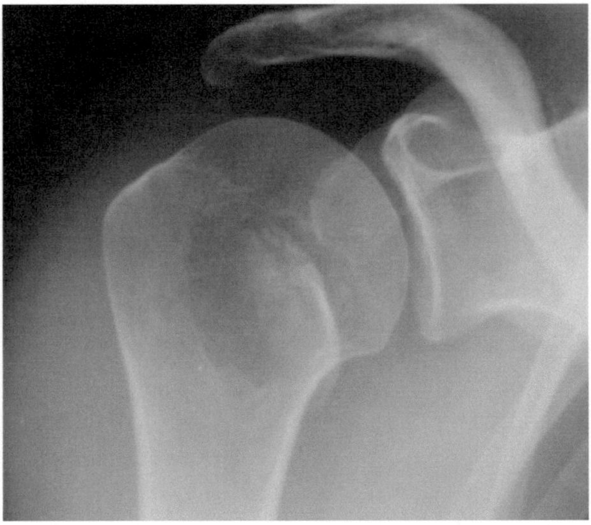

Fig. 21.11 Fracture of the tubercle minor diagnosed on AP shoulder radiograph performed for a persistent pain 10 days after the initial trauma (the initial radiographs were labeled "normal")

21.2 In Conclusion

Beware of apparent normal shoulder radiographs especially when they are of inadequate quality or they diverge with the clinical presentation (subtle deformation, pain, limited ROM, functional disability, etc.)

Always reassess the shoulder after 1 week if the initial evaluation is doubtful or not conclusive.

Routine ultrasound does not present any real advantages. It is prescribed only when a rotator cuff pathology is suspected, especially in patients >45 years.

In young adult, MRI is more pertinent as it is more specific and sensitive in revealing occult fractures, bone contusions, and soft tissue lesions (tendinous and capsulo-ligamentous lesions).

Fractures of the Humeral Shaft 22

Humeral shaft fractures are rare in sports traumatology, except for ski and hang-gliding. In opposition, they are common in road traffic accidents.

22.1 Patho-Anatomy

1. Fractures of the humeral shaft are, by definition, located between the inferior border of the humeral insertion of the pectoralis major tendon and 6 cm proximal to the elbow joint line.
2. They are described according to:
   (a) The fracture configuration or pattern.
      - Simple transverse and short oblique: usually secondary to direct trauma,
      - Spiral and long oblique with or without wedge: usually secondary to indirect trauma, mainly rotational,
      - Segmental, simple or fragmentary: usually secondary to high energy trauma.

   (b) The fracture location.
      - Proximal shaft (proximal 1/4),
      - Mid-shaft (mid 2/4),
      - Distal shaft (distal 1/4).
3. *Radial nerve palsy* is a well-known complication of humeral shaft fractures, more frequent in fractures of the mid-shaft and fractures located at the junction of the mid 2/4 with the distal 1/4 of the shaft.

22.2 Diagnosis

1. Clinical presentation:
   (a) Pain, deformation, functional disability.

D. Saragaglia, A. Hassan Chamseddine, *Traumatology for the Emergency Doctor*, https://doi.org/10.1007/978-3-031-63196-2_22

   (b) Look for associated lesions or complications:
      - Open fracture?
      - Vascular compromise (distal pulses)?
      - Radial nerve palsy (deficit of active extension of the wrist and long fingers, deficit of active abduction of the thumb)?
2. Radiographic diagnosis is obvious:
   (a) Radiographic assessment should include two views (AP and lateral).
   (b) The radiographic views and assessment should always include the shoulder and the elbow (proximal and distal joints).

22.3 Management

- A specialized orthopedic opinion is mandatory.
- As humeral shaft fractures are usually very painful, hospitalization is generally recommended.
- An initial immobilization is required using a sling and swathe (shoulder brace-immobilizer).
- For the orthopedic treatment (when indicated), a "hanging cast" or a Sarmiento cast (or brace) can be applied.
- For the surgical treatment (when indicated): open reduction and internal fixation with plate and screws is the gold standard treatment (Figs.22.1 and 22.2).
- ***In case of associated radial nerve palsy:***
  - "Wait and see" is a common attitude.
  - Spontaneous recovery of the radial paralysis occurs in up to 90% of cases.
  - EMG is neither required nor helpful in the early stage.

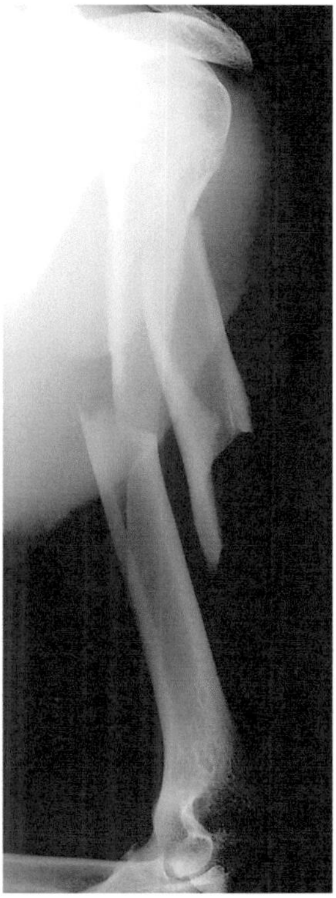

Fig. 22.1 Humerus X-ray showing a comminuted fracture of the proximal half of the humeral shaft

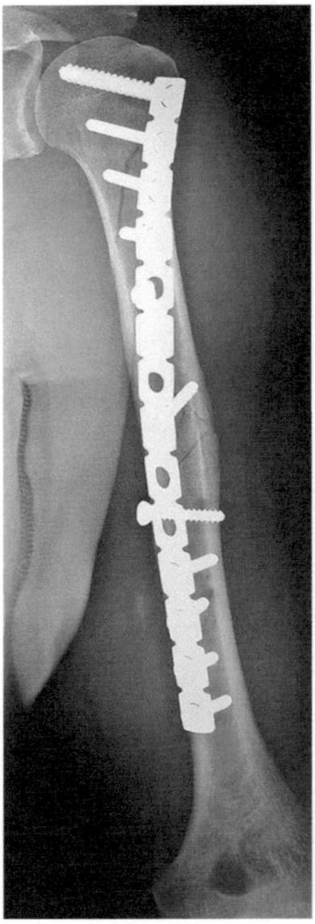

Fig. 22.2 Radiograph of the same fracture as shown in Fig. 22.1 after open reduction and internal fixation with plate and screws

Tendon Injuries in the Arm 23

23.1 Rupture of the Long Head of the Biceps Tendon

It usually occurs in the context of preexisting rotator cuff pathology.

23.1.1 Diagnosis

- The patient commonly reports a sudden moderate pain and audible snap, sometimes with a history of previous shoulder pain and discomfort.
- The clinical presentation is usually obvious with a bulge in the middle of the anterior aspect of the arm (giving the appearance of a "Popeye muscle") (Fig. 23.1).
- A shoulder ultrasound can be helpful in confirming the diagnosis, showing an image of an "empty" bicipital groove.

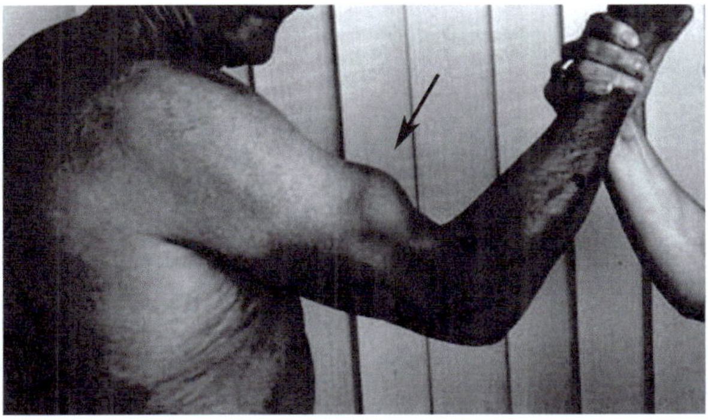

Fig. 23.1 Photo of a patient with rupture of the long head of biceps: "Popeye" sign in elbow flexion against resistance

D. Saragaglia, A. Hassan Chamseddine, *Traumatology for the Emergency Doctor*, https://doi.org/10.1007/978-3-031-63196-2_23

23.1.2 Management

- For patients >50 years.
  - Start functional treatment with rehabilitation,
  - Reassess with Arthro-CT or Arthro-MRI of the shoulder after 2–3 weeks.
- For patients <50 years (especially if they have well developed muscles).
  - Assess the rotator cuff,
  - Early surgery to perform proximal tenodesis (fixation of the proximal stump of the biceps tendon into the Bicipital groove).

23.2 Distal Biceps Avulsion

It is a relatively rare injury which remains unfortunately frequently undiagnosed in the ER (Figs. 23.2 and 23.3).

23.2.1 Diagnosis

- History of a painful audible "pop" of the elbow.
- The diagnosis is clinically obvious when the patient is immediately seen, before the occurrence of swelling and ecchymosis.
- Always make a comparison with the opposite side:
  - Proximal retraction of the biceps belly,
  - Palpable defect and *absence of the distal bicipital "cord"* during active elbow flexion against resistance,
  - *"Hook test":* the patient actively flexes the elbow at 90° with full forearm supination, and the examiner hooks the lateral edge of the distal biceps tendon using their index finger. When the tendon is intact, the examiner's index can be inserted underneath the tendon.

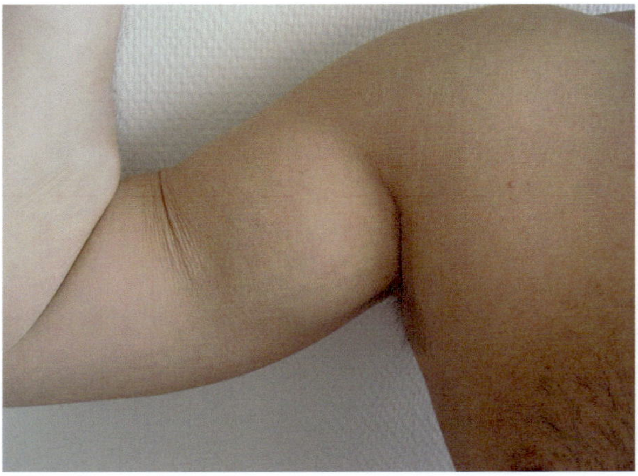

Fig. 23.2 Photo of a patient with a rupture-avulsion of the distal biceps tendon: proximal retraction and bulge of the biceps belly in active elbow flexion

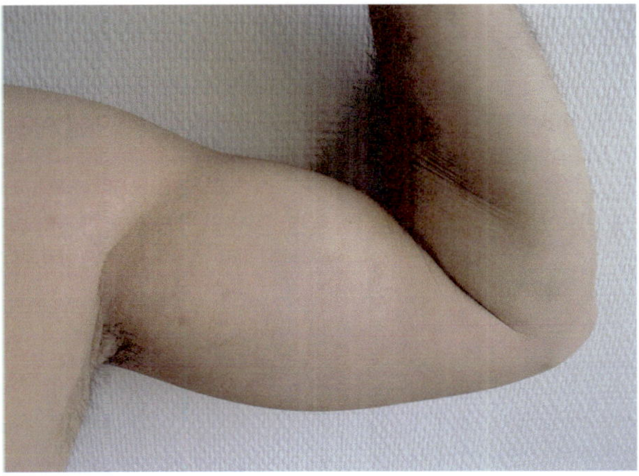

Fig. 23.3 Photo of the opposite side of the same patient as shown in Fig. 23.2 with normal appearance of the arm in elbow flexion

- *"Squeeze test":* with the patient's elbow near to 90° flexion and the forearm in moderate pronation, the examiner squeezes the distal biceps belly (similar to Thompson test for Achilles tendon). Failure to induce supination to the patient's forearm is interpreted as a positive sign for rupture.
- Ultrasound and MRI:
  - They are not indispensable for the diagnosis if the patient is seen immediately after the accident.
  - They are beneficial when the patient is seen a few days later and the physical exam is doubtful.

Treatment is usually surgical by reinsertion of the distal biceps tendon to the bicipital tuberosity of the proximal Radius, or to the anterior brachialis tendon.

23.3 Avulsion of the Distal Triceps Brachii Tendon

It is a relatively rare injury which remains unfortunately frequently undiagnosed in the ER because of the rarity of the injury itself and the lack of adequate physical exam.

23.3.1 Diagnosis

- The injury is commonly secondary to a fall on the outstretched hand with the elbow at 30°–45° flexion.
- Clinical presentation:
  - Painful elbow,
  - Posterior elbow swelling,
  - Passive and active elbow ROM are normal,

- *Active extension against gravity or against resistance is weak* or completely deficient (Fig. 23.4).

- Elbow radiographs frequently reveal (80%) a *bone chip* detached from the posterior aspect of the olecranon process (at the posterior aspect of the elbow) and displaced proximally (2–3 cm) (Fig. 23.5).
- The ultrasound can be useful if it is clinically oriented.
- The MRI confirms the diagnosis if any doubt remains.

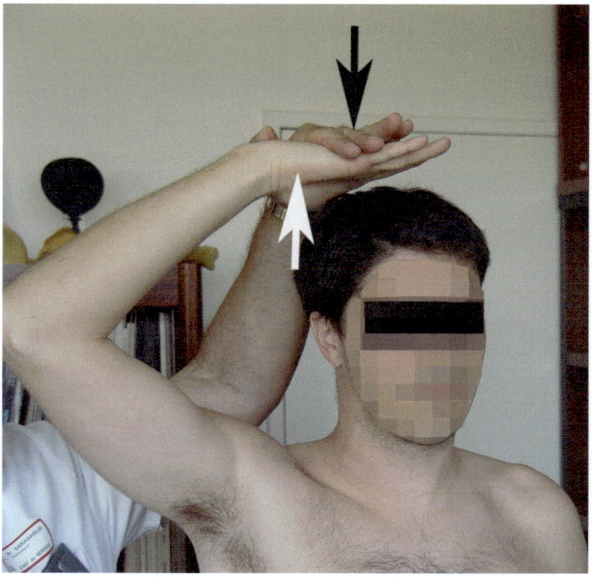

Fig. 23.4 Photo of the elbow active extension test against resistance for the diagnosis of distal triceps rupture (in overhead position of the hand)

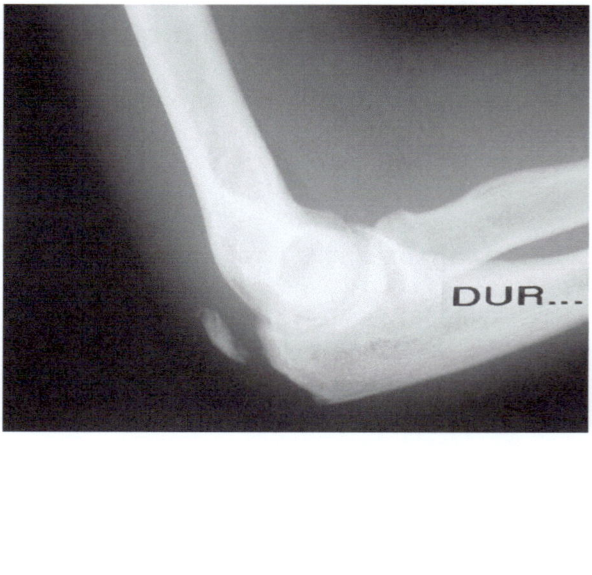

Fig. 23.5 Elbow lateral radiograph for a patient with a distal avulsion-rupture of the triceps brachialis. Note the image of "bone fleck" detached from the posterior aspect of the olecranon process and displaced proximally

23.3.2 Management

- Attention should be made not to miss the diagnosis for "calcified olecranon bursitis."
- Ask for a specialized orthopedic opinion for diagnosis confirmation and further management (reinsertion of the avulsed tendon).

Elbow Fractures in Adult

24

24.1 Fractures of the Distal Humerus

24.1.1 Patho-Anatomy

Fractures of the distal humerus are divided into:

24.1.1.1 Extra-Articular Factures. They Are Categorized Into

- ***Supra-condylar fractures (complete fractures)*** (Fig. 24.1)
  - Rare in adult,
  - They commonly correspond to fractures of the humeral shaft extending to the distal 1/4 of the bone.
- ***Partial fractures***
  - Fracture of the medial epicondyle: relatively more frequent in children (Fig. 24.2),
  - Fracture of the lateral epicondyle: exceptional in both adult and pediatric patients (Fig. 24.3).

D. Saragaglia, A. Hassan Chamseddine, *Traumatology for the Emergency Doctor*, https://doi.org/10.1007/978-3-031-63196-2_24

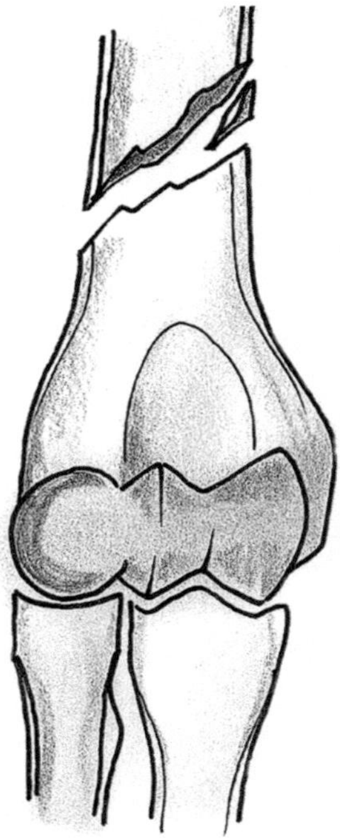

Fig. 24.1 Illustration of a supra-condylar fracture of the distal humerus

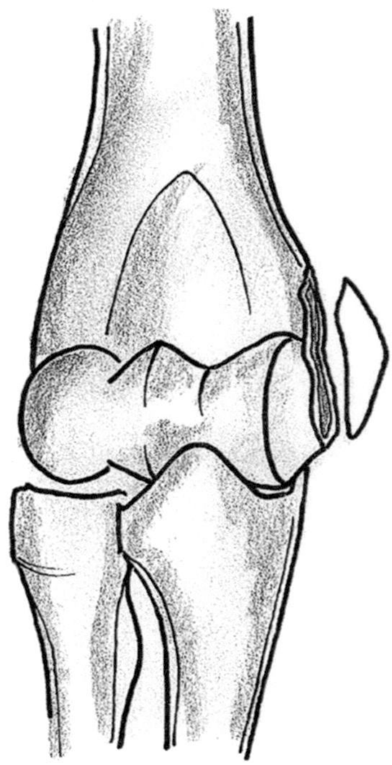

Fig. 24.2 Illustration of a medial epicondyle fracture

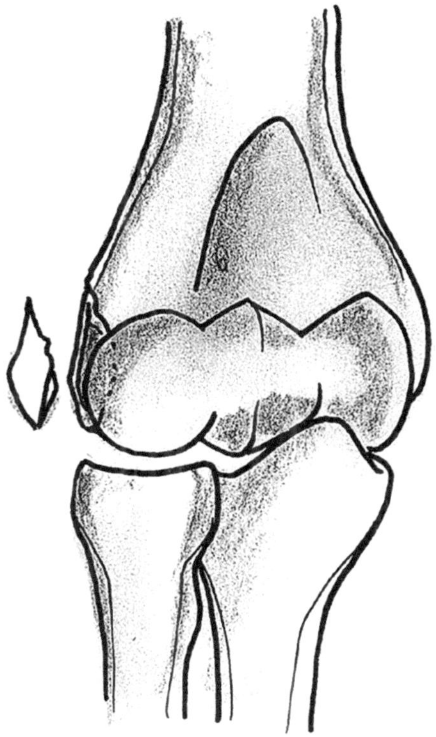

Fig. 24.3 Illustration of a lateral epicondyle fracture

24.1.1.2 Articular Fractures. They Are Categorized Into

- ***Partial sagittal fractures (uni-condylar fractures)***, with the fracture line running in either the sagittal or para-sagittal plane.
  - Fracture of the medial condyle (Fig. 24.4),
  - Fracture of the lateral condyle (Fig. 24.5).
- ***Inter-condylar fractures (complete fractures)***, ranging from the simplest to the most complex fracture pattern (Fig. 24.6). They correspond to supra-condylar fractures with inter-condylar extension.
- ***Partial coronal fractures***: the so-called coronal shear fractures, with the main fracture line running in the coronal plane. They may involve:
  - The capitulum alone (Fig. 24.7),
  - The capitulum with a variable part of the anterior aspect of the trochlea (from lateral to medial) (Fig. 24.8),
  - The capitulum and the anterior part of the whole trochlea (simple or comminuted) (Fig. 24.9).

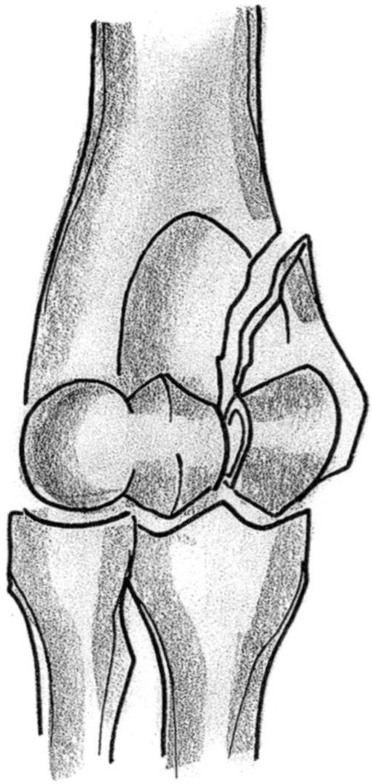

Fig. 24.4 Illustration of a medial condyle fracture (sagittal fracture line)

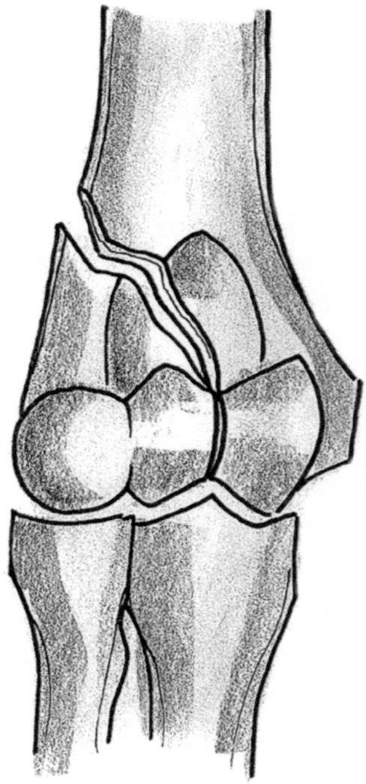

Fig. 24.5 Illustration of a lateral condyle fracture (sagittal fracture line)

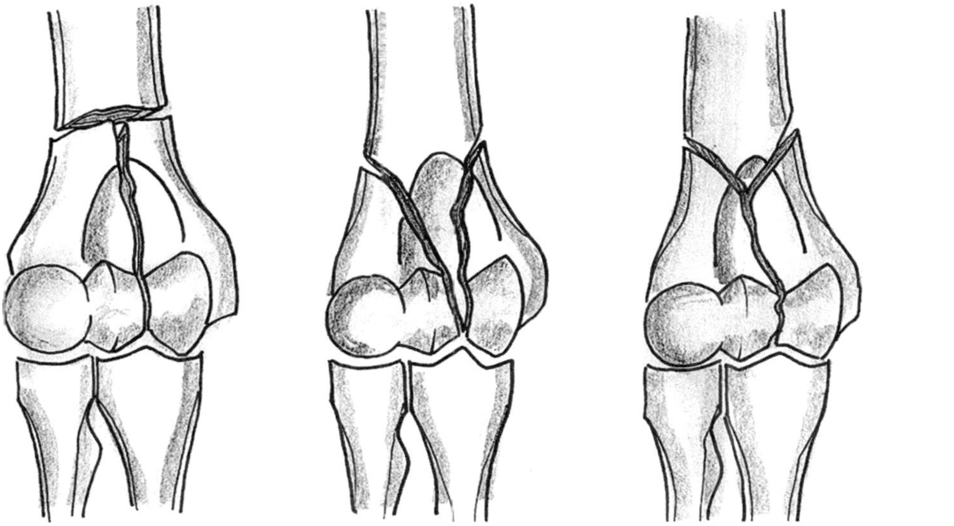

Fig. 24.6 Illustration of different types of complete inter-condylar fractures of the distal humerus (T, V, and Y shapes)

Fig. 24.7 Illustration of an isolated fracture of the capitulum (coronal fracture line)

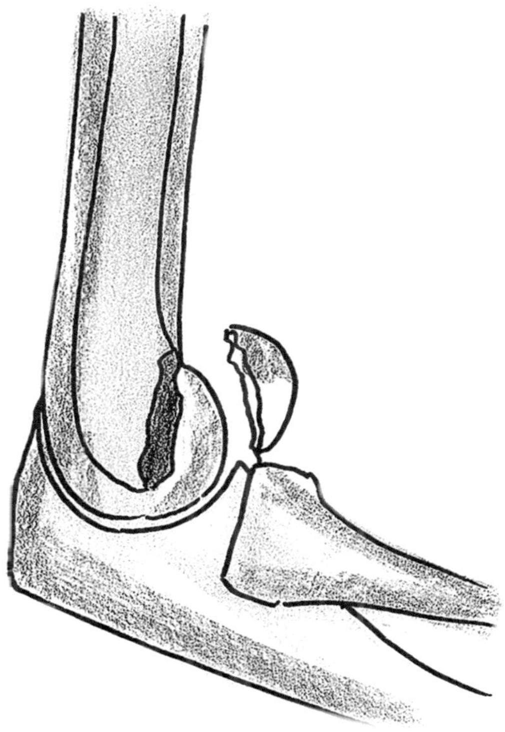

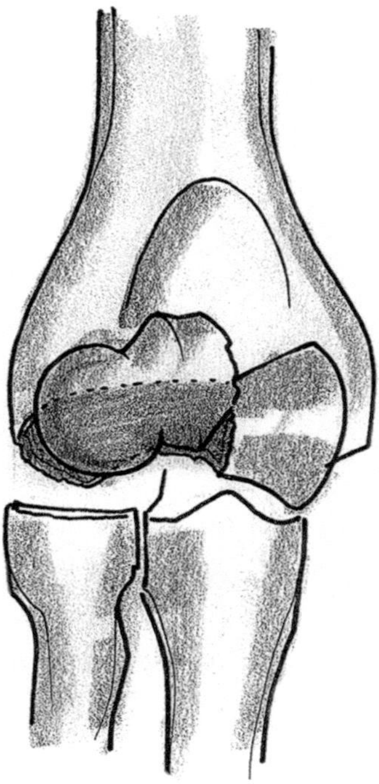

Fig. 24.8 Illustration of a fracture of the capitulum involving the anterior aspect of the lateral part of the trochlea (coronal fracture line)

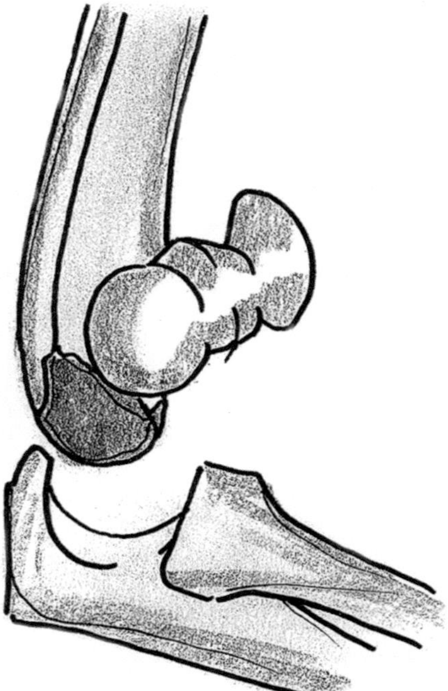

Fig. 24.9 Illustration of a fracture of the capitulum involving the anterior aspect of the whole trochlea in one fragment (coronal fracture line)

24.1.1.3 Associated Lesions

Variable and different lesions can be associated with the fractures of the distal humerus:

- ***Bony***: fracture of the radial head, fracture of the olecranon process, fracture of the coronoid process.
- ***Vascular***: rare (brachial artery injury).
- ***Neurologic***: median nerve, radial nerve, ulnar nerve (more frequent than other nerves).
- ***Skin***: abrasions, open fracture.

24.1.2 Diagnosis

- ***Clinical presentation*****:** elbow pain, swelling, and complete functional disability.
- ***Physical exam*** should look for any associated lesions (distal pulses, capillary refill, distal sensory or motor disturbance).
- ***Radiographic assessment*** typically includes a minimum of two orthogonal views (AP and lateral). This is essential for making an adequate diagnosis and planning the appropriate treatment.
- ***CT scan with 2-D and 3-D reconstruction*** is now considered an indispensable complementary tool for surgical planning.

24.1.3 Management

- A Specialized orthopedic consultation is a must.
- *Orthopedic treatment is rarely indicated.* Non-displaced fractures may benefit from above elbow cast immobilization for 4–6 weeks. Weekly radiographic control is necessary for the first 3 weeks to diagnose secondary displacement promptly.
- *Surgical treatment is very commonly indicated.* Open reduction and stable internal fixation should be performed as soon as possible to allow early rehabilitation and minimize the risk of elbow stiffness (Figs. 24.10, 24.11, 24.12 and 24.13).
- Temporary elbow immobilization with cast or trans-olecranon skeletal traction is recommended if the final surgical treatment is delayed for any reason, such as unavailability of the operating theater, local skin condition and blisters, or the general patient condition.

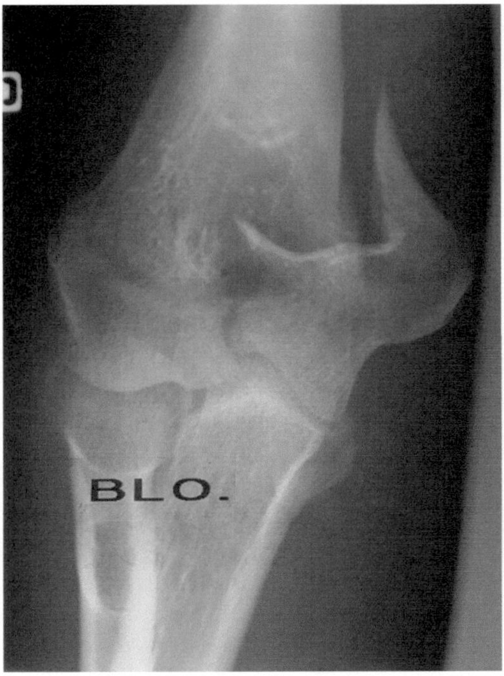

Fig. 24.10 AP radiograph of an inter-condylar fracture of the distal humerus

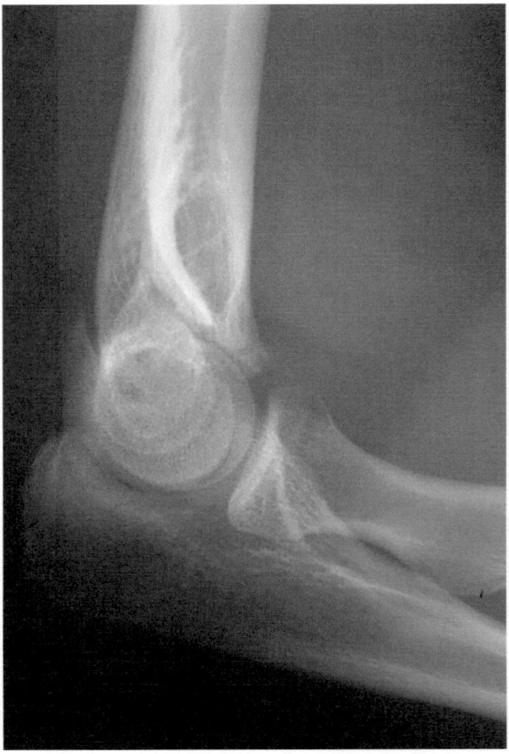

Fig. 24.11 Lateral radiograph of the same fracture as in Fig. 24.10

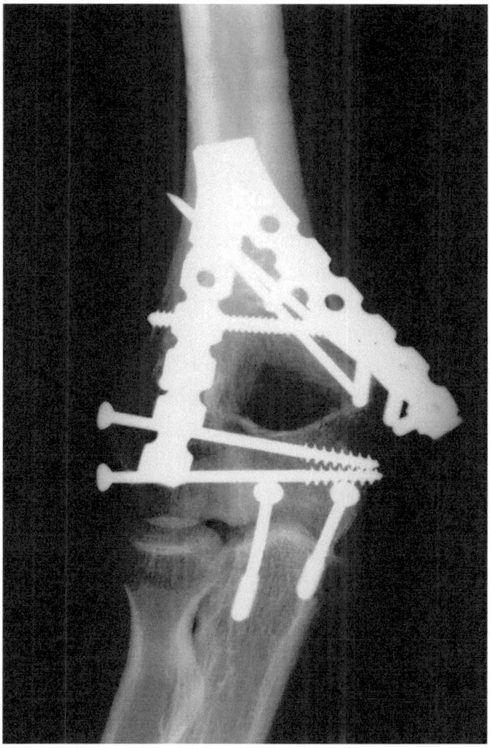

Fig. 24.12 AP radiograph of the same fracture as shown in Fig. 24.10 after open reduction and internal fixation with plate and screws ("Y" plate)

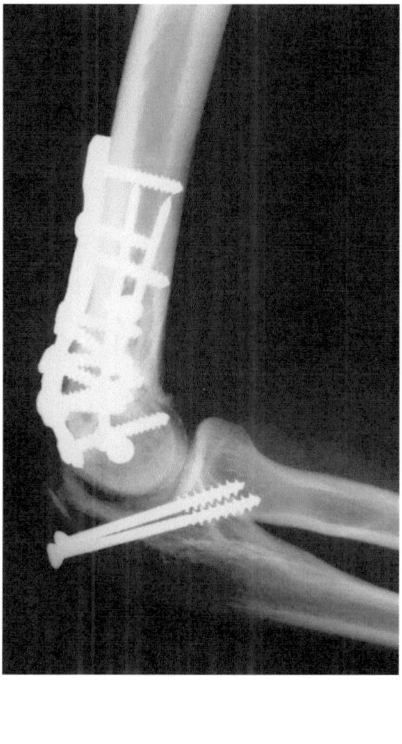

Fig. 24.13 Lateral radiograph of the same fracture as shown in Fig. 24.10 after open reduction and internal fixation

24.2 Fractures of the Olecranon Process

- Fractures of the olecranon process result in *the interruption of the extensor mechanism of the elbow.*
- They may present a simple (Fig. 24.14) or a fragmentary pattern (comminuted).
- *The Clinical presentation* includes:
  - Elbow swelling,
  - Possible skin abrasion or open fracture,
  - Functional disability with deficit of active elbow extension.
- *The Diagnosis* is confirmed by AP and lateral elbow radiographs.
- *Treatment*
  - A Specialized orthopedic consultation is a must.
  - Orthopedic treatment is rarely indicated. Non-displaced fractures are treated with an above elbow cast immobilization for 4–6 weeks. Weekly radiographic control is necessary for the first 3 weeks to diagnose secondary displacement promptly.
  - *Surgical treatment* is commonly indicated using open reduction and stable internal fixation to allow early rehabilitation and minimize the risk of stiffness (Figs. 24.15 and 24.16).

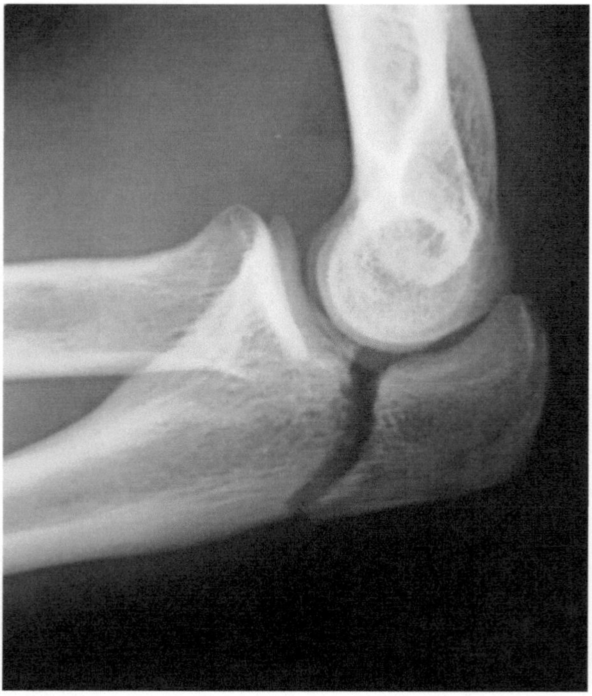

Fig. 24.14 Lateral elbow X-ray showing a simple fracture of the olecranon process

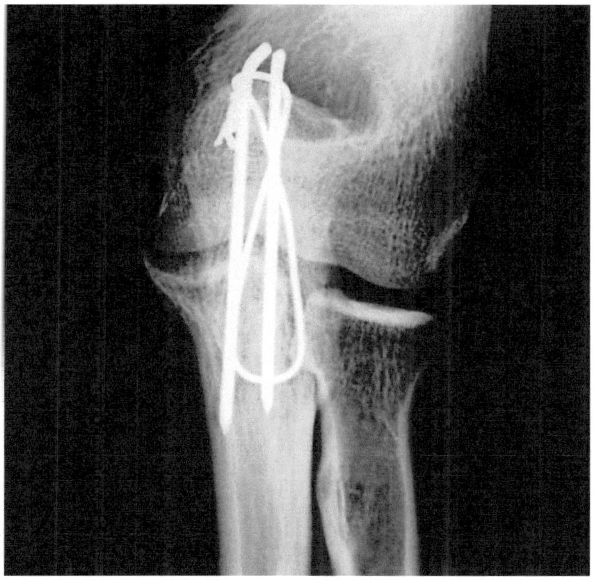

Fig. 24.15 AP radiograph of the same elbow as shown in Fig. 24.14 after open reduction and internal fixation using two pins and metallic wire ("figure of 8" fixation construct)

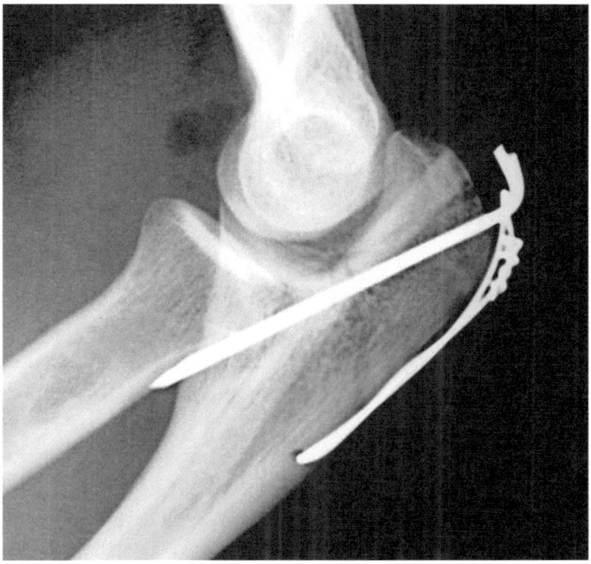

Fig. 24.16 Lateral radiograph of the same elbow as shown in Fig. 24.15 ("figure of 8" fixation construct)

24.3 Fractures of the Radial Head

1. Fractures of the radial head can involve the head alone, the neck (usually commonly in children), or both the head and neck in combination, especially in cases of high-energy trauma.
2. The fracture may be simple or fragmentary (comminuted).
3. Radial head fracture may occur as:
   (a) an isolated fracture,
   (b) or part of a more complex injury pattern, such as:
      - Elbow dislocation with radial head and coronoid process fractures (the so-called *terrible triad of the elbow*),
      - Fracture of the ulna and radial head (equivalent of a Monteggia lesion),
      - Distal radio-ulnar dislocation with radial head fracture and disruption of the inter-osseous radio-ulnar membrane (the so-called *Essex-Lopresti lesion*),
      - Radial head (and or neck) fracture with rupture of the Medial Collateral Ligament of the elbow.
4. Clinical examination reveals:
   (a) Pain and tenderness at the lateral aspect of the elbow (palpation of the radial head) and during passive pronation-supination movement,
   (b) Painful limited active range of pronation-supination movement.
5. The diagnosis is based on the *radiographic assessment*:
   (a) Elbow radiographs with AP, lateral, and oblique views (crucial to disclose subtle fractures).
   (b) Wrist radiographs should always be requested to disclose any associated injuries.
   (c) *CT scan with 2-D and 3-D reconstruction* is a must, especially in doubtful cases and to disclose any associated subtle lesions.
6. Management
   (a) For undisplaced isolated fractures: orthopedic treatment is indicated as follows:
      - *Functional treatment*: early rehabilitation to restore range of motion. NSAID's are usually prescribed for pain control (pain may persist for 4–6 weeks),
      - Or an *above elbow immobilization* (cast or brace for 10–14 days only) for non-compliant patients.
   (b) For displaced fractures: surgical treatment is indicated.
      - Open reduction and internal fixation for fractures that are amenable to fixation (simple fractures),
      - Radial head replacement (prosthesis) for fractures that are not amenable to fixation (fragmentary, comminuted).

24.4 Fractures of the Coronoid Process

- The coronoid process is an important anatomic structure for the primary elbow stability.
- Isolated fractures of the coronoid process are rare.
- Fractures of the coronoid process are typically associated with complex injury patterns, such as elbow dislocation, terrible triad of the elbow, comminuted fracture of the olecranon process, etc.
- The size of the coronoid fractured fragment is predictive of elbow instability, with larger fragments being associated with increased instability.
- Treatment
  - Orthopedic treatment with elbow brace or above elbow cast immobilization (3 weeks) for undisplaced small fractures (tip of the coronoid process).
  - Surgical treatment is indicated for large and displaced fractures: open reduction and internal fixation (especially when the fracture is part of a more complex injury pattern).

25 Management of Elbow Trauma with "Normal" Radiographs

Painful elbow with normal radiographs after trauma is a rare presentation. The quality of the radiographs and the adequacy of the views are crucial for a good judgment and to rule out any subtle fractures ("hairline" or undisplaced radial head fracture, for example).

25.1 Presentation and Clinical Assessment

- The patient may present either immediately or a few days after the trauma for elbow pain or "discomfort."
- The history of the accident helps for diagnosis orientation:
  - Direct trauma,
  - Fall on the outstretched hand,
  - Elbow position at the moment of the trauma: flexion? extension? hyperextension?
- Elbow examination.
  - Mild to moderate pain and, or, functional disability?
  - Tenderness on palpation? (lateral epicondyle? Medial epicondyle? radial head? etc.),
  - Active and passive range of motion in flexion–extension and pronation–supination with and without resistance (limited? Painful?).

25.2 Radiographic Assessment

- The request of the radiographic views is oriented by the result of the clinical examination.
- Ask for multiple and special views for the radial head (standard AP and lateral views and with pronation and supination positions as tolerated).

D. Saragaglia, A. Hassan Chamseddine, *Traumatology for the Emergency Doctor*, https://doi.org/10.1007/978-3-031-63196-2_25

- The CT scan is very helpful in revealing "subtle" fractures in the presence of unexplained pain or disability.
- The MRI is an important tool for diagnosing capsulo-ligamentous injuries, such as medial collateral ligament, lateral collateral ligament, etc.

25.3 Diagnosis

The differential diagnosis of a "traumatic elbow with normal radiographs" includes a wide variety of injuries:

- *Subtle or non-displaced radial head fracture* (diagnosed on CT scan),
- *Medial collateral ligament injury* (diagnosed on MRI),
- *Lateral collateral ligament injury* (diagnosed on MRI),
- *Avulsion of the triceps brachii tendon* (presence of a bone fleck at the posterior aspect of the olecranon process misdiagnosed as "calcification" of the distal triceps tendon),
- *Avulsion of the distal biceps brachii tendon* (well seen on MRI),
- *Fracture of the tip of the coronoid process* during elbow dislocation with spontaneous reduction,
- *Subtle fracture of the olecranon process*,
- *Simple elbow contusion.*

25.4 Management

- *If the elbow is severely painful* with no definite diagnosis:
  - An above elbow cast immobilization is applied for 2 weeks (for pain control),
  - Rehabilitation is started after cast removal if the pain subsides or the elbow is reassessed with MRI if the pain persists.
- *If the elbow is mildly painful* with no definite diagnosis:
  - Prescribe NSAID's and start functional rehabilitation (restore and maintain range of motion).
  - The patient is then reassessed after 2 weeks for further investigation if he remains symptomatic.

26 Elbow Dislocations

There are three anatomic types of elbow dislocation: posterior, postero-lateral, and postero-medial.

Red Flag:

- In children, elbow dislocation is commonly associated with fracture of the medial epicondyle. This association may be source of complication: intra-articular entrapment of the medial epicondyle during elbow relocation.
- In adult, fracture of the radial head and/or the coronoid process may be associated with elbow dislocation. Terrible triad of the elbow is a very unstable injury pattern defined by the association of the three injuries together.

26.1 Diagnosis

- The diagnosis is suspected in a patient presented to the ER after a fall on the outstretched hand with elbow pain, swelling, deformity (posterior prominence of the olecranon process), and functional disability.
- The physical exam should always check for any associated neuro-vascular impairment.
- The diagnosis is made on elbow radiographs (AP and lateral views) (Figs. 26.1 and 26.2).
- Oblique elbow views may help in revealing associated bone injuries (radial head, coronoid process, etc.).

D. Saragaglia, A. Hassan Chamseddine, *Traumatology for the Emergency Doctor*, https://doi.org/10.1007/978-3-031-63196-2_26

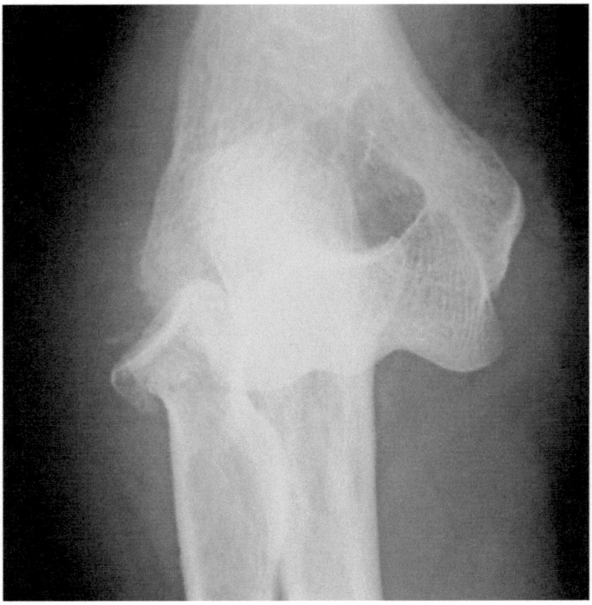

Fig. 26.1 AP elbow X-ray: postero-lateral elbow dislocation with radial head fracture

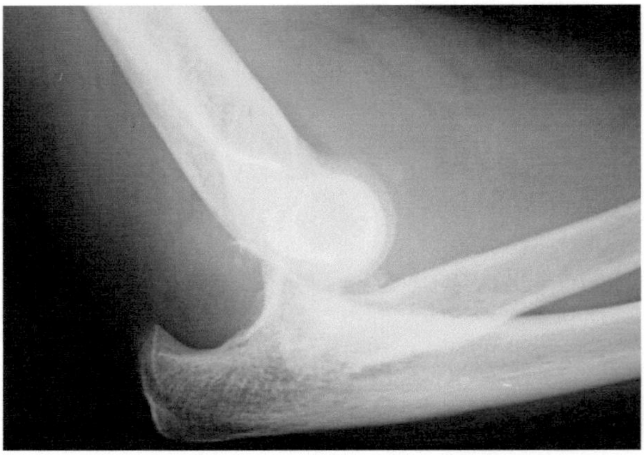

Fig. 26.2 Lateral X-ray of the same elbow as shown in Fig. 26.1 showing the same fracture–dislocation pattern

26.2 Management

- Elbow relocation is considered as an emergency procedure.
- It can be performed either under general anesthesia or simple sedation with analgesia.
- Elbow relocation maneuver is performed using traction along the axis of the forearm with concomitant elbow flexion (> 90°).
- Above elbow cast immobilization is then applied (elbow flexed at 100°) for 2–3 weeks.

- ***Red flag***
  - Re-dislocation into cast may occur (especially in the case of severe associated capsulo-ligamentous injuries).
  - Radiographic control is mandatory after elbow relocation, after cast application, and 3–5 days later.
- A specialized orthopedic consultation and management are required in the presence of:
  - Associated fracture,
  - Instability after reduction (immediate or into cast),
  - Irreducible dislocation.
- Elbow rehabilitation,
  - is started after cast removal for the restoration of the range of motion,
  - should be gentle and progressive,
  - massage and aggressive manipulation are prohibited (risk of peri-articular ossifications).
  - Recovery is usually expected after 3–6 months.
  - Mild lack of full extension (5–20°) may occur.
- Recurrent dislocations are exceptional. However, Judoka (athletes who practice judo) are prone to develop this type of complication.

Forearm Fractures

27

Radius and ulna fractures are common injury induced by either direct or indirect trauma.

Fracture line is located in the part of the shaft between the bicipital tuberosity of the proximal radius and 4 cm above the radio-carpal joint line (wrist joint line). Beyond these two limits, they are considered as elbow fractures and wrist fractures, respectively.

27.1 Patho-Anatomy

Forearm fractures are categorized into:

- **Isolated fracture** of one bone: radius or ulna.
- **Fracture of both bone**: radius and ulna.
- Fracture of one bone associated with dislocation of the head of the other bone:
  - **Monteggia lesion** (Fig. 27.1a, b): corresponds to a fracture of the ulna associated with dislocation of the radial head (radio-humeral joint). The dislocation of the radial head follows the direction of the apex of the angulation of the displaced ulnar fracture; it may be anterior (Fig. 27.1a, b), posterior (Fig. 27.2a–c), or lateral.
  - **Galeazzi lesion** (Figs. 27.3 and 27.4): corresponds to a fracture of the radius associated with dislocation of the ulnar head (distal radio-ulnar joint).

The fracture line may be transverse, oblique, spiral, wedge, or fragmentary (comminuted).

D. Saragaglia, A. Hassan Chamseddine, *Traumatology for the Emergency Doctor*, https://doi.org/10.1007/978-3-031-63196-2_27

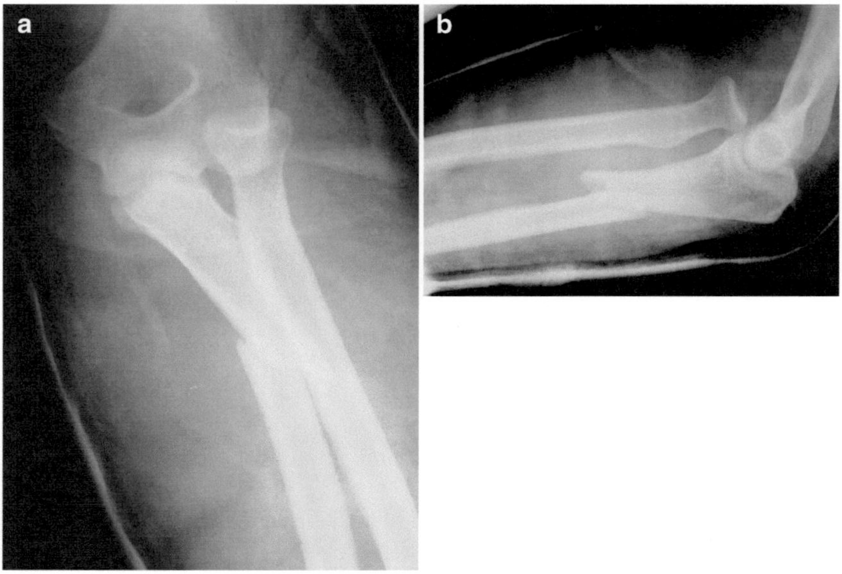

Fig. 27.1 (**a**) AP radiograph of a Monteggia fracture. (**b**) Lateral view of the same elbow as shown in Fig. 27.1a

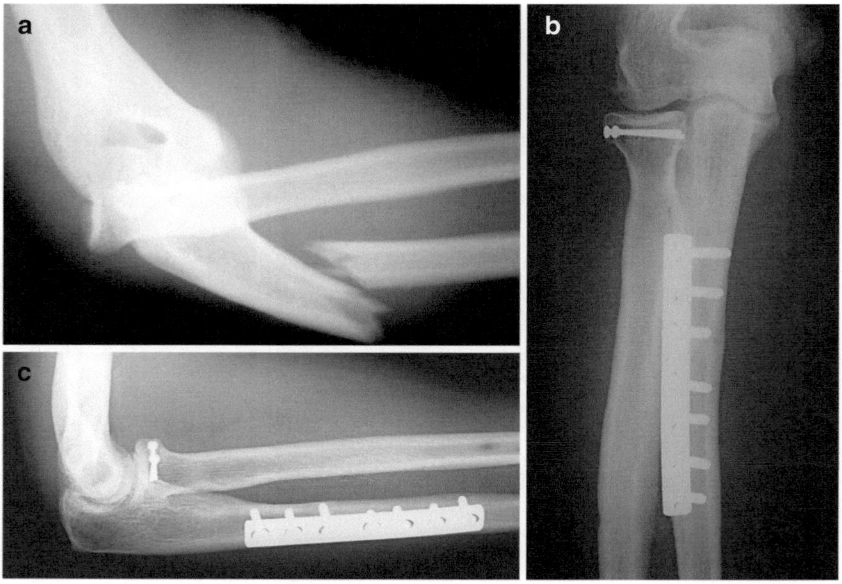

Fig. 27.2 (**a**) Lateral elbow X-ray showing a particular type of Monteggia lesion (reversed Monteggia fracture) with combination of ulnar fracture (dorsal angulation), posterior radial head dislocation (same direction as the ulnar fracture angulation), and partial radial head fracture. (**b**) AP X-ray of the same Monteggia lesion as shown in Fig. 27.2a after open reduction and internal fixation of the ulna (plate and screws) and the radial head (two screws). (**c**) Lateral elbow X-ray of the same patient as shown in Fig. 27.2b: note the reduction of the radial head dislocation

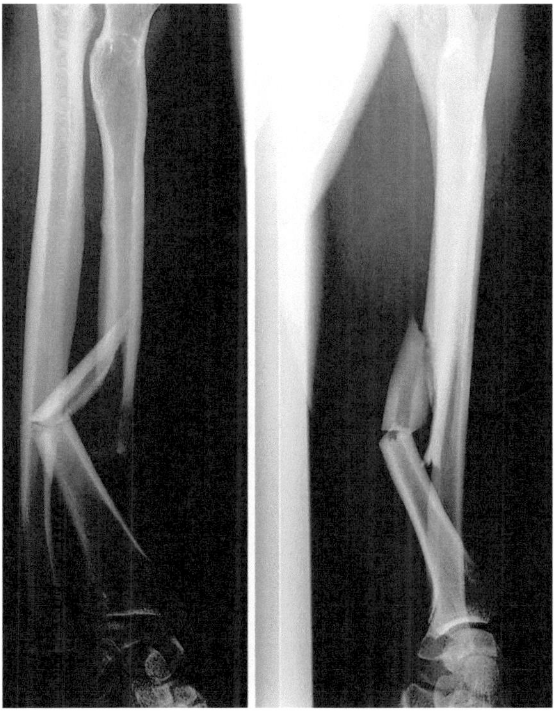

Fig. 27.3 AP and lateral forearm radiographs showing a Galeazzi lesion (fracture of the radial shaft with dislocation of the distal radio-ulnar joint)

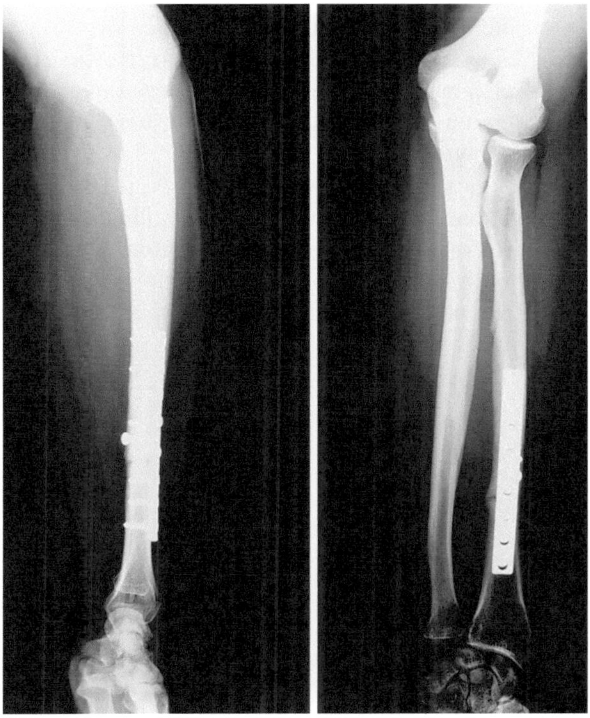

Fig. 27.4 AP and lateral radiographs of the same injury as shown in Fig. 27.3 after open reduction and internal fixation of the radial shaft fracture with plate and screws. Note the spontaneous reduction of the distal radio-ulnar joint dislocation without any direct surgical action

27.2 Diagnosis

- Clinical presentation and examination:
  - Pain, swelling, and deformation,
  - Functional disability of the forearm,
  - Examine for neurovascular complications (distal pulses and sensation),
  - Examine for the potential development of compartment syndrome, especially in cases of high energy trauma or crush injury. Compartment syndrome is characterized by spontaneous severe exorbitant pain, tense swelling of the forearm, pain in the volar aspect of the forearm during passive extension of the fingers, distal sensory impairment, and delayed capillary refill. The measurement of the compartment pressure is helpful in confirming the diagnosis if there is any doubt.
- The diagnosis is made on forearm radiographs (two orthogonal views: AP and lateral) including the adjacent joints (elbow and wrist) to prevent missing any associated dislocation of the radial or ulnar head.

27.3 Management

- ***Orthopedic treatment*** is exceptional in adult. Only non-displaced fractures of the ulna may benefit from orthopedic treatment using an above cast immobilization for 2 months.
- ***Surgical treatment***
  - is the gold standard for fractures of the radius and ulna (open reduction and internal fixation with plate and screws).
  - fracture reduction should restitute the radial curvature and the anatomical relationship between the two bones to prevent malunion. Malunion, or fracture union with malalignment, disturbs the pronation–supination movement of the forearm.
  - surgical treatment is usually performed as soon as possible, to avoid complications associated with severe swelling.
  - if surgery is delayed for any reason, a temporary immobilization using an above elbow cast or splint is performed while waiting for the final surgical treatment. This is accompanied by close clinical observation for compartment syndrome.

Fractures of the Distal Radius 28

Distal radius fractures are very frequent injuries in the ER. They are common in patients from the elderly age group. Young adult may also be affected during sports, domestic, work, and road traffic accidents.

28.1 Mechanism

- The most common mechanism is a fall on the outstretched hand (with the wrist in extension position). The fracture is produced by compression-extension mechanism.
- A less common mechanism is a fall on the dorsal aspect of the hand with the wrist in flexion position. The fracture is produced by compression-flexion mechanism.

28.2 Patho-Anatomy

Fractures of the distal radius can be divided into three major varieties:

28.2.1 Extra-Articular Fractures

They are categorized into two types based on the direction of the displacement of the distal fragment:

- ***Dorsal displacement*** (53%): typically represented by the so-called Colles' fracture (Figs. 28.1 and 28.2), induced by a compression-extension mechanism. Dorsal metaphyseal comminution (fragmentation) and cancellous bone compression (or impaction) may occur in elderly patients after a simple fall, and in

D. Saragaglia, A. Hassan Chamseddine, *Traumatology for the Emergency Doctor*, https://doi.org/10.1007/978-3-031-63196-2_28

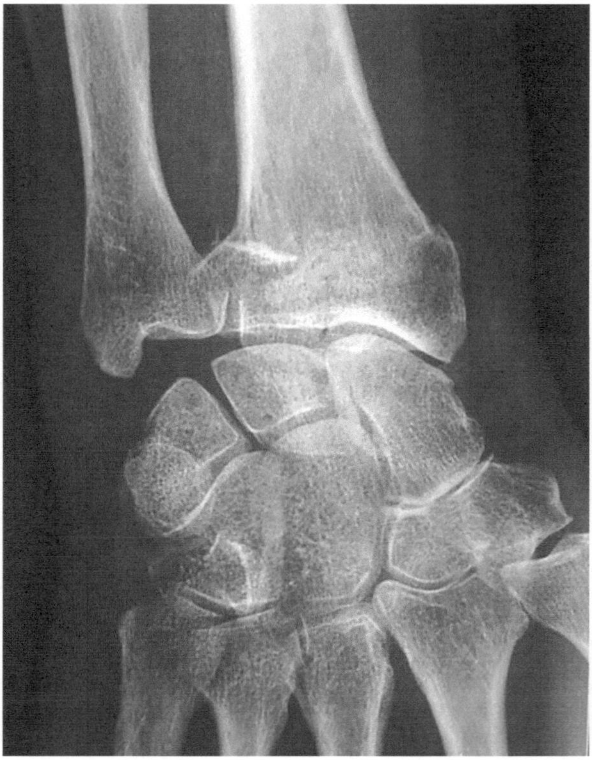

Fig. 28.1 AP wrist X-ray showing a so-called Colles' fracture of the distal radius

young patients after a high energy trauma. Both metaphyseal dorsal comminution and cancellous impaction represent patterns of fracture instability.
– ***Volar displacement*** (2.5%): typically represented by the so-called Smith's fracture (Fig. 28.3), induced by a compression-flexion mechanism. The fracture displacement follows the opposite direction of that of "Colles' fracture."

28.2.2 Articular Fractures

Characterized by the involvement of the articular surface of the distal radius. Multiple types are categorized:

- ***Fracture of the radial styloid***, the so-called Chauffer's fracture.
- Fracture-compression of the lunate fossa of the distal radius, the so-called ***Die-punch fracture***,
- ***Extra-articular fractures radiating to the articular surface of the distal radius*** (25%):

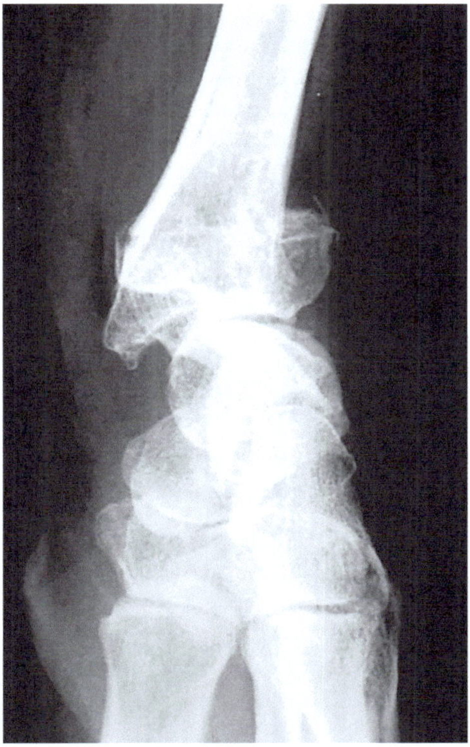

Fig. 28.2 Lateral wrist X-ray showing a so-called Colles' fracture of the distal radius

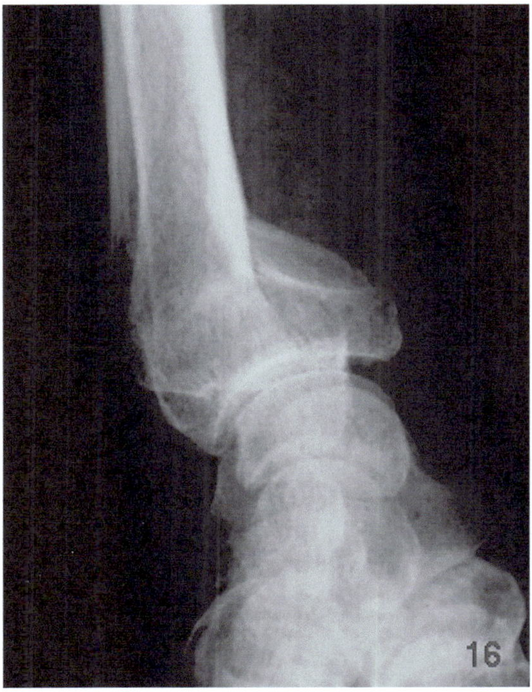

Fig. 28.3 Lateral wrist X-ray showing a so-called smith's fracture of the distal radius

   - the extra-articular fracture line is similar to Colles' fracture and extends into the articular surface of the distal radius; the fracture line runs into the frontal plane and, or the sagittal plane.
   - These fractures are commonly unstable and encompass a high risk of secondary displacement (Figs. 28.4 and 28.5).
- ***Comminuted (fragmentary) fractures*** (5%).
   - They may occur in both young and elderly patients usually following high energy and domestic fall, respectively.
   - Fracture pattern commonly involves severe impaction and comminution of the epiphysis and metaphysis of the distal radius (Fig. 28.6).

28.2.3 Marginal Fractures

- They may involve either the ***volar or the dorsal lip*** of the distal radial epiphysis (the so-called Volar Barton and dorsal Barton fracture, respectively) (Figs. 28.7 and 28.8).
- The fracture pattern corresponds to a ***fracture–dislocation*** of the radio-carpal joint: the carpal bones are usually displaced with the marginal fragment of the distal radius (volar or dorsal displacement according to the fracture location).

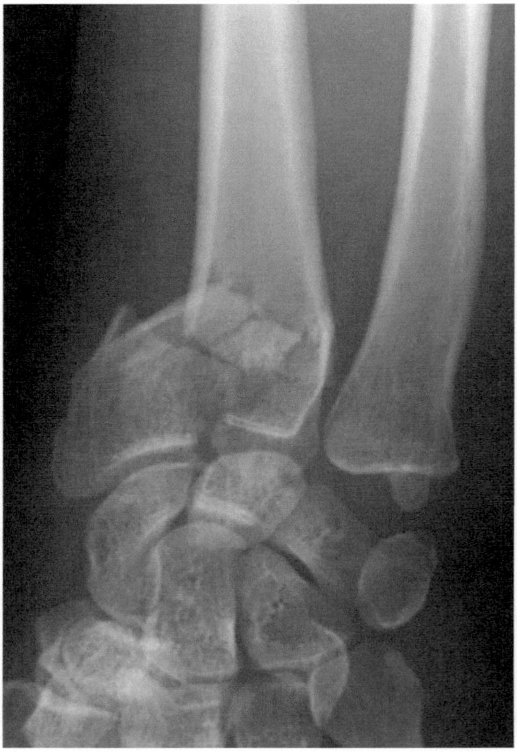

Fig. 28.4 AP wrist X-ray of a displaced articular fracture of the distal radius

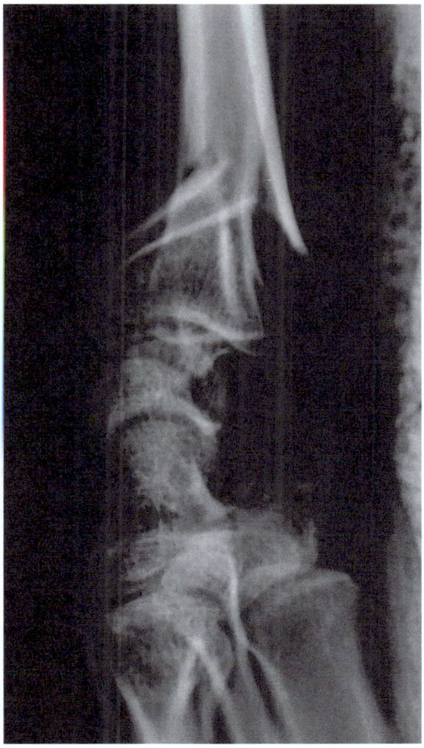

Fig. 28.5 Lateral wrist X-ray of a displaced articular fracture of the distal radius

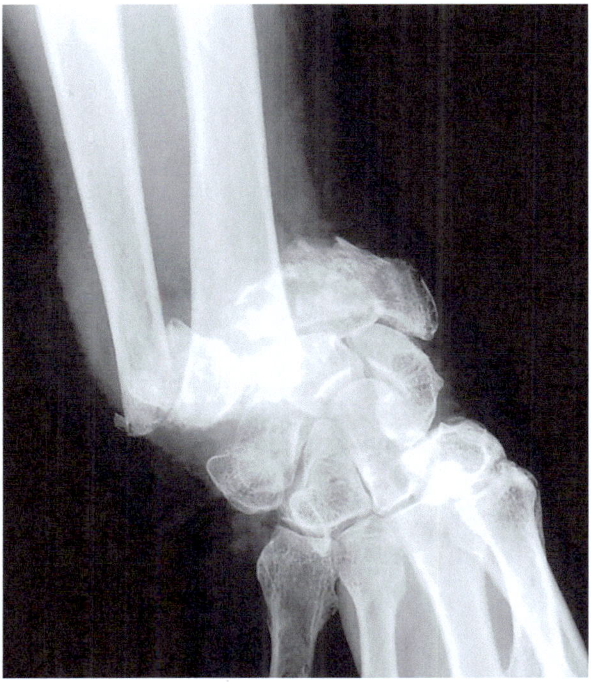

Fig. 28.6 Wrist radiograph showing a comminuted fracture of the distal radius with ulnar head fracture

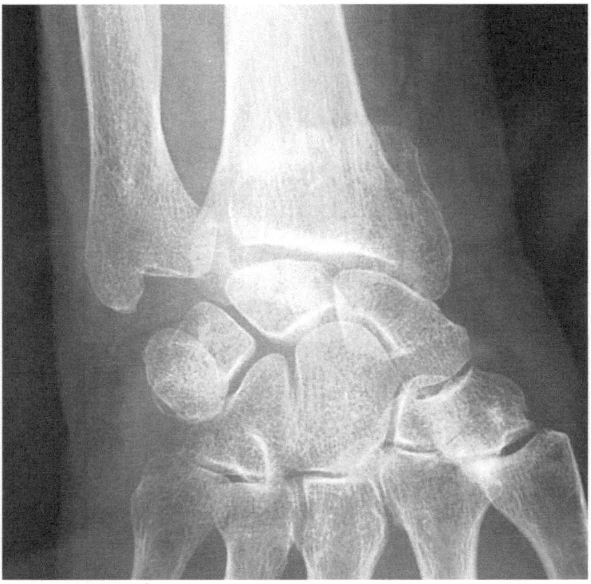

Fig. 28.7 AP wrist radiograph showing an ill-defined fracture pattern of the distal radius

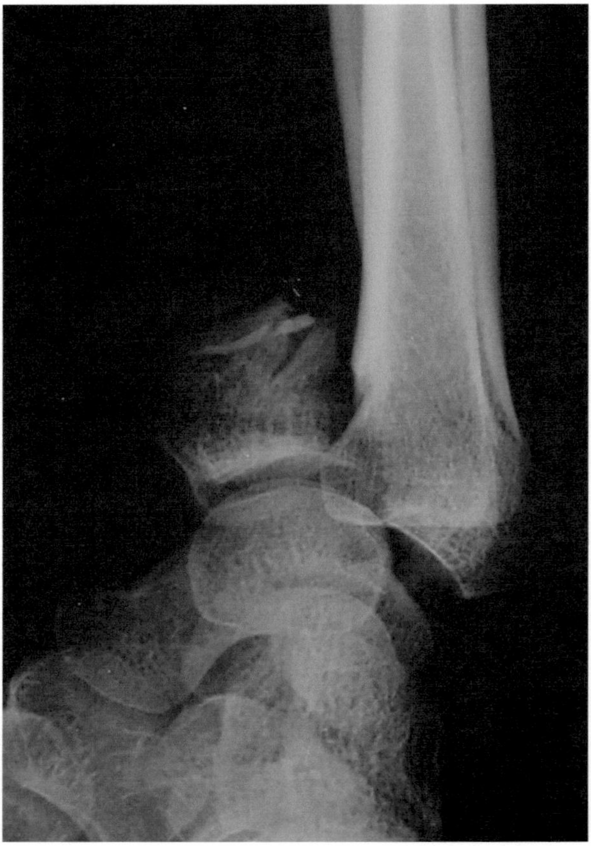

Fig. 28.8 Lateral wrist radiograph of the same patient as shown in Fig. 28.7 showing more precise characteristics of the fracture pattern: marginal fracture involving the volar lip of the distal radius with volar displacement of the carpal bones along with the radial marginal volar fragment (the so-called volar Barton fracture)

28.2.4 Associated Lesions

- Fracture of the *ulnar styloid* is common (50%). It rarely influences the final treatment.
- *Distal radio-ulnar joint dislocation.*
- Other less common associated injuries: fracture of the carpal scaphoid, perilunate dislocation, scapholunate ligament injury.

28.3 Clinical Presentation and Examination

- Wrist pain, swelling, and deformity.
- Dorsal or volar shift of the hand according to the direction of the displacement.
- Examine for potential neurovascular impairment: radial and ulnar pulses, capillary refill, and distal sensation.
- Check for open fracture.

28.4 Radiographic Assessment

- *Wrist radiographs* (AP and lateral views) are fundamental for the diagnosis.
- Additional oblique views are helpful for a better analysis of the fracture pattern.
- ***CT scan*** is not a routine request in emergency. It helps for surgical planning in complex fractures.

28.5 Management

Treatment is either non-operative or operative based on the fracture pattern, and the patient's age and demands.

28.5.1 Non-Operative Treatment

Closed reduction and cast immobilization.

- Under adequate anesthesia,
- External maneuvers with traction and gentle dorso-volar push on the distal fragment (for the initially dorsally displaced fractures),
- Cast immobilization for 6 weeks.
  - Well molded cast,
  - Position of immobilization: Moderate wrist flexion and ulnar deviation,
  - An above elbow cast gives better immobilization of the fracture.

- Weekly radiographic control for 3 weeks to check for any secondary displacement into cast (the initially very displaced and unstable pattern fractures are more predisposed to secondary displacement).
- Secondary displacement is almost impossible to restore by closed maneuvers after 3 weeks.

28.5.2 Operative Treatment

Surgical treatment can be achieved using one of the three following methods:

- Closed reduction and percutaneous pinning (with K-wires) using either:
  - Intra-focal pinning (Kapandji technique) (Figs. 28.9 and 28.10),
  - or direct trans-fracture pinning (from the epiphyseal fragment, through the fracture, to the distal diaphyso-metaphyseal junction).
- Open reduction and internal fixation using volar plate and screws (Fig. 28.11),
- External fixator (using distraction ligamentotaxis) (Fig. 28.12).

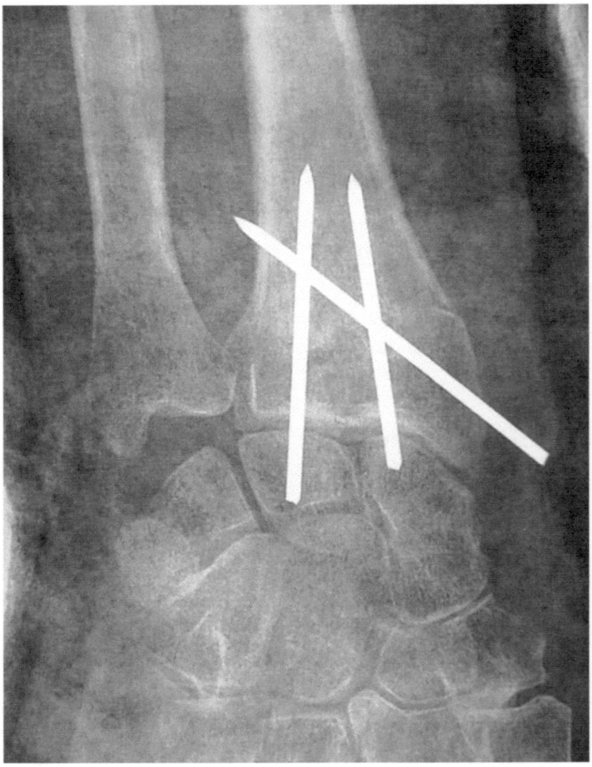

Fig. 28.9 AP wrist radiograph showing an intra-focal pinning fixation (Kapandji technique) of an initially displaced Colles' fracture (satisfactory reduction with restitution of the radial inclination and the radial height)

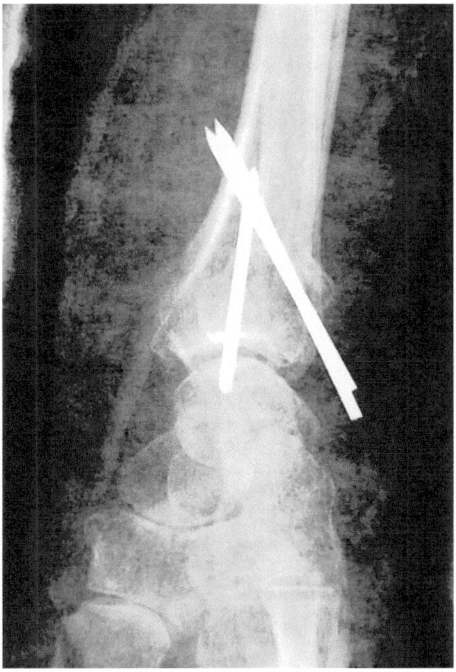

Fig. 28.10 Satisfactory reduction with restitution of the radial volar tilt on the lateral radiograph of the same wrist as shown in Fig. 28.9

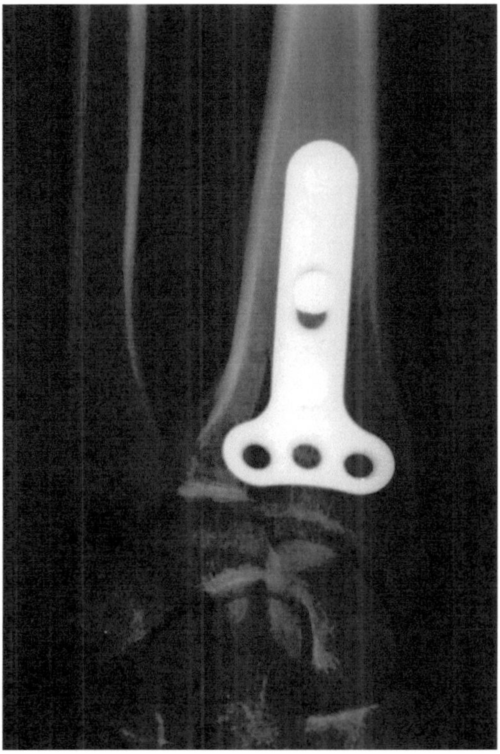

Fig. 28.11 Post-operative AP wrist X-ray of a marginal volar fracture treated with open reduction and internal fixation using the "buttress plating" technique

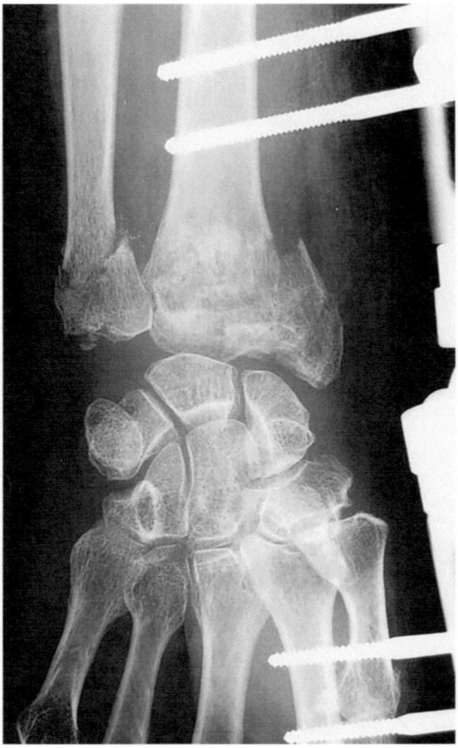

Fig. 28.12 AP radiograph of the same comminuted distal radius fracture with a distal ulnar fracture as shown in Fig. 28.6 after treatment with an external fixator (using distraction ligamentotaxis reduction technique)

Criteria of satisfactory reduction.

- Reduction maneuvers and fixation (or immobilization) should result in restoration of the normal anatomic configuration and relationships of the distal radius (assessed on AP and lateral radiographs):
- AP view
  - Radial inclination (normal value 23°, acceptable if loss of less than 5°),
  - Radial height (normal value 13 mm, acceptable if shortening of less than 5 mm).
- Lateral view
  - Volar tilt (normal value 15°, acceptable if dorsal tilt of less than 5° or within the limits of 20° of dorsal angulation, from the initial value of 15° volar tilt).
  - Excessive volar tilt is not well tolerated.

28.5.3 Indications

- Indications are based on:
  - the fracture's pattern (stable/unstable, simple/comminuted),
  - the patient's age (young/elderly),
  - the patient's functional demands.
- Stable fractures are usually treated non-operatively and can be managed by the ER physicians.
- Unstable fractures are usually managed operatively by orthopedic-trauma surgeons.

28.6 Prognosis

- *Algodystrophy or complex regional pain syndrome* (the so-called reflex sympathetic dystrophy syndrome) is characterized by a functional impairment associated with edema, pain, hyperalgesia, and, or allodynia. It is more likely to occur after external fixation (distraction ligamentotaxis), immobilization, and delayed restoration of the range of motion of the wrist and hand.
- *Carpal tunnel syndrome* secondary to distal radius fractures is a well-known complication.
- *Satisfactory functional outcomes* are associated with,
  - The restitution of the anatomical configuration and relationships of the distal radius,
  - A satisfactory reduction of the articular radial surface,
  - An early restoration of the range of motion of the wrist and hand.
- *Poor outcomes* are associated with,
  - Fracture malunion with alteration of the shape, alignment, and anatomical relationships of the distal radius (which may require corrective osteotomy in young patients),
  - The occurrence of algodystrophy,
  - The presence of osteoporosis,
  - Worker's compensation.

Fractures, Dislocations, and Fracture–Dislocations of the Carpal Bones

29

Carpal bones injuries are common in road traffic accidents, domestic trauma, sports practice, and work accidents. Radiographs of good quality along with appropriate views are crucial for the diagnosis.

29.1 Radiographic Views of the Carpal Bones

29.1.1 Standard Radiographic Views

- PA view (hand facing the film) with alignment of radial shaft-third metacarpal (Fig. 29.1).
- Lateral view: is delicate to perform (elevate the ulnar border of the wrist and align the dorsal aspect of the radius with the dorsal aspect of the third metacarpal). It serves for the measurement of the scapholunate angle (Fig. 29.2).

29.1.2 Special or « Oriented Views »

- PA view with 20° elevation of the ulnar border of the wrist. It perfectly shows the scapholunate joint line,
- PA oblique view with 45° pronation: useful to visualize the triquetrum,
- PA oblique view with 45° supination: useful to visualize the hamate and hook,
- PA view with ulnar and radial inclination,
- Lateral view with wrist flexion and extension.

29.1.3 Scaphoid Views

- PA view with ulnar inclination,
- Fist view with ulnar inclination,

D. Saragaglia, A. Hassan Chamseddine, *Traumatology for the Emergency Doctor*, https://doi.org/10.1007/978-3-031-63196-2_29

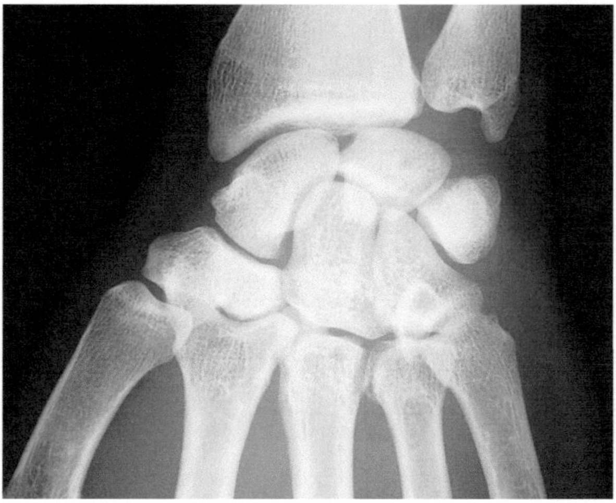

Fig. 29.1 PA wrist view for the carpal bones: normal presentation

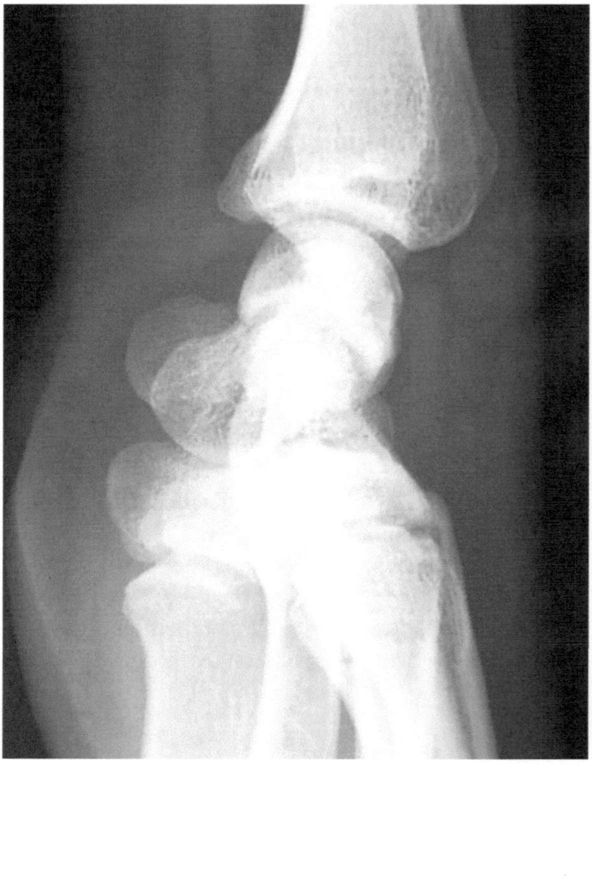

Fig. 29.2 Lateral wrist view for the carpal bones: normal presentation

- PA view with fingers 20° elevated (extended): useful to visualize the capitate and the proximal pole of the scaphoid.
- PA view with the hand well applied on the film (writing position): useful to visualize the capitate and the scaphoid tubercle.

29.2 Clinical Presentation and Diagnosis

The history taken from the patient and their entourage helps clarifying the mechanism and circumstances of the injury.

The patient usually presents with a variable degree of wrist pain and functional disability. The wrist may or not present deformity.

29.2.1 Wrist Trauma with Deformity

The clinical aspect of the deformity may predict the diagnosis which is then confirmed after the radiographic assessment:

- **Distal radius fracture** is the most common wrist injury (refer to chapter fractures of the distal radius).
- **Carpal dislocations:** history of high-energy trauma, pain, local swelling, ecchymosis, and deformity. The dislocation may occur according to one of the following types:
  - ***Perilunate dislocation***: dorsal dislocation of all carpal bones excepting the lunate (which remains in position under the articular surface of the distal radial epiphysis),
  - ***Trans-scaphoid perilunate fracture-dislocation*** (Fig. 29.3a): fracture of the scaphoid bone associated with perilunate dislocation of the carpal bones (with the lunate remaining in position),
  - **Trans-radial styloid fracture-dislocation,**
  - **Trans-scaphoid trans-capitate peri-lunar fracture-dislocation,**
  - **Lunate dislocation**: volar or dorsal dislocation of the lunate (the other carpal bones remain united and displace together proximally) (Fig. 29.3b).
- **Radiographic assessment**
  - PA view: widening of the scapholunate space and triangular shape appearance of the lunate bone (with distal apex) (Fig. 29.3c),
  - Lateral view: confirms the direction of the dislocation (Fig. 29.4).

29.2.2 Wrist Trauma Without Deformity

1. **Fracture of the scaphoid bone** (Fig. 29.5).
   (a) Is the most common carpal fracture.
   (b) The clinical examination usually demonstrates two signs:

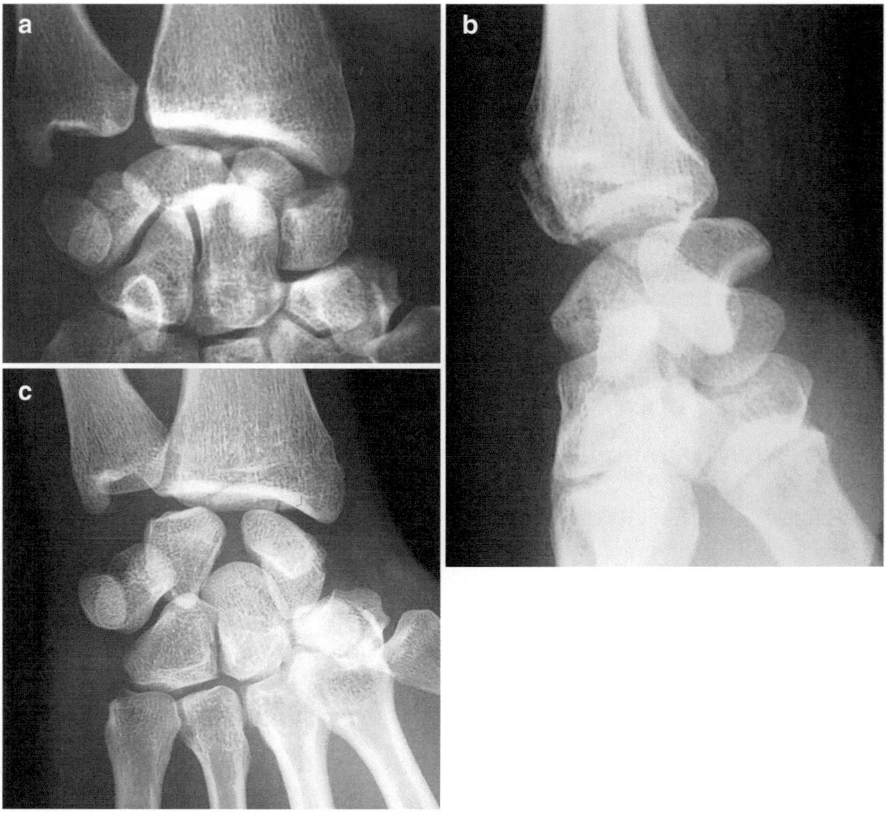

Fig. 29.3 (**a**) PA wrist radiograph showing a trans-scaphoid perilunate fracture-dislocation. Note the important displacement of the scaphoid fracture with the proximal migration of the capitate bone to the level of the first carpal row. (**b**) Lateral wrist view showing a volar dislocation of the lunate. Note that the rest of the carpal bones remain united and proximally displaced together. (**c**) PA wrist radiograph showing a volar dislocation of the lunate. Note the triangular shape with distal apex of the lunate bone

- Tenderness on palpation of the "snuffbox,"
- Pain on axial traction-compression load along the axis of the thumb.

(c) Radiographic assessment:

- Ask for the radiographic scaphoid views.
- Usually demonstrates the fracture pattern:
  - Fracture location (proximal pole, waist, base),
  - Simple vs. comminuted,
  - Undisplaced vs. displaced.
- If the facture is clinically suspected and the fracture line is not visible on the initial radiographic assessment, the radiographs should be repeated *10–21 days* later (after a temporary cast immobilization using a thumb spica).

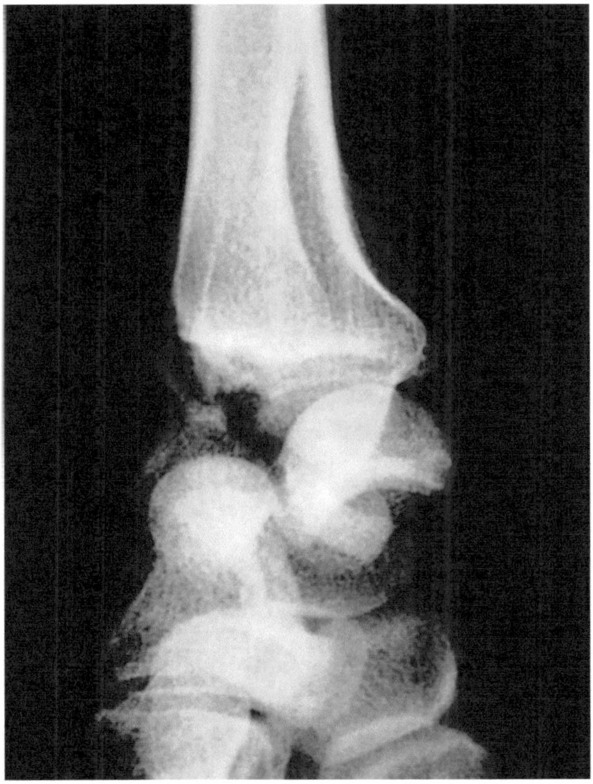

Fig. 29.4 Lateral wrist X-ray of a trans-scaphoid perilunate fracture-dislocation. Note the unchanged location of the lunate bone in relation to the articular surface of the distal radius, and the dorsal location of the capitate bone in relation to the lunate

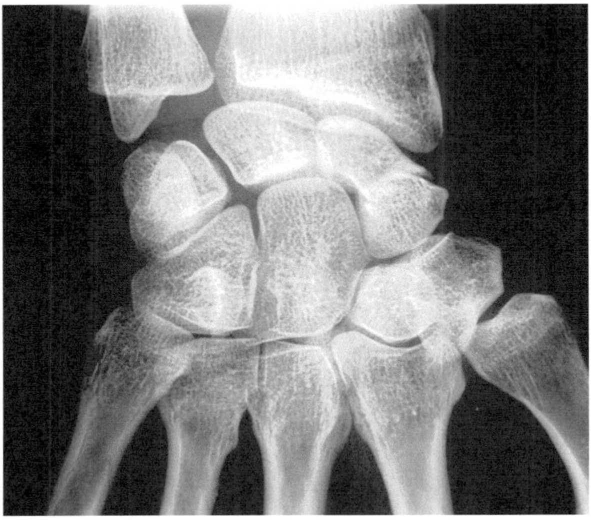

Fig. 29.5 PA wrist radiograph of a scaphoid fracture

  - If doubt persists: *ask for MRI.*
2. **Other carpal bones fractures**: the clinical presentation is unspecific and the fracture is commonly seen on a random radiographic evaluation (incidental finding). CT scan is very helpful in demonstrating the fracture pattern:
   (a) ***Lunate fracture***: risk of necrosis if displaced fracture.
   (b) ***Triquetrum fracture*** (Figs. 29.6, 29.7, and 29.8): usually associated with intra-carpal ligamentous injuries.
   (c) ***Capitate fracture***: can be associated to perilunate dislocation.
   (d) ***Trapezium fracture***: rare injury.
   (e) ***Hamate fracture***: fracture of the hook of the hamate is a well-known injury in golfers and racket players (tennis, badminton, etc.).
3. **Scapholunate dissociation**
   (a) The clinical presentation encompasses,
      - dorsal wrist pain, clicking, and sensation of instability,
      - Tenderness on palpation of the dorsal wrist aspect (at the scapholunate space).
   (b) The radiographic diagnosis may be subtle in the early phase.
      - PA view showing,
        – *A widening* of the scapholunate space >3 mm (Fig. 29.9),
        – *The ring sign* (resulting from the spontaneous horizontal / flexion position of the scaphoid),

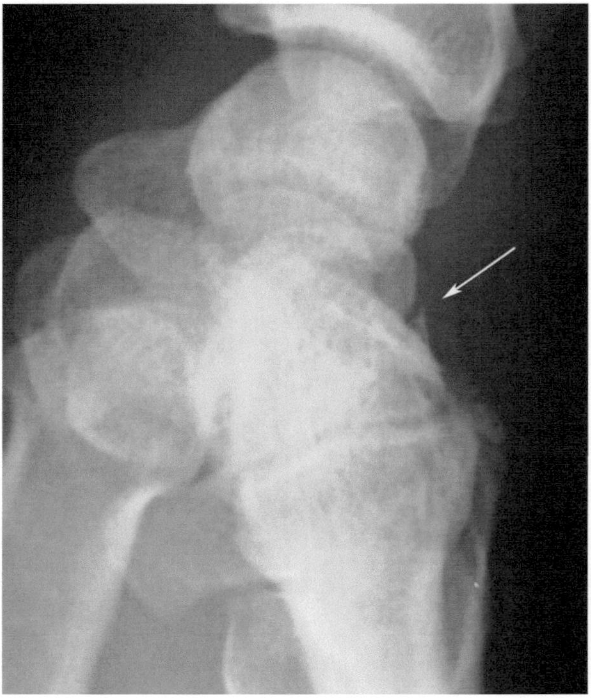

Fig. 29.6 Lateral wrist radiograph of a triquetral bone fracture

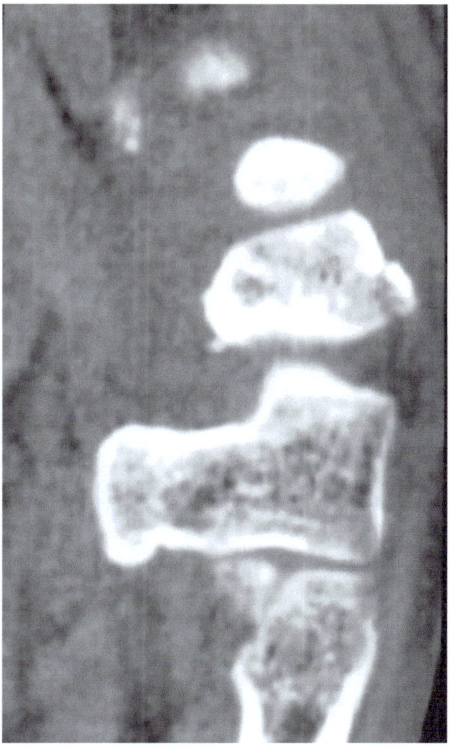

Fig. 29.7 Sagittal CT scan cut showing the same triquetral bone fracture as shown in Fig. 29.6

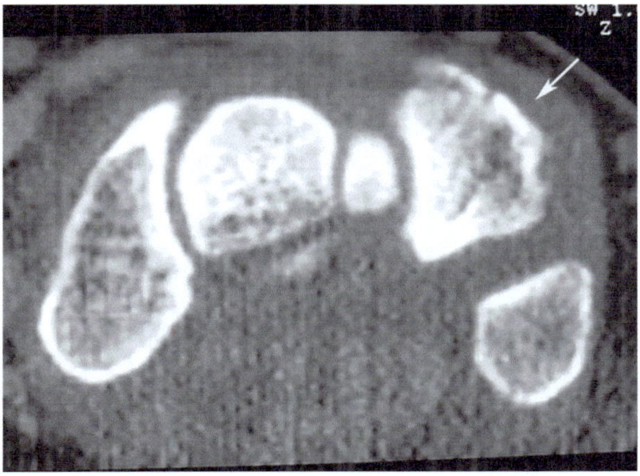

Fig. 29.8 Axial CT scan cut showing the same triquetral bone fracture as shown in Fig. 29.6

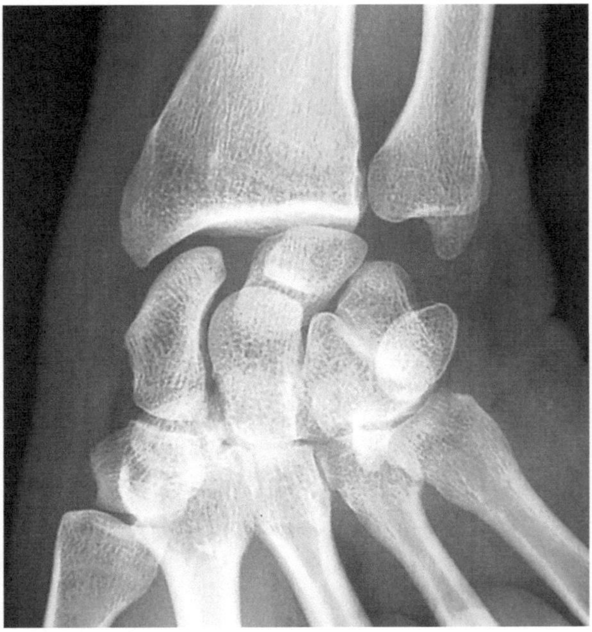

Fig. 29.9 PA wrist radiograph of a scapholunate dissociation. Note the widening of the space between the scaphoid and the lunate

  - An appearance of shortened scaphoid.
- Lateral view (Fig. 29.10) showing:
  - *An increased scapholunate angle* > 70°, secondary to the spontaneous horizontal positioning (flexion) of the scaphoid associated with a dorsal tilt of the lunate (extension),
  - An image of DISI deformity (with dorsal tilt of the lunate).

4. **Wrist sprain**
   (a) *Is an exceptional injury.*
   (b) "Wrist sprain" is commonly a preliminary diagnosis in the ER if no other diagnosis could be made.
   (c) Final diagnosis of "wrist sprain" is only made at a later stage after all previous injuries have been ruled out.

29.2.3 Management

1. **Carpal dislocations**
   (a) Relocation is recommended in emergency because of neurovascular threats.
   (b) Treatment should be done by an orthopedic or hand surgeon under anesthesia:
   - The reduction maneuver involves a continuous axial traction for 10–15 min (5–7 kg using finger traps is helpful).
   - Post-reduction cast immobilization while waiting for the final open treatment (ligament repair and fixation).

Fig. 29.10 Lateral wrist radiograph of the same patient as shown in Fig. 29.9. Note the spontaneous horizontalization of the scaphoid with the dorsal tilt of the lunate (DISI)

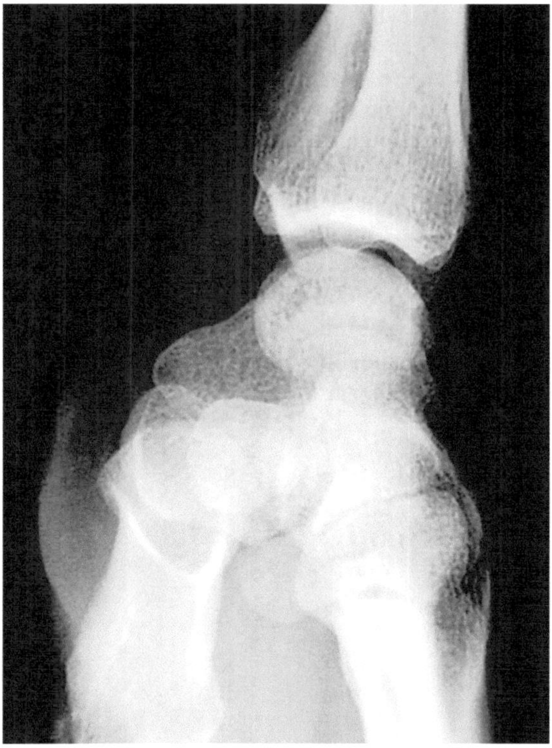

- Final surgical repair.
  - Fixation of the associated fractures (scaphoid, radial styloid, capitate, etc.).
  - Scapholunate ligament repair (with common use of anchor suture) associated to protective pinning,
  - Lunotriquetral ligament repair associated to protective pinning.

2. **Scaphoid fractures**
   (a) *For stable non-displaced fractures,* which correspond to the large majority of cases, an orthopedic closed treatment is indicated.
   - A below elbow cast, including the metacarpo-phalangeal joint of the thumb ("thumb spica"), is applied in position of mild flexion and radial inclination of the wrist for 3 months.
   - Radiographic control is made at the end of immobilization with additional 1 month into cast if no signs of complete healing are seen.

   (b) *For displaced fractures*: ask for a specialized orthopedic consultation for surgical treatment planning.
3. **Other carpal bones fractures**
   (a) The majority are treated non-operatively, except for the displaced fractures and the fractures that are associated with carpal dislocation: a cast

immobilization is applied for 6–8 weeks without need for radiographic controls into cast (no risk of secondary displacement).
   (b) Fractures of the hook of the hamate bone commonly progress to non-union and commonly require secondary excision.

4. **Scapholunate dissociation**
   (a) *Red Flag*: Do not miss it!
   (b) Treatment is usually operative: open reduction of the dissociation with scapholunate ligament repair (anchor suture) and protective pinning.
5. **Wrist sprain**
   (a) Diagnosis of "wrist sprain" is considered only if all other possible injuries have been ruled out.
   (b) A wrist immobilization is performed for 3 weeks.
   (c) Reassessment and specialized consultation are required if pain persists after cast removal.

Hand Injuries

30

30.1 Fractures

30.1.1 Fractures of the First Ray (Thumb)

30.1.1.1 Fractures of the First Metacarpal

1. ***Patho-anatomy*** (Fig. 30.1)

   The first Metacarpal articulates with the trapezium and has a wide range of motion.

   First metacarpal fractures are divided into,

   (a) Diaphyseal fractures: the fracture pattern is usually transverse, short oblique, or long oblique,

   (b) Fractures of the base: which are either extra-or intra-articular.

   - Extra-articular fractures: the fracture line is commonly transverse and leads to a significant displacement in adduction (Fig. 30.2).
   - Intra-articular fractures. They are categorized into,
     - *Bennett fracture* (partial articular): it consists of a fracture dislocation of the base of the first metacarpal, with a basal volar ulnar fragment of variable size that remains attached to the base of the second metacarpal (Fig. 30.3).
     - *Rolando fracture* (complete articular): with a "T" or "Y" shape articular fracture pattern of the base of the first metacarpal (Fig. 30.4).
     - Fragmentary (comminuted) fractures.

2. ***Clinical presentation***: pain and functional disability of the thumb.
3. ***Radiographic assessment***: AP, lateral, and oblique views of the base of the thumb.
4. ***Treatment***

   (a) For non-displaced fractures: A non-operative treatment is applied, using a "thumb spica" cast for 4–6 weeks. It may be done by the ER physician, before transferring the patient for follow-up in the orthopedic (or hand surgery) OPD.

D. Saragaglia, A. Hassan Chamseddine, *Traumatology for the Emergency Doctor*, https://doi.org/10.1007/978-3-031-63196-2_30

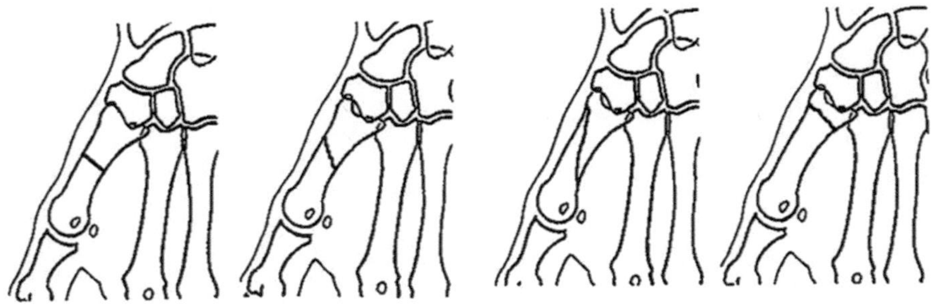

Fig. 30.1 Illustration of the different types of fractures of the first metacarpal bone

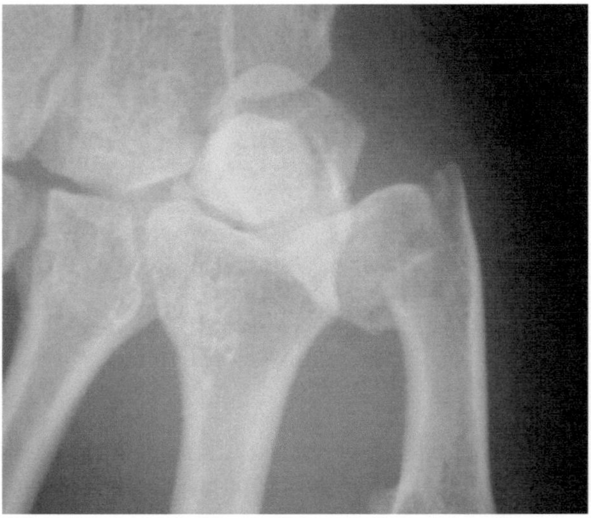

Fig. 30.2 Radiograph of the base of the thumb showing an extra-articular fracture of the base of the first metacarpal bone. Note the spontaneous closure of the first space induced by the displacement of the first metacarpal in adduction

(b) For displaced fractures: A surgical treatment is applied, using one of the following methods:
   - Closed reduction with a percutaneous inter-metacarpal pinning (M1-M2) for Bennett fractures (commonly indicated in the presence of small basal fragment),
   - Open reduction with internal fixation,
     - Screw fixation for Bennett fracture (commonly indicated in the presence of large basal fragment),
     - Plate and screws fixation for Rolando fracture and/or diaphyseal fractures.

5. ***Complication***: the most redoubtable complication is the closure or contracture of the first space because of an irreducible or fixed adduction of the first metacarpal secondary to fracture malunion.

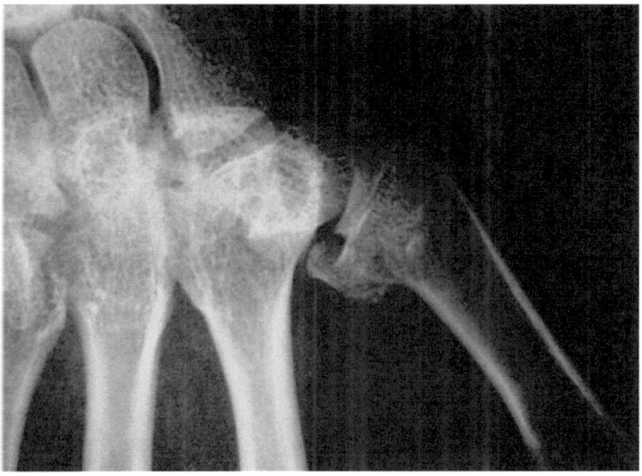

Fig. 30.3 Radiograph of the base of the thumb showing a Bennett fracture

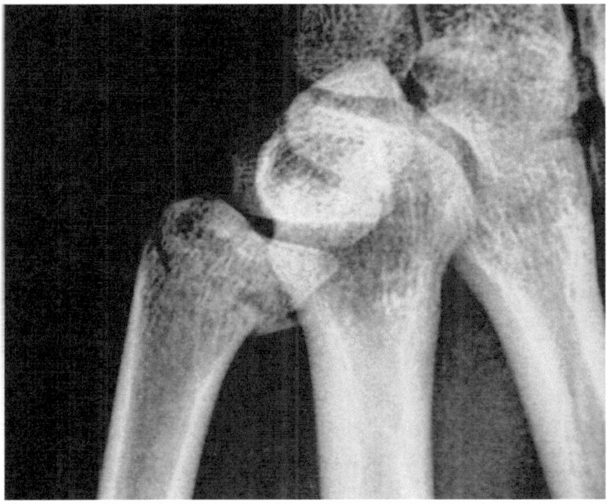

Fig. 30.4 Radiograph of the base of the thumb showing a Rolando fracture

30.1.1.2 Fractures of the First Phalanx (P1) of the Thumb

1. They are categorized into,
   (a) Diaphyseal fractures (transverse, short oblique, or long oblique),
   (b) Articular fractures of the base of P1 with,
      - dorsal fragment (inducing volar metacarpophalangeal subluxation),
      - volar fragment (inducing dorsal metacarpophalangeal subluxation).
   (c) Fractures of the head of P1 with usually "L" or "T" shape pattern resulting in a "uni" or "bicondylar" fracture, respectively.
2. Treatment
   (a) A non-operative treatment is commonly indicated for the closed extra-articular fractures that are initially non-displaced or stable after a closed

reduction, performed under digital nerve bloc: it consists of applying a thumb spica cast including the first phalanx for 1 month.
(b) An operative treatment is indicated for the all other types of fractures.
(c) In all cases, the patient should be transferred to the care of a specialized orthopedic or hand surgery team.

30.1.1.3 Fractures of the Second Phalanx (P2) of the Thumb

- They are categorized into,
  - Fractures of the base, which may be intra-or extra-articular.
  - Fractures of the tuft: simple vs. comminuted, and closed vs. open.
- Treatment
  - Evacuation of the subungual hematoma (when it exists), by opening a small window into the nail (Fig. 30.5).
  - Reconstruction-fixation of the nail when it is avulsed (Fig. 30.5).
  - Tubular dressing of the distal phalanx when there is a comminuted fracture of the tuft.
  - Axial pinning for realignment of a displaced fracture of the base of P2 (when it exists).
  - The operative treatment should be done by a specialized orthopedic or hand surgeon.

30.1.2 Fractures of the Lateral Fingers (Second to Fifth Finger)

30.1.2.1 Fractures of the Lateral Metacarpals (M2 to M5)

1. ***Patho-Anatomy***

   The lateral metacarpals have different range of motion: the second and third are fixed, while the fourth is semi-mobile and the fifth is mobile.

   Fractures of the lateral metacarpals may affect the base, the shaft, the neck, or the head of the metacarpal.

   (a) *Fractures of the base*: articular fractures of the base of the fifth metacarpal correspond to an equivalent of Bennett fracture (of the first metacarpal) and should be treated accordingly (although with less functional consequences).
   (b) Fractures of the shaft (Fig. 30.6a): the fracture pattern may be transverse, short oblique, long oblique, wedge, or fragmentary. The fracture is

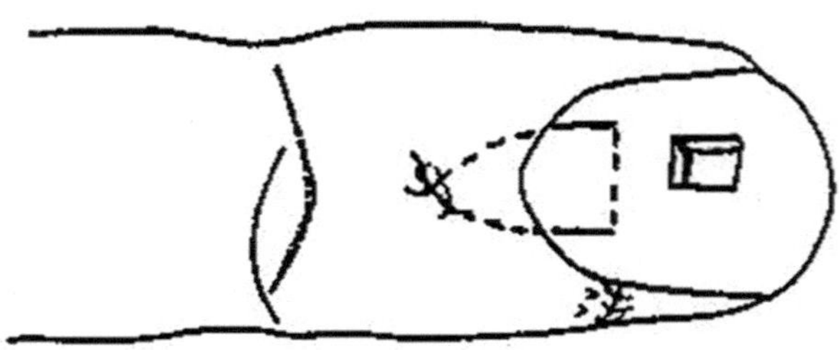

Fig. 30.5 Illustration of a subungual hematoma evacuation (window in the nail) with a suture-fixation of the base of the nail

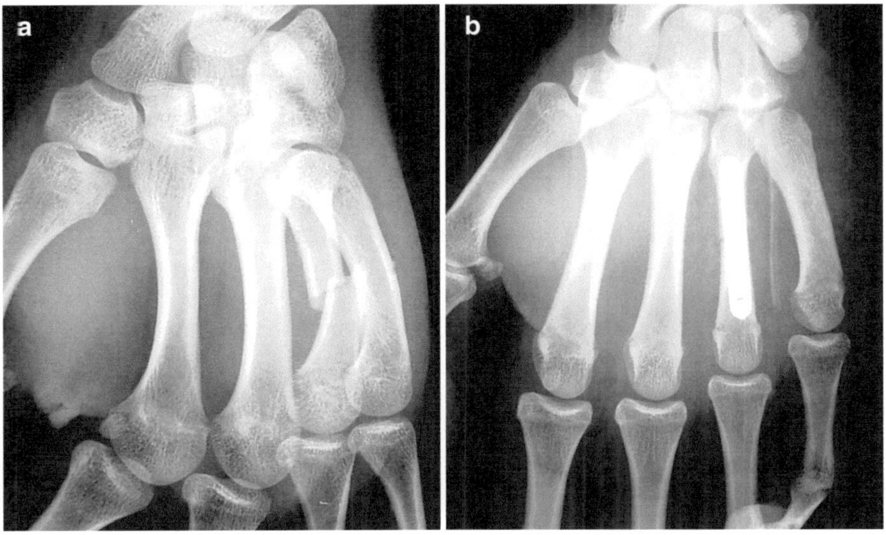

Fig. 30.6 (**a**) Hand X-ray showing a displaced transverse fracture of the shaft of the fourth metacarpal bone. (**b**) Post-operative hand radiograph of the same patient as shown in fig. 30.6a showing internal fixation with mini-plate and screws

commonly displaced with variable association of dorsal angulation, shortening, and rotation.

(c) *Fractures of the neck*: the most common is the fracture of the neck of the fifth metacarpal. The measurement of the angulation of the fracture site is important for the therapeutic decision. Less angulation is accepted for the less mobile metacarpals (20° for the second, third, and 4th) than for the fifth metacarpal (30–40°).

(d) *Fractures of the head*: they are commonly secondary to a crush injury and are therefore often comminuted and associated with soft tissue damage (open fracture).

2. ***Radiographic assessment:*** Multiple views are required for a better visualization of the fractured metacarpal (elimination of radiographic image of superposition) and the fracture pattern.
3. ***Treatment***

(a) For non-displaced fractures (no excessive angulation, no shortening, no malrotation),

- A non-operative closed treatment is applied, using a rigid metacarpal protective splint (or brace) and temporary syndactylization with the adjacent fingers, to promote early motion of the metacarpophalangeal and interphalangeal joints.
- The duration of the protective splinting is 4–6 weeks.

(b) For displaced fractures with malrotation, excessive angulation, and shortening (Fig. 30.6b), a specialized surgical consultation is required for surgical

planning and management (closed reduction with percutaneous pinning, open reduction with internal fixation, special brace, etc.).
4. The ER physician should be able to initially manage non-displaced metacarpal fractures with close follow-up in cooperation with a competent rehabilitation team (early restoration of the range of motion, and follow-up for early detection of any secondary displacements).

30.1.2.2 Phalanx Fractures of the Lateral Fingers (Second to Fifth Finger)

1. ***Patho-Anatomy***

   The fracture may affect the base, the shaft, or the head of the proximal (P1), middle (P2), or distal (P3) phalanx.
2. *P3 fractures*
   (a) They are the most common and are often associated with soft tissue injury.
   (b) They are categorized into,
   - Comminuted fractures with minimal or no displacement (as the fracture is well contained by the finger pad and the nail),
   - Fractures of the base that may either involve a volar fracture-avulsion of the insertion of the flexor digitorum profundus tendon (*Jersey finger*) or a dorsal fracture-avulsion of the insertion of the extensor tendon (*mallet finger*).

   (c) *P2 fractures* (Fig. 30.7)
   - The displacement of the proximal fractures is controlled by the insertions of the flexor digitorum superficialis and the extensor tendon.
   - Only distal fractures may be unstable and displaced.

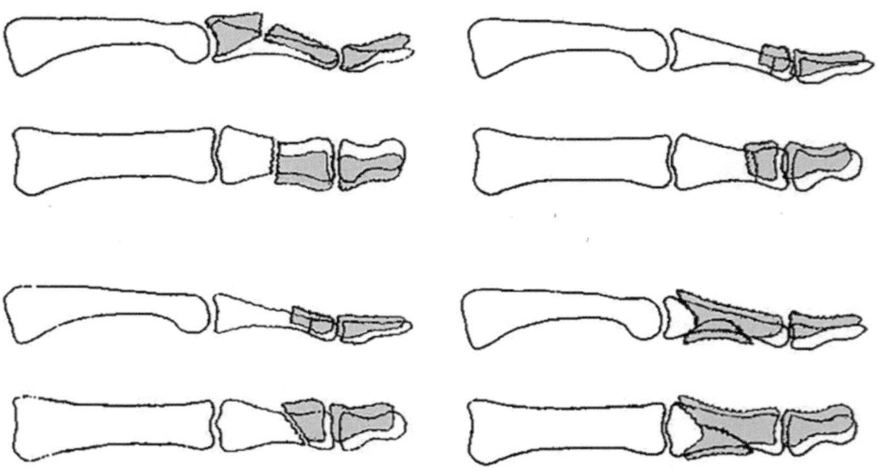

Fig. 30.7 Illustrations of the different types of fractures of P2 (of the lateral fingers) with their potential displacements

   (d) *P1 fractures* are more often displaced than P2 and P3 fractures (because of the absence of large tendinous insertions).
3. ***Treatment***
   (a) P3 fractures and non-displaced P2 and P1 fractures can be initially managed by the ER physician:
      - For P3 fractures: an evacuation of the subungual hematoma is performed.
      - For P2 and P1 non-displaced fractures: a syndactylization is performed, and is followed by early range of motion.
4. Stiffness is a common complication of phalangeal fractures whether treated surgically or not.
5. Ask for a specialized orthopedic or hand surgery consultation, for further management and follow-up.

30.2 Sprains and Dislocations

30.2.1 Sprain of the Metacarpophalangeal Joint (MPJ) of the Thumb

The ulnar collateral ligament (UCL) is ten times more commonly injured than the radial collateral ligament (RCL). A direct trauma to the extremity of the thumb in abducted position may result in UCL injury.

1. **Imaging**
   (a) ***Radiographic assessment*** (AP and lateral views of the MPJ).
      - It should be done before any clinical testing (because of the risk of inducing a displacement of an initially undisplaced fracture).
      - It looks for the presence of,
        - P1 subluxation,
        - Fracture-avulsion of the base of P1 (equivalent to a ligamentous injury of the MPJ).
   (b) ***Ultrasound***
      - May help in demonstrating the rupture of the ligament,
      - Is operator-dependent.
   (c) ***MRI***
      - valuable in doubtful cases,
      - 100% specific and sensitive.
2. **Clinical assessment**
   (a) Inspection: presence of hematoma / ecchymosis at the dorsal aspect of the MPJ is suggestive of capsulo-ligamentous rupture.
   (b) Palpation
      - Tenderness of the ulnar or radial aspect of the MPJ (according to the injured ligament).

  - Possible palpation of the Stener lesion (small mass representing the tip of the avulsed UCL retracted proximally and lying superficial to the adductor aponeurosis of the thumb).

(c) Testing
  - Is only performed after the radiographic assessment and if the radiographs are normal (absence of fracture or bony avulsion).
  - It examines the presence of laxity (defined by the absence of an "end point" during the stress test).
  - It may be done with local anesthesia for pain relief and elimination of the patient's resistance and guarding.
  - It involves stress in extension position and at 30° flexion of the MPJ.
  - It is performed for the UCL and the RCL.
    - UCL testing: is performed with application of a radial stress.

      A laxity at 30° flexion of the MPJ indicates an injury of the proper UCL,

      A laxity in extension of the MPJ indicates an injury of the accessory UCL +/− the volar plate.
    - RCL testing: is performed with application of an ulnar stress.

(d) Grade of injury
  - Grade 1: is a simple benign sprain, which is manifested as pain without laxity during the testing.
  - Grade 2: is manifested as a moderate laxity of a few degrees, with presence of an early end point during the testing.
  - Grade 3: is manifested as a significant laxity, with virtually no end point, and 30–40° of joint line opening during the testing.

3. **Treatment**

(a) Methods
  - Functional treatment. It consists of a protected active range of motion, with strapping of the MPJ for 3 weeks.
  - Orthopedic treatment. It consists of a rigid cast for 4 weeks (the hand cast includes the MPJ and the first phalanx of the thumb).
  - Surgical treatment. It depends on the patho-anatomy of the injury and may consist of one of the following: a direct suture of a mid-substance rupture of the ligament, a trans-osseous fixation of the ligament, or a fixation of a bony avulsion of the ligament (using a screw or a K-wire). The surgical repair is followed by 4 weeks of rigid cast immobilization.
  - A rehabilitation program is prescribed after the cast removal to restore the range of motion and the function of the thumb.

(b) Indications

The ER physician should be able to make the diagnosis and to identify the degree of severity of the injury. The treatment depends on the degree of severity of the sprain:

- Grade 1 injury: functional treatment,
- Grade 2 injury: orthopedic treatment,
- Grade 3 injury: surgical treatment.

30.2.2 Dislocation of the Metacarpophalangeal Joint (MPJ) of the Thumb (Fig. 30.8)

1. The volar dislocation is rare.
2. The most common type is the ***dorsal dislocation*** (Fig. 30.9).
   (a) The diagnosis is often clinically evident.
   (b) Radiographs of the thumb are made to confirm the diagnosis and to rule out any associated fractures.
   (c) Treatment.
      ER physician should be able to make the diagnosis and start the treatment.
      - Closed reduction under local anesthesia.
         – Reduction maneuver: direct push applied to the dorsal aspect of the base of the first phalanx (P1) to slide it over the dorsal aspect of the metacarpal neck and head.
         – The goal of the maneuver is to force the phalanx to cross the dorsal aspect of the MPJ by pushing the sesamoid bones from the dorsal aspect of metacarpal neck to their anatomic location at the volar aspect of the MPJ.
         – *Red Flag:* traction maneuver is dangerous and is prohibited, as it may induce an incarceration (entrapment) of the sesamoid bones inside the

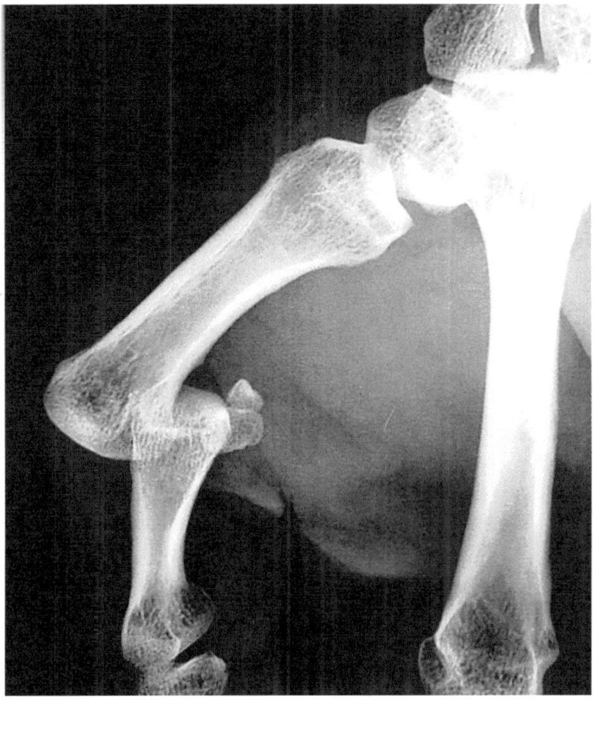

Fig. 30.8 Radiographic presentation of a volar dislocation of the MPJ of the thumb

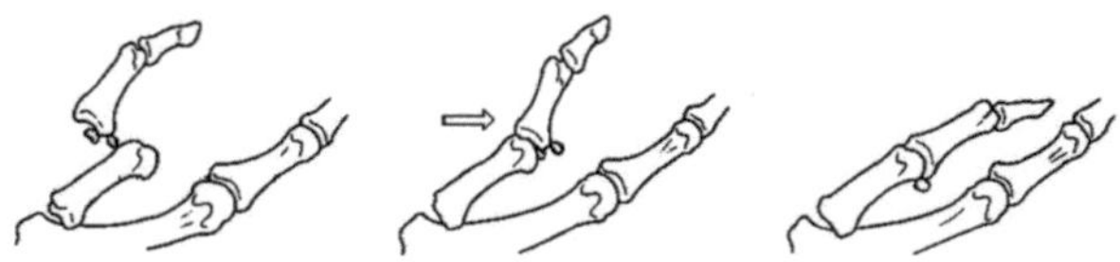

Fig. 30.9 Illustration of a dorsal dislocation of the MPJ of the thumb and its corresponding maneuver for closed reduction

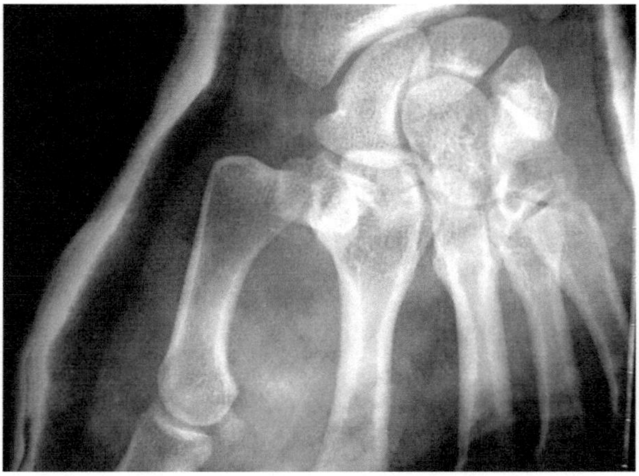

Fig. 30.10 Radiographic evidence of a trapezio-metacarpal dislocation immobilized in a cast: the injury was initially overlooked during the patient's first visit to the ER where the cast was applied for an unrelated injury

MPJ, resulting in irreducible dislocation (which requires a surgical reduction).

- After reduction,
  - A testing of the collateral ligaments of the MPJ is performed (UCL and LCL).
  - A residual post-reduction laxity (ulnar or radial) should be treated as detailed above.

30.2.3 Thumb Carpometacarpal (CMC) or Trapezio-Metacarpal Dislocation

- The trapezio-metacarpal joint (or carpometacarpal CMC) is a saddle-type joint with a large range of motion.
- The traumatic dislocation of CMC joint is rare (1% of hand injuries).
- The mechanism of injury is often an axial force applied to the thumb in a flexion-abduction position.
- The severity of the injury ranges from ***the sprain to the dislocation*** in high-energy trauma (Fig. 30.10).
- The radiographic assessment confirms the diagnosis of dislocation (AP, lateral, and oblique views of the base of the thumb).
- Treatment.

- For CMC sprains: the ER physician should be able to make the diagnosis and to initiate the treatment, using a below elbow cast that includes the P1 of the thumb (for 4 weeks).
- For CMC dislocations: the treatment is surgical and should be performed by a specialized hand surgery team. It consists of reduction, repair, and stabilization of the CMC dislocation.

30.2.4 Sprain and Dislocation of the Long Rays (Second to Fifth)

30.2.4.1 Carpometacarpal (CMC) Dislocation

- The dislocation may involve,
  - Only one ray: the fifth ray is the most common site,
  - 2 or 3 rays together (Fig. 30.11),
  - All rays together.
- The clinical presentation is suggestive of the injury when the patient is seen early after the accident,
  - Pain,
  - Deformity: appearance of "stair-step" of the dorsal aspect of the hand.
- Radiographic assessment
  - The AP, lateral, and oblique views confirm the diagnosis of dislocation and show the number of dislocated rays.
  - CT scan with 2-D and 3-D reconstruction is very helpful in the doubtful cases.

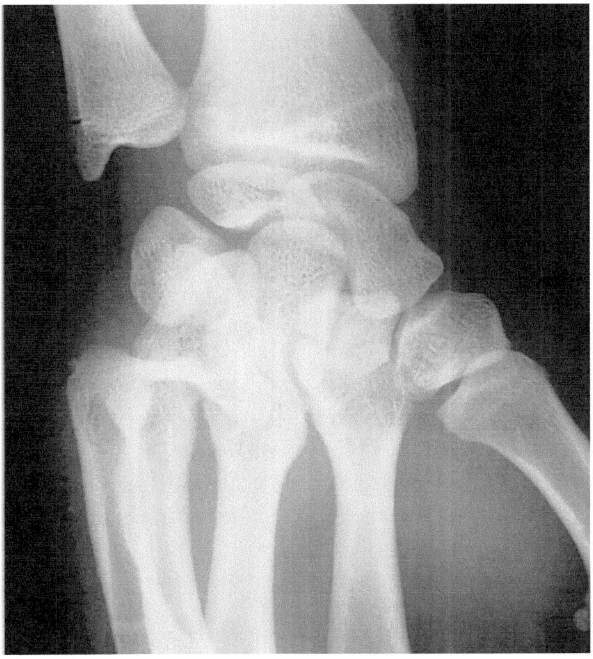

Fig. 30.11 Radiographic presentation of a carpometacarpal dislocation of the third, fourth, and fifth rays of the hand

- Treatment: transfer to the care of hand surgery team is requested for management (a surgical fixation is often needed after a closed or an open reduction).

30.2.4.2 Metacarpophalangeal Joint (MPJ) Sprain and Dislocation

- The MPJ injuries are rare.
- The sprain of the MPJ involves injury of the collateral ligaments (radial or ulnar) with variable degrees of severity.
- The dislocation of the MPJ is often dorsal (hyperextension mechanism).
- The dislocation may be simple or complex.
  - Simple dislocation is an incomplete dislocation (or subluxation) in which the base of P1 remains in partial contact with the head of the corresponding metacarpal. There is no soft tissue incarceration or entrapment into the MPJ.
  - Complex dislocation is a complete dislocation with interposition of the volar plate (with or without the sesamoid bones) into the MPJ. The metacarpal head is usually entrapped into a tendino-ligamentous buttonhole and caught into a volar position, with the index finger being the most common site. The injury is commonly irreducible by external maneuvers.
- Radiographic assessment. The AP, lateral, and oblique views confirm the diagnosis of dislocation and allow to disclose any associated lesions.
- Treatment
  - Sprains are treated with temporary syndactylization and early rehabilitation. A residual pain may persist for several months.
  - Dislocations of MPJ are transferred to the care of the hand surgery team.

30.2.4.3 Inter-Phalangeal Joint (IPJ) Sprain and Dislocation

1. The injuries of the proximal inter-phalangeal joint (PIPJ) are the most common hand injuries.
2. They often occur in the context of balloon sports (volley ball, basket ball, hand ball).
3. Clinical presentation includes,
   (a) Finger swelling and pain,
   (b) Possible hematoma and ecchymosis.
   (c) Type of injuries.
      - Simple sprains involve a benign capsulo-ligamentous injury of the PIPJ,
      - Severe sprains involve a capsulo-ligamentous rupture of the PIPJ, which often results in,
        - Pain and ecchymosis,
        - Laxity on physical examination (radio-ulnar and/or dorso-volar laxity).
      - Dislocation of the PIPJ (most commonly dorsal).
4. Radiographs of the finger in two orthogonal views are used to disclose any associated bony injuries, such as,
   (a) fracture-avulsion of the volar plate of the PIPJ (a source of secondary deficit of extension),
   (b) articular fracture of the PIPJ.

Fig. 30.12 Photo of a temporary syndactylization (fourth and fifth fingers)

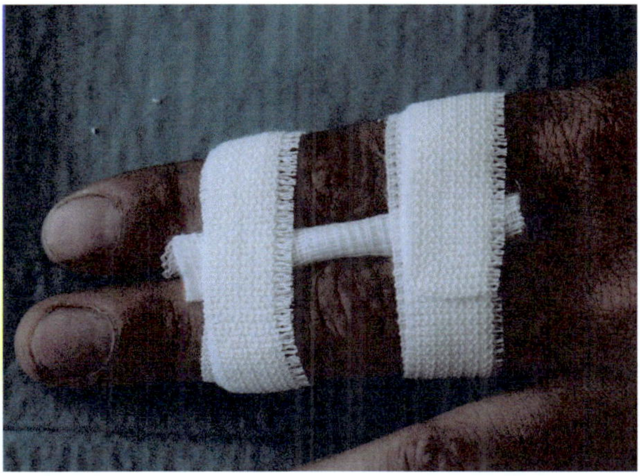

5. Treatment
   (a) Functional treatment using temporary syndactylization and early restoration of the range of motion (Fig. 30.12) under the supervision of a physiotherapist. Residual swelling and pain are common for several weeks after treatment.
   (b) Surgical treatment using open reduction and internal fixation.
   (c) Indications for treatment are as follows:
      - Surgical treatment is indicated for an associated fracture with a displaced or large fragment,
      - Functional treatment is indicated for the other cases.

The ER physician should be able to reduce the PIPJ dislocation under digital bloc anesthesia and initiate treatment (syndactylization).

30.3 Tendon Injuries

30.3.1 Extensor Tendon Injuries

Injuries to the extensor tendon can occur as a result of either a laceration (cut) or closed trauma.

30.3.1.1 Anatomy Review

1. The extensor tendons of the fingers are thin and flat tendons running at the dorsal aspect of the wrist, hand, and fingers (Fig. 30.13). They are not enclosed in a synovial sheet.
2. At the wrist, the extensor tendons run under the extensor retinaculum and are positioned into six osteo-fibrous compartments made by the retinaculum, the bones of the forearm, and the fibrous septa joining the retinaculum to the bones.

Fig. 30.13 Illustration of extensor mechanism anatomy of the fingers

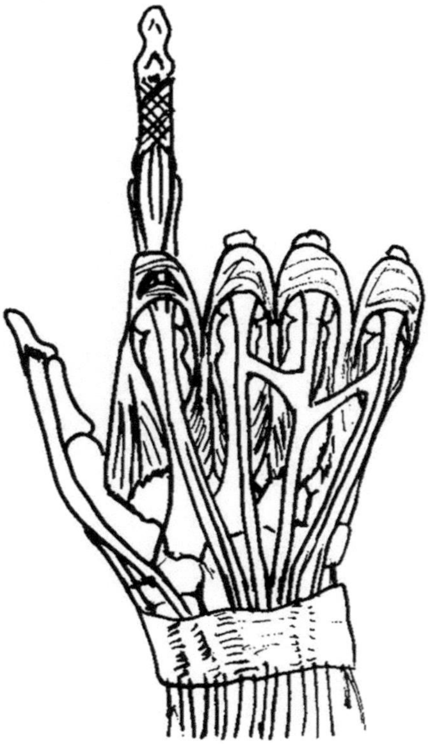

The extensor retinaculum prevents bowstring of the tendons at the dorsal aspect of the wrist.

3. At the dorsum of the metacarpophalangeal joint (MPJ),
   (a) The extensor digitorum is a relatively large tendon stabilized by the sagittal band,
   (b) The extensor digitorum tendon of the second and fifth fingers is reinforced by the confluence of the extensor indicis tendon and the extensor digiti minimi tendon respectively.
4. At the level of P1,
   (a) The extensor digitorum receives insertion of the lumbricals and the interossei muscles.
   (b) The tendon then divides into three slips or parts: one central and two lateral (ulnar and radial).
      - The central slip bridges over the proximal inter-phalangeal joint (PIPJ), and then inserts onto the dorsal aspect of the base of P2,
      - The lateral slips run laterally (ulnar and radial) over the dorsal aspect of P1, PIPJ, and P2 and merge together proximal to the distal inter-phalangeal joint (DIPJ) to form one dorsal tendon which inserts onto the dorsal aspect of the base of P3.

30.3.1.2 Clinical Presentation

1. A complete deficit of finger extension indicates a complete interruption or discontinuity of the extensor mechanism.
2. A partial extension deficit may coexist with a quasi-complete interruption of the tendon.
3. In the case of laceration, a surgical exploration of the wound is warranted to confirm and treat the injury, along with the associated lesions (e.g., digital nerve).
4. The site or the level of the extensor injury can be specified or described according to eight zones (Z) for the long fingers and six zones for the thumb (T) (Fig. 30.14).
   (a) *Long fingers*: Z1 over DIPJ; Z2 over P2; Z3 over PIPJ; Z4 over P1; Z5 over MPJ; Z6 over metacarpal bone; Z7 at the wrist; and Z8 at the distal forearm.
   (b) *Thumb*: T1 over the IPJ; T2 over P1; T3 over MPJ; T4 over metacarpal bone; T5 over the CMC joint; T6 over the wrist.
5. Particular sites of injury
   (a) *Mallet finger*
      - Clinical presentation: deficit of extension of the DIPJ (P3 over P2).

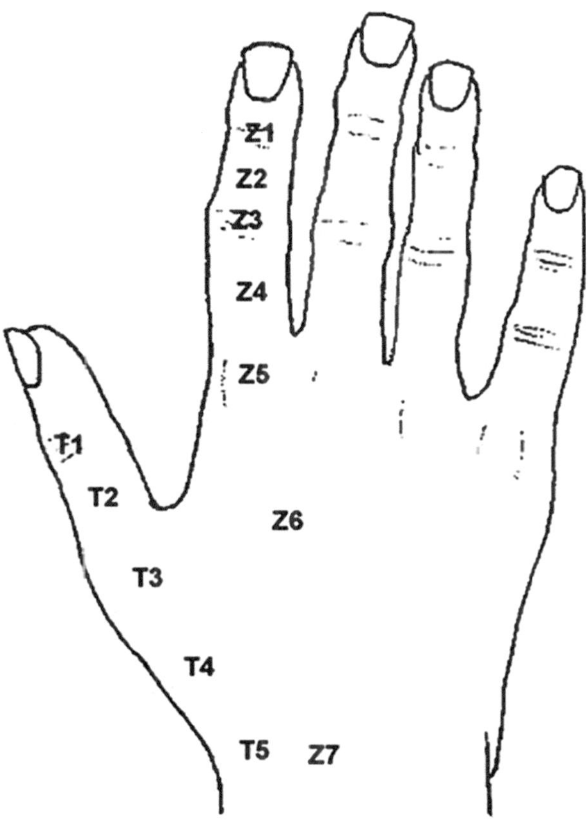

Fig. 30.14 Illustration of the extensor zones

  - The injury can be either a pure rupture or a fracture-avulsion of the terminal part of the extensor mechanism at the base of P3.

(b) *Boutonniere deformity*
  - The central slip of the extensor mechanism is disrupted at the level of the PIPJ,
  - The head of P1 protrudes dorsally through a "buttonhole" between the two lateral slips.
  - The finger is deformed, with flexion of the PIPJ and extension of the DIPJ.

6. Radiographs of the finger are usually requested for closed injuries to rule out a potential bony fragment avulsion.

30.3.1.3 Treatment

- *The surgical repair* is the only treatment.
  - It is indicated for the extensor injuries secondary to lacerations.
  - It is performed using a central Kessler suture (4/0) associated with a peripheral continuous running suture (6/0).
  - A special brace is applied after the surgical repair, for suture protection (6 weeks).
  - Early rehabilitation is highly recommended under the supervision of a physiotherapist to prevent any deficit of the ROM, secondary to local adhesions.
- *Mallet finger*
  - Closed mallet finger is treated with a special hyperextension splint of the DIPJ for 8 weeks (Fig. 30.15).
  - Open and displaced bony avulsion of the extensor at the base of P3: surgical repair is recommended.
- *Boutonniere deformity*: a specialized hand surgery consultation is required.

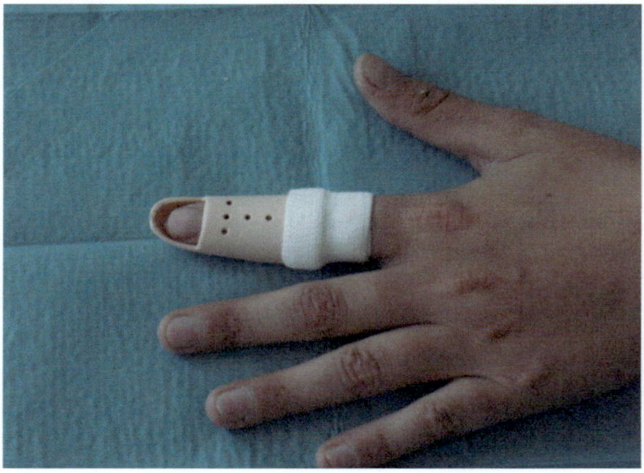

Fig. 30.15 Photo of a hyperextension splint of the DIPJ for the treatment of mallet finger

The ER physician should be able to identify the zone of the injury and to perform an exploration of the wound under local anesthesia to determine whether the extensor disruption is complete or not.

30.3.2 Flexor Tendon Injuries

Flexor tendon injuries can be secondary to lacerations or trauma. It may affect one or both tendons of each finger (flexor digitorum superficialis and flexor digitorum profundus).

30.3.2.1 Anatomy Review

- Each finger has two flexor tendons: the flexor digitorum profundus (FDP) and the flexor digitorum superficialis (FDS).
- They are surrounded by a synovial sheet and stabilized into the digital canal by a pulley system.

30.3.2.2 Clinical Presentation

- When a patient presents with a laceration of the palmar aspect of the hand, a *surgical exploration is warranted.*
- An incomplete flexor interruption can progress into a complete interruption if it was initially undiagnosed.
- *Testing of the FDS of the affected finger.*
  - The examiner first manually blocks the adjacent fingers in extension, and then asks the patient to perform an active flexion of the PIPJ of the affected finger. The presence of active flexion of P2 over P1 in the affected finger corresponds to the presence of continuity of the FDS. The absence of active flexion of P2 over P1 means a disruption of the FDS.
- *Testing of the FDP of the affected finger.*
  - The examiner first manually blocks the PIPJ of the affected finger by holding P2, and then asks the patient to perform an active flexion of the DIPJ. The presence of active flexion of P3 over P2 corresponds to the presence of continuity of the FDP. The absence of active flexion means a disruption of the FDP of the affected finger.
- *The site or the level of the flexor injury* may be specified or described according to five zones (Fig. 30.16):
  - Z1 is distal to the FDS insertion (DIPJ and P3),
  - Z2 is the digital canal (MPJ, P1, PIPJ, and P2),
  - Z3 is the palm of the hand (from the MPJ to the distal border of the transverse carpal ligament),
  - Z4 is the carpal tunnel,
  - Z5 is proximal to the carpal tunnel (wrist and forearm).
- A particular type of injury corresponds to the so-called *Jersey finger.*
  - It is a closed traumatic distal avulsion of the FDP (from the base of P3).

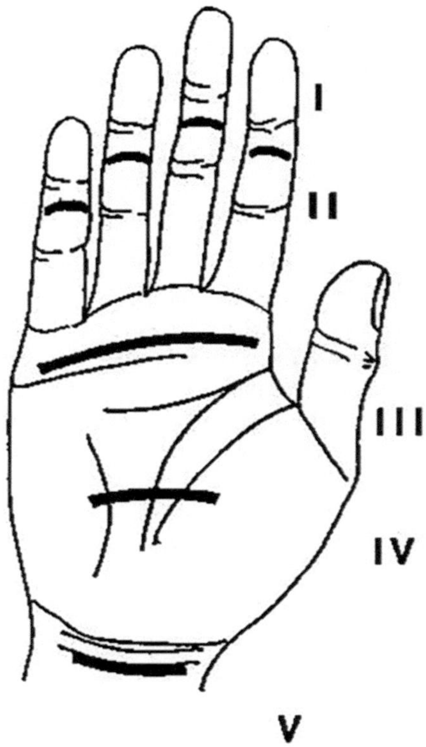

Fig. 30.16 Illustration of the flexor zones

- It is secondary to a forced flexion of the DIPJ against resistance (radiographs are required to disclose any possible bony avulsion of the FDP).
- The proximal stump of the FDP is usually retracted proximally.
- The treatment is surgical.

30.3.2.3 Treatment

- The treatment of flexor tendon injuries is surgical.
- The surgical exploration should always look for any associated lesions, e.g., collateral neuro-vascular bundles of the digit.
- It should be done by a specialist in hand surgery. It is a technically demanding procedure, as it encompasses a risk of adhesions which often results in a limited ROM and secondary stiffness of the finger.

30.4 In Conclusion

- **Any laceration located over the trajectory of a tendon, a neuro-vascular bundle, or a joint should be surgically investigated, especially if its clinical presentation or manifestation is ambiguous.**

- **In the hand, the joints of the fingers are superficial (especially at the dorsal aspect), and there are multiple crossroads for numerous tendons and neurovascular bundles: surgical debridement and exploration of any hand laceration is a must.**
- **Any wound of the hand with ambiguous clinical presentation should be washed, sutured, and dressed while waiting for the final surgical treatment by a specialist in hand surgery.**

Part III

Traumatic Injuries of the Lower Limb

Traumatic Injuries to the Pelvic Ring

31

The pelvis is a bony ring structure consisting of anterior, posterior, and lateral parts. Traumatic injuries may affect any part of the ring, resulting in either isolated or combined bony injuries. In polytrauma patients, pelvic injuries can correspond to a life-threatening condition. Fractures of the acetabulum, which forms the lateral part of the ring, are discussed in the subsequent chapter entitled "Hip Trauma."

31.1 Patho-Anatomy

31.1.1 Injuries to the Anterior Pelvic Ring

- Symphysis pubis dislocation or disruption (Fig. 31.1).
- Fractures of the superior pubic ramus (ilio-pubic) and/or inferior pubic ramus (ischio-pubic), including unilateral and bilateral fractures.

31.1.2 Injuries to the Posterior Pelvic Ring

- Sacro-iliac joint dislocation (Fig. 31.1).
- Fractures of the sacrum.
- Associated fracture-dislocations.

31.1.3 Combined Injuries to the Anterior and Posterior Parts of the Pelvic Ring

- These injuries often induce a major instability of the pelvic ring and may lead to a complete displacement with "dislocation" of the affected hemi-pelvis.
- Urinary complications are common with these injuries: rupture of the urethra and urinary bladder injury.

D. Saragaglia, A. Hassan Chamseddine, *Traumatology for the Emergency Doctor*, https://doi.org/10.1007/978-3-031-63196-2_31

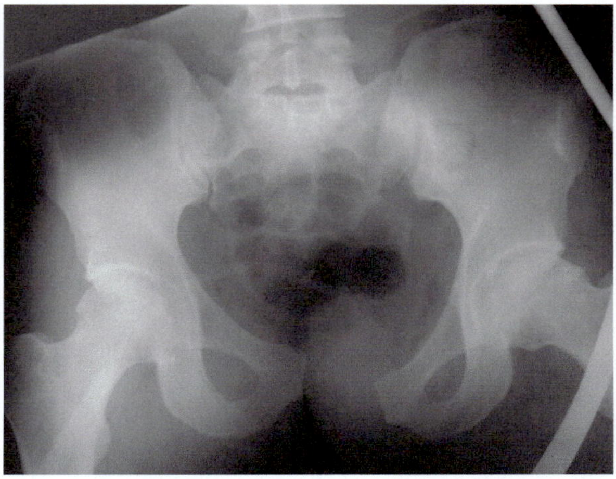

Fig. 31.1 AP pelvis radiograph showing a symphysis pubis disruption with left sacro-iliac joint dislocation

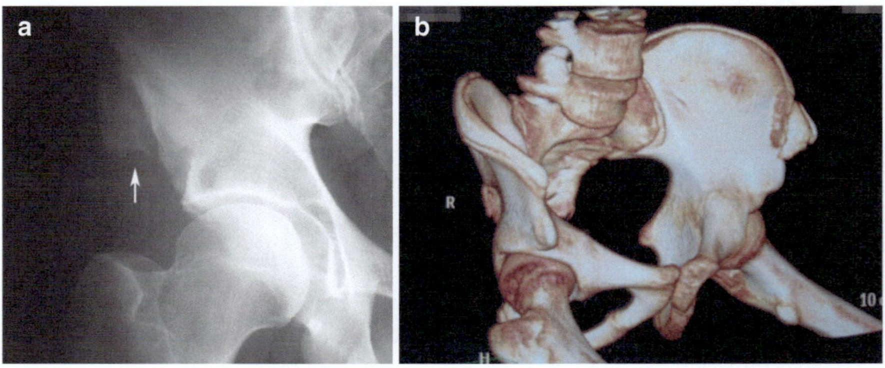

Fig. 31.2 (**a**) Fracture-avulsion of the right antero-superior iliac spine. (**b**) 3D CT scan of an avulsion of the anterior superior iliac spine

31.1.4 Bilateral Pelvic Injuries Corresponding to "Floating Pelvis"

31.1.4.1 Partial Fractures Without Rupture of the Pelvic Ring

1. ***Fracture of the ilium and iliac crest*** secondary to direct trauma.
2. ***Fracture-avulsions*** (Fig. 31.2a and b):
   (a) These injuries usually occur during sports activities, especially in adolescent patients.
   (b) They correspond to a fracture-avulsion of:
   - The anterior superior iliac spine,
   - The anterior inferior iliac spine,
   - And the ischial tuberosity.

31.2 Management

1. **Pelvic injuries, secondary to high-velocity or high-energy trauma,** are commonly seen in polytrauma patients. These injuries may contribute to a life-threatening condition such as in hemodynamically unstable patient, multiple fractures, multiple organ injuries (brain, chest, abdomen, etc.). These patients should be urgently managed according to the trauma life support principles with active participation of the reanimation team.
2. **Pelvic injuries, secondary to low-velocity or low-energy trauma,** are usually benign and do not pose a life threat. A *Basic radiographic assessment* should include an antero-posterior view of the pelvis, alar, and obturator oblique views of the affected hip, as well as inlet and outlet views.
3. ***CT scan with 2D and 3D*** reconstruction is considered indispensable for the evaluation of pelvic injuries. It has practically replaced the oblique views (Fig. 31.3a and b).
4. **A Surgical consultation is recommended for the following fracture patterns:**
   (a) Sacro-iliac joint dislocation or disjunction,
   (b) Symphysis pubis separation,
   (c) Combined anterior and posterior ring injuries (Fig. 31.4),
   (d) Fracture-avulsion with more than 2 cm displacement.
5. **Medical (non-surgical) management is indicated for:**
   (a) *Undisplaced and minimally displaced superior and inferior pubic rami fractures.*
   - hospitalization for 3–4 days, as these patients are usually elderly patients,
   - non-weight or partial weight bearing as tolerated, using a walking assistance device for 4–6 weeks,
   - and special geriatric care as needed.

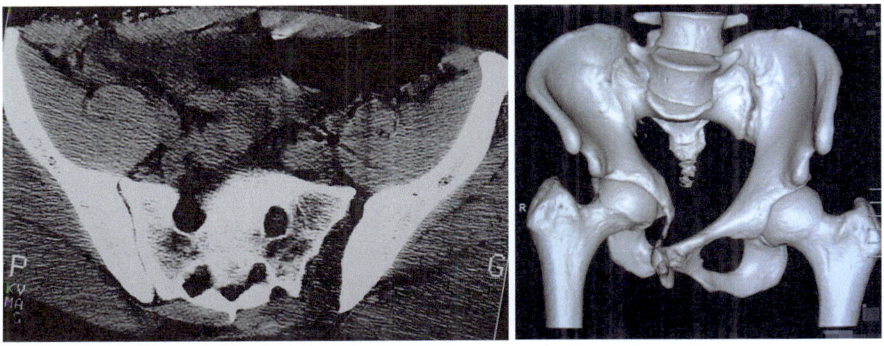

Fig. 31.3 (**a**) Axial CT scan cut showing a left sacro-iliac joint dislocation. (**b**) 3D CT scan of a malunion of the pelvic ring

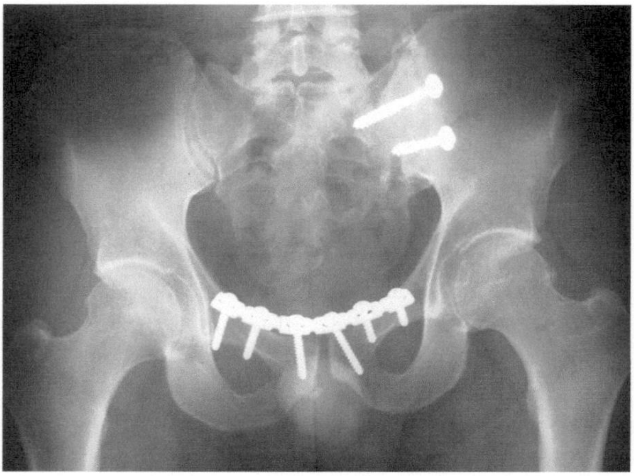

Fig. 31.4 Post-operative AP pelvis radiograph of the same patient as shown in Fig. 31.1 after open reduction and internal fixation of the symphysis pubis with plate and screws associated with reduction-fixation of the left sacro-iliac joint with two screws

(b) *Fracture-avulsion with minimal displacement (<2 cm).*
   - non-weight or partial weight bearing as tolerated, using a walking assistance device for 4–6 weeks,
   - resume of sports activities after 3 months.

(c) *Fractures of the iliac wing* usually heal without complications. A period of relative rest is recommended with the use of analgesics and NSAIDs for pain control.

Hip Trauma

32

32.1 Fractures of the Acetabulum

Fractures of the acetabulum are intra-articular fractures that can jeopardize hip function. They can occur either as isolated fractures or in association to other fractures or injuries, particularly in polytrauma patients. In such cases, a multidisciplinary team approach is required, involving teams from different specialties such as anesthesia, reanimation, ortho-trauma, urology, general surgery, neurosurgery, etc.

32.1.1 Patho-Anatomy

Acetabular fractures can be categorized into:

- Fractures of the anterior wall and/or column,
- Fractures of the posterior wall and/or column,
- Fractures of both columns (Fig. 32.1),
- Complex fracture patterns.

32.1.2 Radiographic Assessment

1. **Plan radiographs:** antero-posterior pelvis view, alar oblique view, and obturator oblique view of the affected hip.
2. **CT scan with 2D and 3D reconstruction:** considered indispensable for the evaluation of pelvic injuries. It has practically replaced the oblique views.
3. **The imaging assessment is crucial for,**
   (a) identifying the fracture type and pattern,
   (b) evaluating the displacement,
   (c) assessing the coxo-femoral congruence,

D. Saragaglia, A. Hassan Chamseddine, *Traumatology for the Emergency Doctor*, https://doi.org/10.1007/978-3-031-63196-2_32

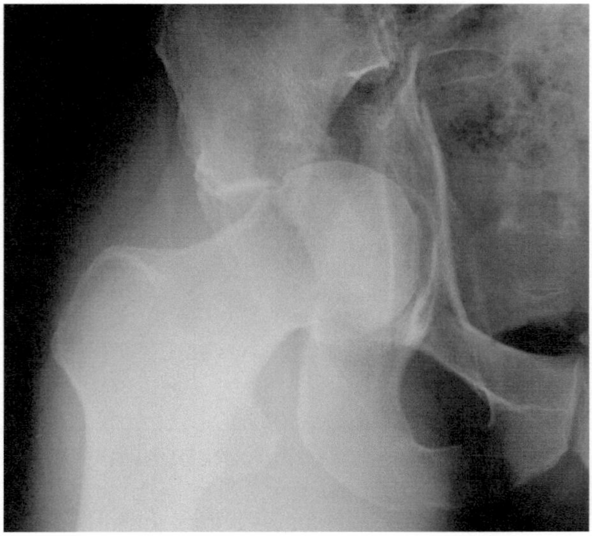

Fig. 32.1 AP hip radiograph showing a displaced fracture of both columns of the acetabulum (anterior and posterior)

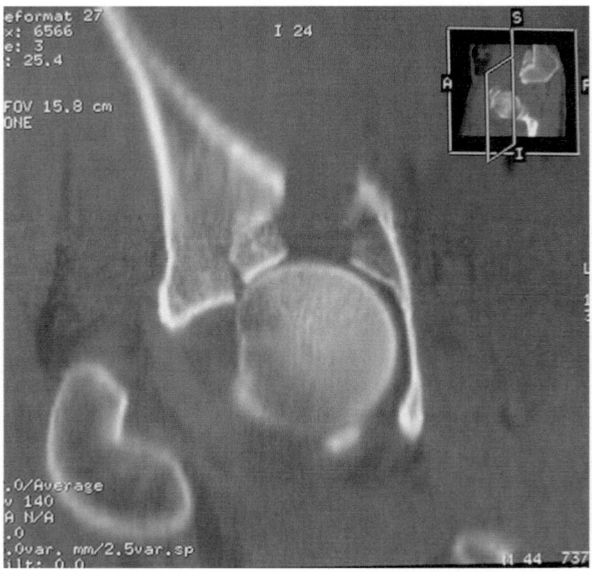

Fig. 32.2 Coronal CT scan cut of the same hip as shown in Fig. 32.1

(d) disclosing,
- associated posterior ring injuries,
- antero-posterior incongruence (sub-luxation),
- intra-articular "incarcerated" osteo-cartilaginous loose body,
- osteo-cartilaginous articular impaction (Fig. 32.2).

All acetabular fractures require a *specialized surgical consultation* for appropriate management and indication (Fig. 32.3).

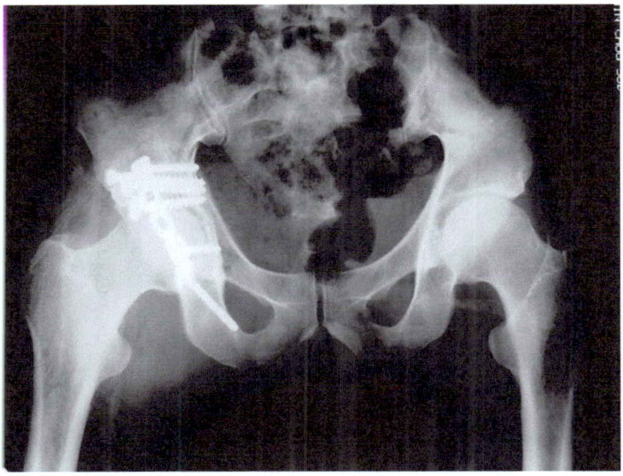

Fig. 32.3 AP pelvis X-ray of the same patient as shown in Fig. 32.1 after open reduction and internal fixation of the acetabular fracture (using plate and screws)

32.1.3 Initial Management in the ER

- Skeletal (trans-osseous) traction:
  - Trans-tibial for undisplaced fractures.
  - Trans-femoral for displaced fractures.
- Final therapeutic decision (by the ortho-trauma team) after CT scan assessment.

32.2 Hip Dislocations

32.2.1 Patho-Anatomy

Two types of Hip dislocations are categorized based on the direction of the displacement:

32.2.1.1 Posterior Dislocation (Figs. 32.4 and 32.5)

- It is the most common type (75%).
- The dislocation position may be "superior" (iliac position) or "inferior" (ischial position).
- It is frequently associated with a fracture of the posterior wall of the acetabulum (Fig. 32.6) with an increased risk of avascular necrosis of the femoral head (>25% versus <5% for isolated posterior dislocation).

32.2.1.2 Anterior Dislocation

- It is less common (25%).
- The dislocation position may be "superior" (pubic position) or "inferior" (obturator position) (Fig. 32.7).

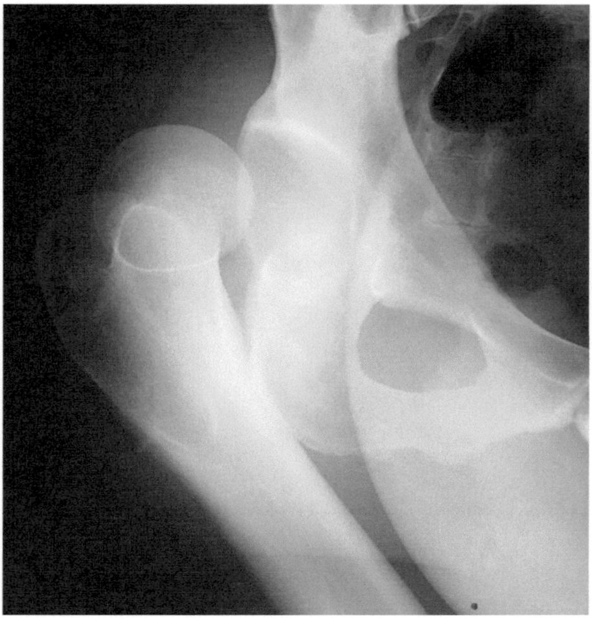

Fig. 32.4 AP radiograph of a right hip with a posterior dislocation

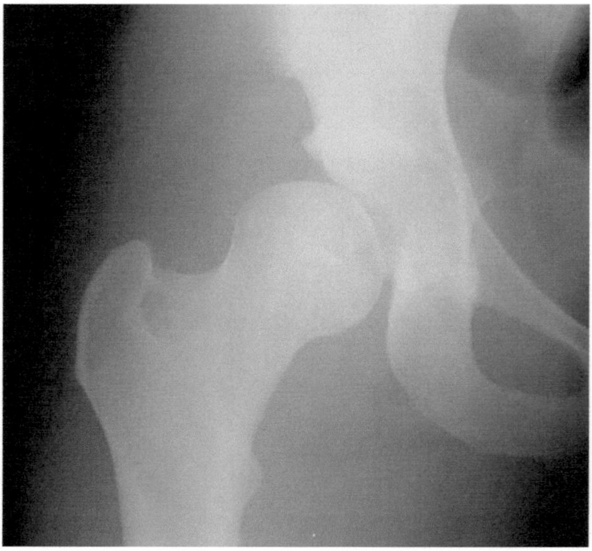

Fig. 32.5 AP radiograph of a right hip showing a posterior sub-luxation: note the widening of the hip joint space

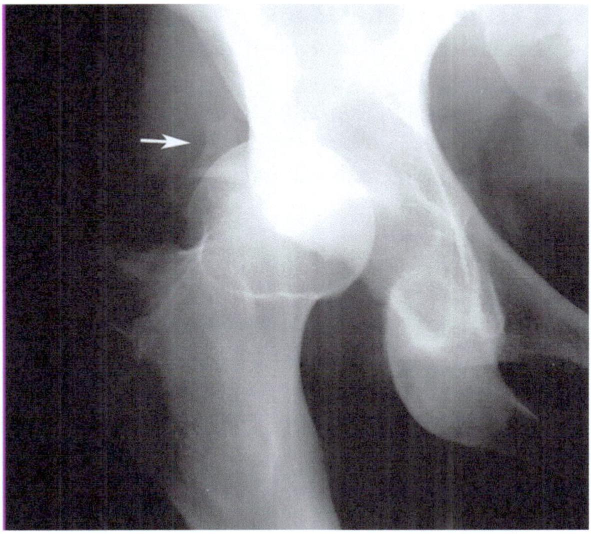

Fig. 32.6 AP X-ray of a right hip showing a posterior dislocation with fracture of the posterior acetabular wall

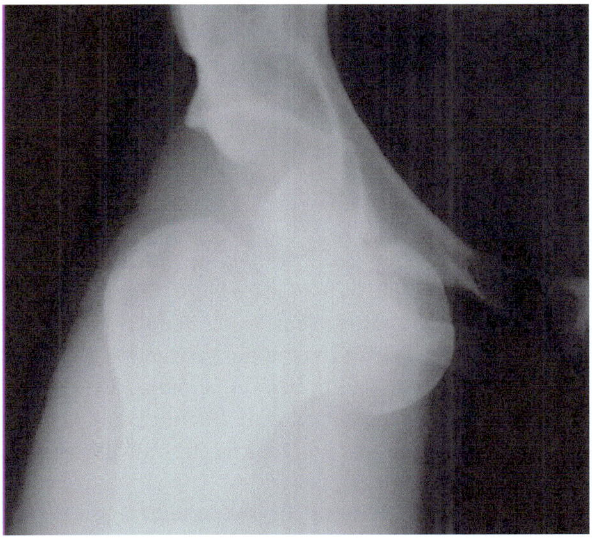

Fig. 32.7 AP X-ray of a right hip showing an antero-inferior dislocation (obturator dislocation position)

32.2.1.3 Associated Injuries

- Acetabulum posterior wall fractures (commonly associated to posterior dislocations),
- Fractures of the *femoral head*, that results in a less favorable prognosis,
- Injury to the *sciatic nerve*, especially the fibular nerve, which should always be tested before the reduction maneuvers.

32.2.2 Clinical Presentation

The clinical diagnosis of hip dislocation is often evident because of the typical and characteristic deformity position of the lower limb in,

- Irreducible abduction-external rotation for the anterior dislocations,
- Irreducible adduction-Internal rotation for the posterior dislocations.

32.2.3 Assessment

- An antero-posterior pelvis radiograph is necessary to confirm the diagnosis.
- A CT scan is usually performed after the reduction of the dislocation to disclose any associated bony injuries.

32.2.4 Management

- The traumatic hip dislocation is an "orthopedic emergency": the relocation of the hip should be *performed during the first 6 h* to reduce the risk of femoral head avascular necrosis (the earlier the reduction, the lower the risk of necrosis).
- For isolated dislocations: a post-reduction skin traction for 7 days, followed by progressive full weight bearing ambulation (authors' preference).
- For associated posterior wall fractures: a surgical treatment is often indicated (open reduction and internal fixation of the posterior wall fragment, especially for large fragments).
- For associated femoral head fracture: a surgical treatment is often indicated, especially for displaced fractures.

32.3 Fractures of the Proximal Femur

Fractures of the proximal femur are common domestic injuries in the elderly patients. They usually often occur after a simple fall from their height.

32.3.1 Patho-Anatomy

Proximal femoral fractures are categorized into:

- Cervical or femoral neck fractures (intra-capsular),
- Pertrochanteric and intertrochanteric fractures (extra-capsular),
- Partial fractures involving either the greater or the lesser trochanter.

32.3.1.1 Femoral Neck Fractures

They are described according to the location of the fracture, the displacement of the fracture, and the orientation of the fracture line. These fractures carry a risk of avascular necrosis of the femoral head and fracture nonunion.

1. ***Location of the fracture***
   (a) Sub-capital (junction head-neck),
   (b) transcervical (through the neck),
   (c) basicervical (base of the neck, at the junction with the trochanteric area).
2. ***Displacement of the fracture***
   (a) *The Garden classification* is commonly used for the description of the fracture displacement.
   (b) It includes four types and helps predict the risk of avascular necrosis of the femoral head, with the risk increasing with the initial displacement of the

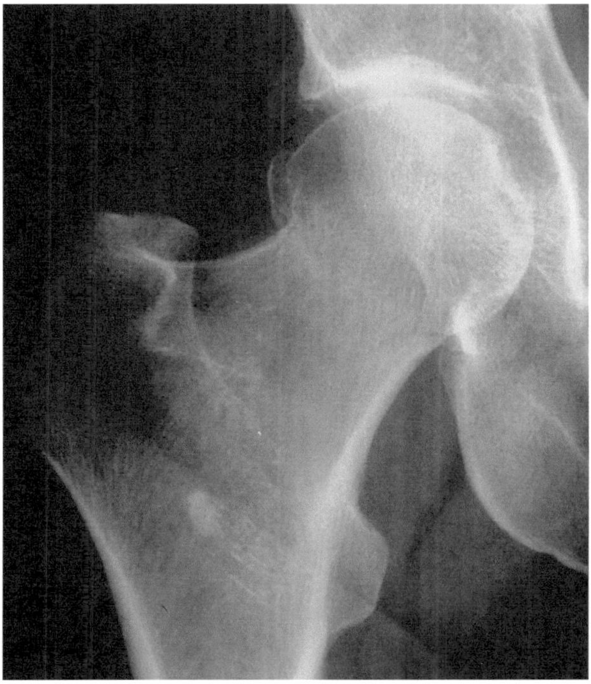

Fig. 32.8 X-ray of a subcapital femoral neck fracture Garden 1, Pauwels 1

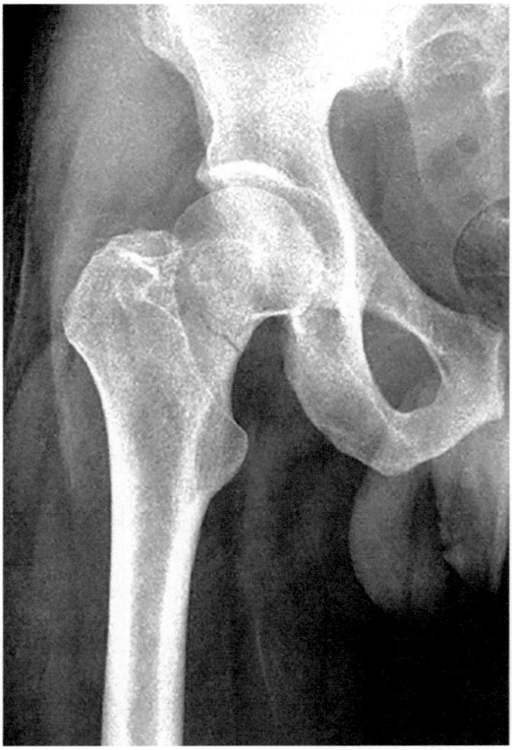

Fig. 32.9 X-ray of a transcervical femoral neck fracture Garden 2, Pauwels 3

fracture. For daily use in the ER, the Garden classification is simplified into two types:

- undisplaced: this includes Garden I (valgus impacted, Fig. 32.8) and Garden II (undisplaced fractures, Fig. 32.9).
- Displaced: this includes Garden III (varus, incomplete displacement of the fracture, with remaining contact between the 2 fragments, Fig. 32.10) and Garden IV (complete displacement of the fracture, with no contact between the two fragments, Fig. 32.11).

3. ***Orientation of the fracture line***
   (a) The identification and description of the fracture line orientation is only possible after reduction of the fracture (usually performed with traction and moderate internal rotation maneuver); it helps predict the mechanical stability of the fracture itself and consequently the risk of nonunion:
   - the more horizontal the fracture, the more stable it is, and the more likely it is to heal.
   - the more vertical the fracture, the more unstable it is, and the less predictable its healing becomes.

   (b) *The Pauwels classification* is commonly used to describe the fracture line orientation. It includes three types based on the angle formed between the fracture line and the horizontal line.

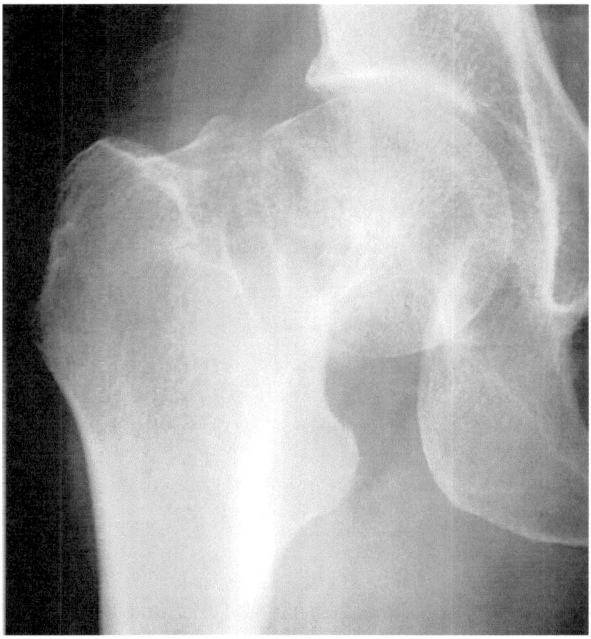

Fig. 32.10 X-ray of a transcervical femoral neck fracture Garden 3, Pauwels 3

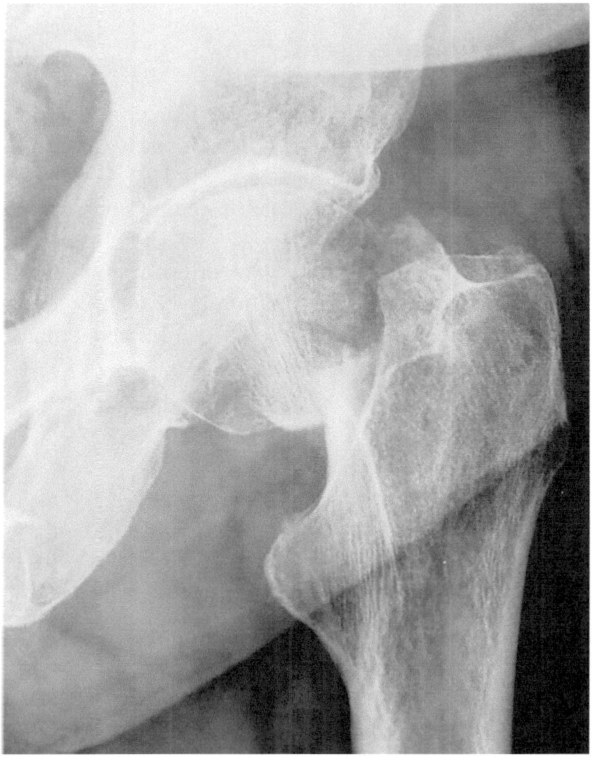

Fig. 32.11 X-ray of a transcervical femoral neck fracture Garden 4, Pauwels 3

(c) For daily use in the ER, the Pauwels classification can simply be described as follows:
   - Type I: the fracture line is closer to the horizontal line,
   - Type II: the fracture line is oblique,
   - Type III: the fracture line is closer to the vertical line.

32.3.1.2 Pertrochanteric (Extra-Capsular) Fractures

- They are commonly categorized into:
  - simple stable fractures (Fig. 32.12),
  - and unstable fractures, with three or four parts, and comminution of the medial pillar (Fig. 32.13). Fractures including pattern of "thin" or fractured "lateral trochanteric wall" are considered unstable.
- They theoretically do not carry a secondary risk of avascular necrosis of the femoral head.
- They present a risk of malunion (varus-shortening) and nonunion, especially for unstable fractures.

32.3.1.3 Partial Fractures

They correspond to either isolated fractures of the greater trochanter or fractures of the lesser trochanter.

32.3.2 Clinical Presentation

- The diagnosis is often evident and is commonly made in the following context:
  - An elderly patient (but not exclusively) after a fall from their height.
  - Pain.
  - Functional disability, such as being unable to walk or elevate the heel from the bed.
  - Typical deformity of the lower limb: shortening and external rotation.
- The above clinical presentation is frequently lessened or absent in the cases of valgus impacted femoral neck fracture and isolated partial fractures (greater or lesser trochanter fracture).

32.3.3 Radiographic Assessment

- Antero-posterior pelvis and hip radiographs are usually appropriate for making the diagnosis.
- An antero-posterior hip radiograph with moderate traction and internal rotation is required to disclose the fracture type and pattern.
- In cases of doubtful femoral neck fracture, an MRI is more helpful than a CT scan.

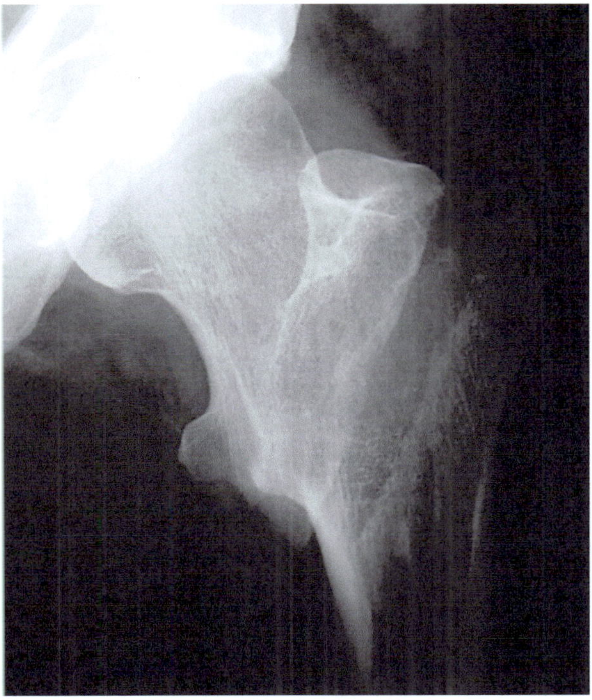

Fig. 32.12 X-ray of a pertrochanteric simple stable fracture of the left hip in a young adult patient (40 years old)

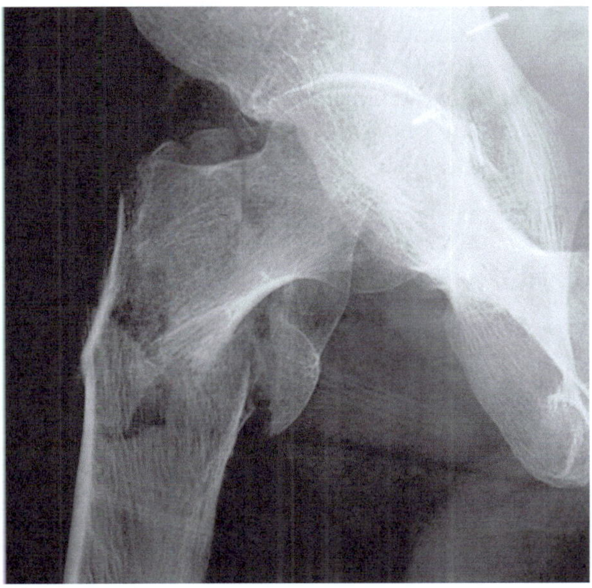

Fig. 32.13 X-ray of a pertrochanteric unstable fracture of the right hip in an elderly patient (88 years old)

32.3.4 Management

In all cases, a specialized orthopedic consultation is required.

The following management is usually recommended:

1. **For partial fractures**
   (a) Surgical treatment is rarely indicated, except for displaced fractures of the greater trochanter in young people.
   (b) A functional treatment is usually performed: weight bearing as tolerated with a walking assistance device for 4–6 weeks.
2. **For valgus impacted femoral neck fractures**
   (a) Traction is neither recommended nor needed.
   (b) The treatment varies according to the personal preferences and experience of the surgeon:
      - A functional treatment with regular weekly radiographic controls to depict any secondary displacement,
      - Or a preventive internal fixation (in situ).
3. **For displaced femoral neck fractures**
   (a) ***In young patients*** (<60–65 years):
      - The treatment is regularly surgical, using reduction and internal fixation (Fig. 32.14).
      - Skeletal traction is only indicated when the surgical treatment is delayed.
      - A temporary skeletal trans-tibial traction (6–8 kg) is installed for fracture reduction and pain relief, only while waiting for the final surgical treatment.
      - The skeletal traction helps in reducing the fracture and decreasing the risk of avascular necrosis of the femoral head.
      - An orthopedic bed with special traction-suspension accessories is required when traction is performed (refer to Chap. 13).

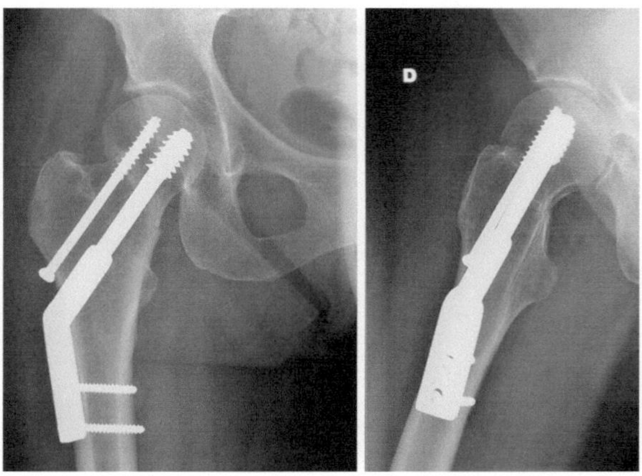

Fig. 32.14 AP and lateral radiographs of the same hip as shown in Fig. 32.9 after open reduction and internal fixation with a dynamic hip screw (DHS) and an isolated cannulated screw

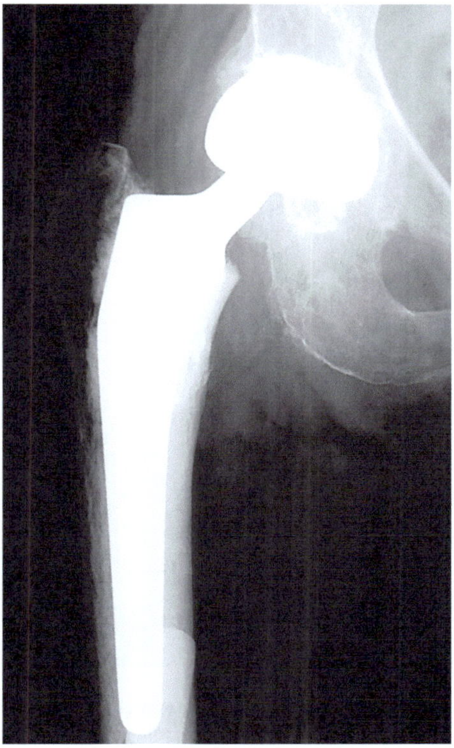

Fig. 32.15 AP X-ray of a hip replacement (bipolar prosthesis) for a transcervical femoral neck fracture in an elderly patient (80 years old)

(b) ***In elderly patients***
- The treatment is regularly surgical (using hip replacement) (Fig. 32.15).
- Skin traction is usually performed with cautious (be careful not to induce skin damage) while waiting for the final surgical treatment.

4. **For pertrochanteric fractures**

(a) ***In a young patient***
- Skeletal trans-tibial traction (with approximately 10 kg) is applied when the final treatment is delayed,
- Radiographs are repeated after the traction-reduction for better identification of the fracture pattern (stable, unstable, comminuted, medial pillar, postero-medial fragment, etc.).
- The final treatment usually corresponds to reduction and internal fixation: extra or intra-medullary fixation according to the fracture type and surgeon's preferences (Fig. 32.16).

(b) ***In an elderly patient***
- Reduction and internal fixation is the best option for stable fractures.
- Hip replacement is a viable option for unstable and osteoporotic fractures (Fig. 32.17), especially for patients who cannot walk with partial or no weight bearing in the immediate post-operative period (due to the risk of secondary displacement of unstable fractures treated with osteosynthesis).

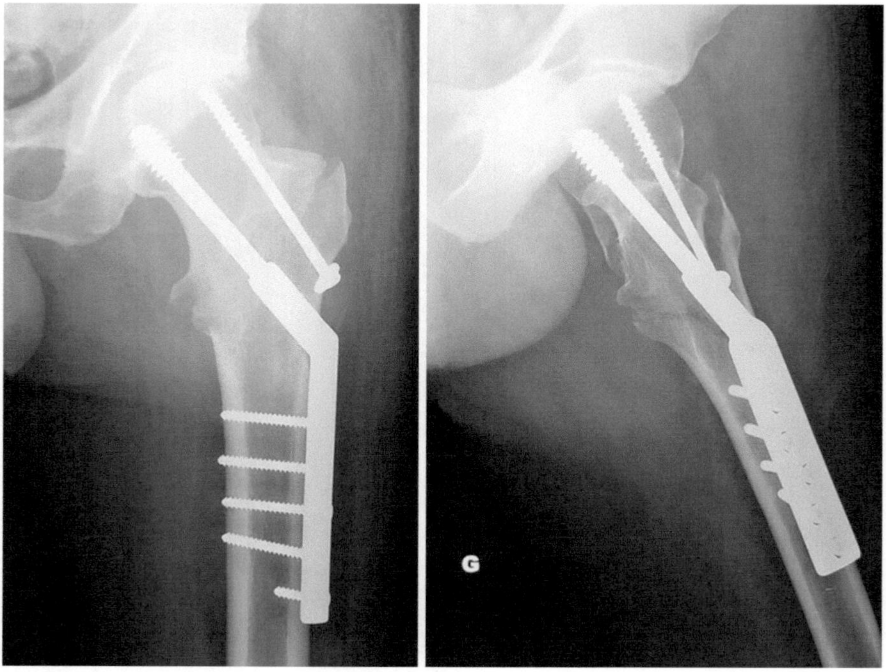

Fig. 32.16 AP and lateral radiographs of the same hip as shown in Fig. 32.12 after open reduction and internal fixation with dynamic hip screw (DHS) and an isolated cancellous screw

Fig. 32.17 AP hip radiograph of a bipolar hip prosthesis with calcar replacement for an unstable intertrochanteric fracture extended to the proximal femoral shaft (trochantero-diaphyseal fracture) in an elderly patient

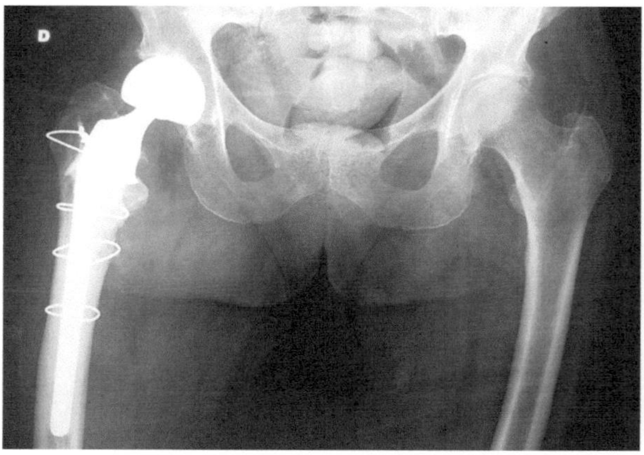

32.4 Assessment of Post-Traumatic Symptomatic Hip and Pelvis with "Normal Radiographs"

- Post-traumatic symptomatic hip conditions with normal radiographs are not a rare presentation.
- Any patient with post-traumatic hip pain or functional disability and "normal radiographs" should not be cleared from the ER before a full workup is performed. They should be informed of the possible presence of an "occult" fracture not revealed by conventional radiographs.
- Post-traumatic hip pain or functional disability with "normal radiographs" should not be considered, under any circumstance, as a "psychosomatic" condition.
- Hip pain or disability can be related to three types of injuries:

32.4.1 Occult Bony Pelvic Injuries

- They correspond to "hair-line" fractures (fissures) of the sacrum, superior pubic ramus, inferior pubic ramus, acetabulum, or iliac wing.
- An *MRI* is the best and more efficient early diagnostic tool for these injuries.
- The use of bone scintigraphy has been supplanted by the MRI. Scintigraphy requires 10–14 days to show hyperfixation ("hot spot") at the fractured site, leading to longer hospitalization time.

32.4.2 Occult Bony Lesions of the Proximal Femur

- They can affect:
  - The greater or the lesser trochanter (partial fractures),
  - The Femoral neck (intra-capsular),
  - The trochanteric area (pertrochanteric: extra-capsular).
- A post-traumatic *hip pain during weight bearing* should be considered as a "Red Flag" for an occult proximal femur fracture. This should always lead to hospital admission, complete bed rest, and a request of an *MRI* (Figs. 32.18 and 32.19).
- Post-traumatic hip pain of a few days duration with normal radiographs may benefit from *bone scintigraphy* (Figs. 32.20, 32.21 and 32.22). However, this exam has been completely supplanted by the MRI.
- Secondary displacement of initially undiagnosed undisplaced proximal femur fracture is not a rare situation (Figs. 32.23 and 32.24); it may lead to medico-legal conflict.
- Surgical treatment using internal fixation is usually performed as soon as the diagnosis is made in order to avoid any secondary displacement of the fracture.

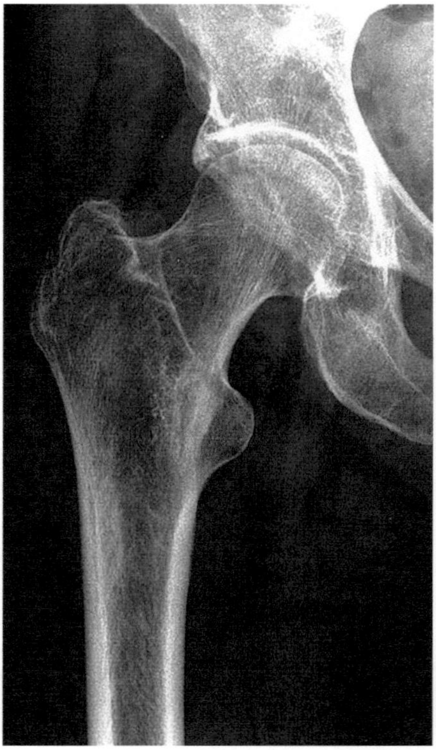

Fig. 32.18 AP hip radiograph labeled "normal" for a patient presented to the ER with "hip contusion" and functional disability

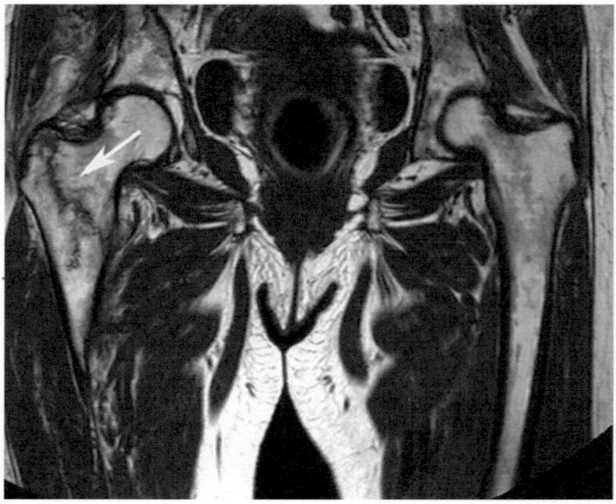

Fig. 32.19 MRI of the same hip as shown in Fig. 32.18 showing an undisplaced pertrochanteric fracture

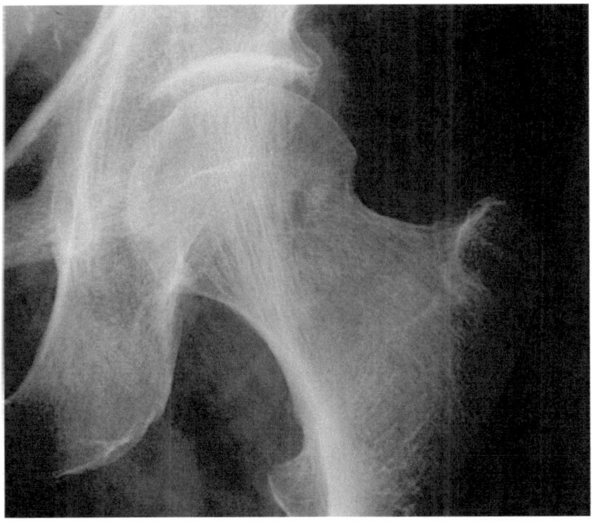

Fig. 32.20 AP hip X-ray labeled as "normal" in a patient who sought medical attention 10-days post-fall due to ongoing hip pain, functional impairment, and pain upon weight bearing

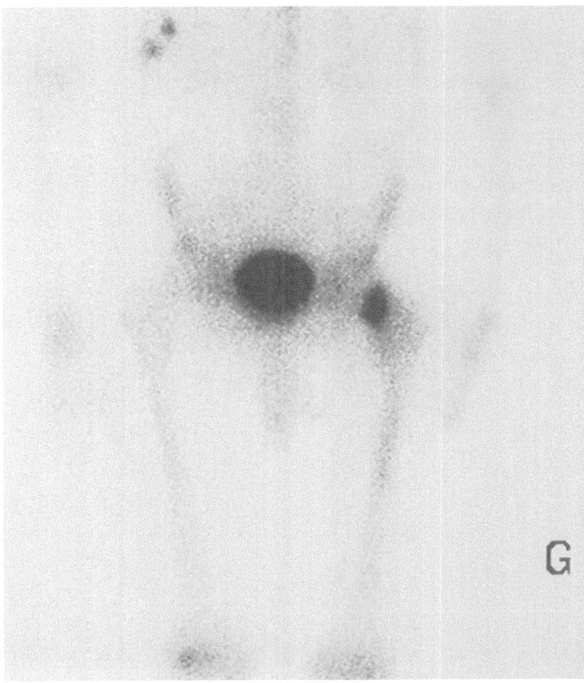

Fig. 32.21 Bone scintigraphy of the same patient as shown in Fig. 32.20 showing a localized hyperfixation (hot spot) in the left femoral neck, suggestive of a fracture

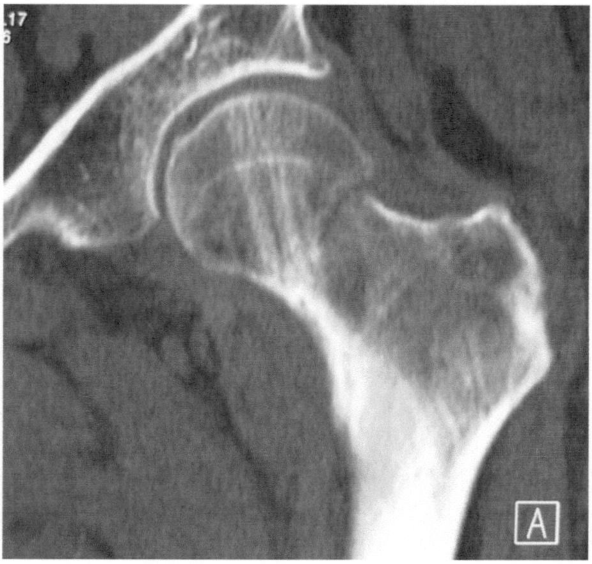

Fig. 32.22 Coronal CT scan cut of the same hip as shown in Figs. 32.20 and 32.21 confirms the diagnosis of an undisplaced transcervical femoral neck fracture

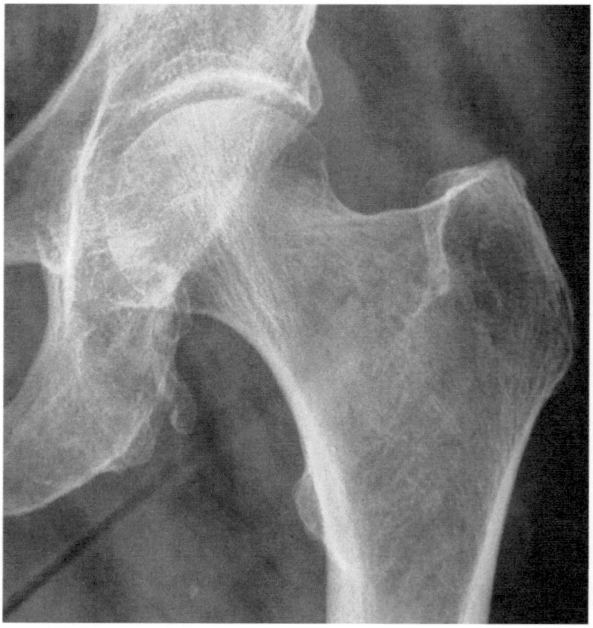

Fig. 32.23 AP left hip X-ray labeled as "Normal" in a patient who presented to the ER with left hip pain after a fall. The patient was discharged without any precautions or follow-up advice

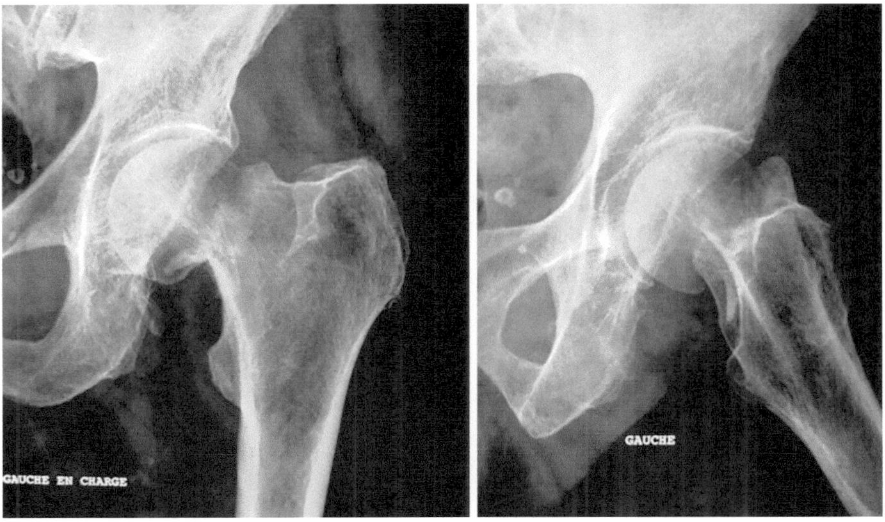

Fig. 32.24 Subsequent AP and lateral radiographs of the same hip as shown in Fig. 32.23 revealed a displaced sub-capital femoral neck fracture. The patient returned 10-days post-initial trauma with severe hip pain and complete functional disability of the left lower limb

32.4.3 Musculo-Tendinous Lesions

- These are usually seen in sports practice.
- They typically correspond to an avulsion of the bony insertion of the:
  - Hamstrings origin (ischial tuberosity—refer to Chap. 44),
  - Adductors origin (pubic bone).

Femoral Shaft Fractures

33

Sub-trochanteric fractures (Fig. 33.1) and supra-condylar fractures (Fig. 33.2a, b) are not included with fractures of the femoral shaft. However, the assessment and management of all these fractures are similar for an ER physician.

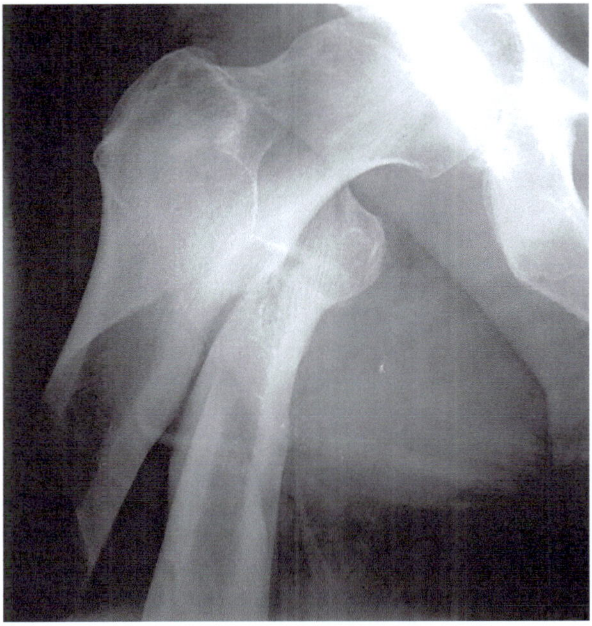

Fig. 33.1 AP hip X-ray showing a sub-trochanteric wedge fracture with large medial fragment involving the lesser trochanter

D. Saragaglia, A. Hassan Chamseddine, *Traumatology for the Emergency Doctor*, https://doi.org/10.1007/978-3-031-63196-2_33

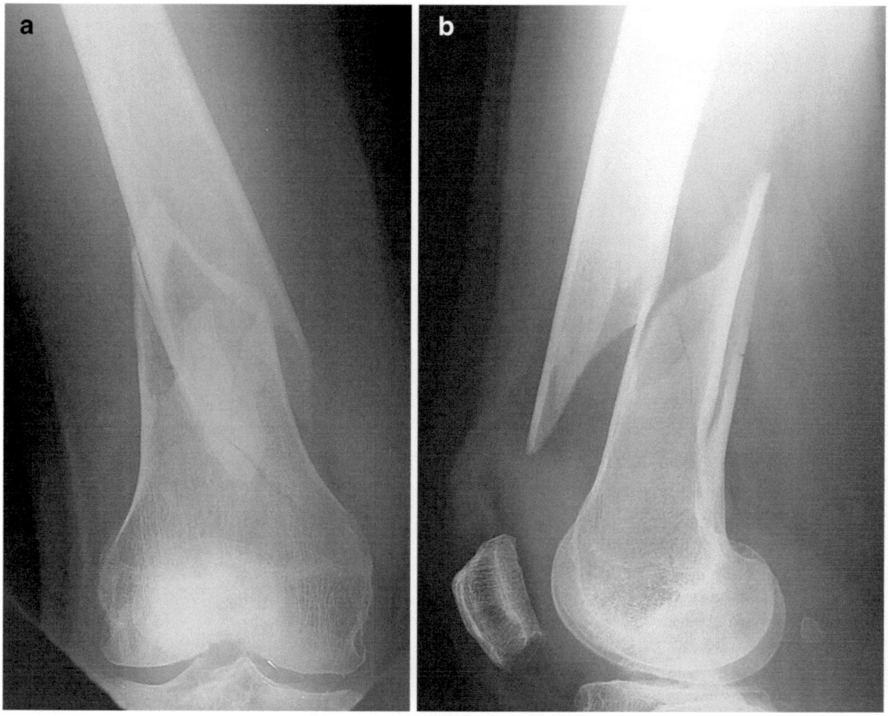

Fig. 33.2 (**a**) AP radiograph of a distal right femur showing a spiral oblique supra-condylar fracture. (**b**) Lateral radiograph of the same fracture depicted in Fig. 33.2a, clearly showing the fracture pattern

33.1 Patho-Anatomy

Femoral shaft fractures can be distinguished into:
- Simple transverse and short oblique fractures (Fig. 33.3),
- Simple spiral and long oblique fractures,
- Wedge fractures (Fig. 33.4),
- Fragmentary wedge fractures (with a comminuted wedge fragment),
- Segmental fractures (with an intact intercalated fragment),
- Fragmentary segmental fractures (with a comminuted intercalated fragment),
- Peri-prosthetic fractures (around or near to a prosthetic femoral stem),
- Associated femoral shaft and neck fractures.

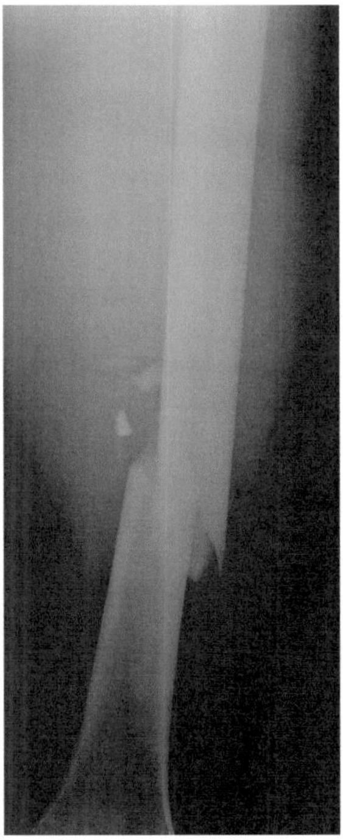

Fig. 33.3 AP left femur X-ray showing a mid-shaft short oblique fracture

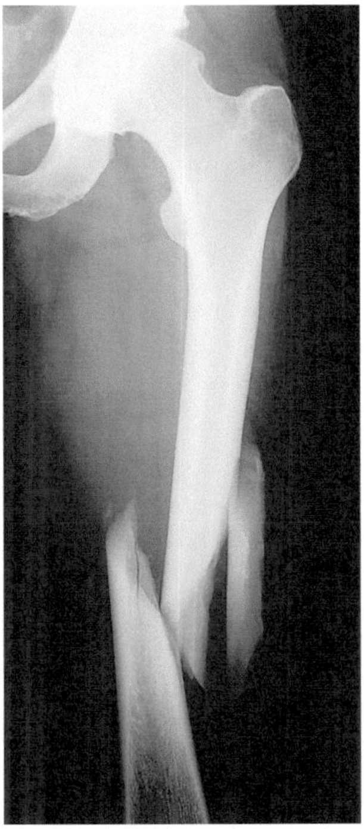

Fig. 33.4 AP left femur X-ray showing a mid-shaft wedge fracture with a complete longitudinal rotation of the wedge fragment

33.2 Assessment and Management

- The clinical presentation is evident: pain, complete functional disability, lower limb deformity, and shortening, etc.
- A general assessment is crucial when the fracture is secondary to high energy trauma (such as a road traffic accident); it should rule out any local, regional, or general associated injuries (open fracture, neuro-vascular impairment, pelvic fracture, spinal injury, head trauma, thoraco-abdominal injury, etc.).
- Temporary skin traction is installed to reduce pain and deformity, while waiting for the radiographic evaluation.
- An intra-venous line is opened for fluids and medication administration (blood and vasopressors for hypovolemic shock, analgesics for pain, etc.).
- After clinical clearance and radiographic assessment, a *skeletal trans-tibial traction* is positioned (10–20% of the body weight) if the patient cannot be operated on soon.
- *Reduction and internal fixation is the gold standard treatment* for femoral shaft fractures; it can be done using an intra-medullary nail (Fig. 33.5) or plate and screws (Figs. 33.6, 33.7a, b) according to the fracture's location and profile and the surgeon's preferences.

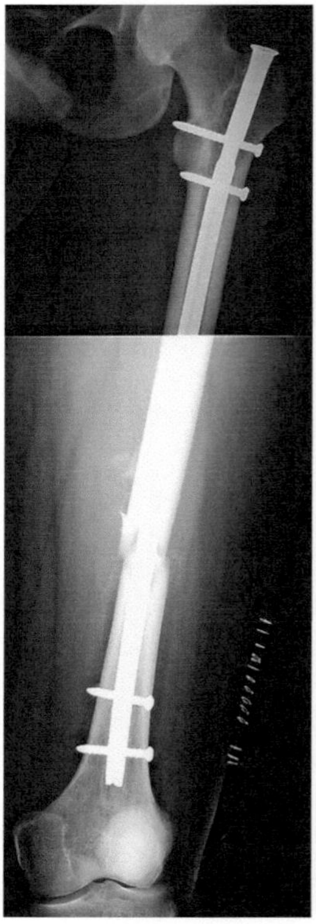

Fig. 33.5 AP left femur radiograph showing an intra-medullary interlocking nail fixation of a short oblique femoral shaft fracture

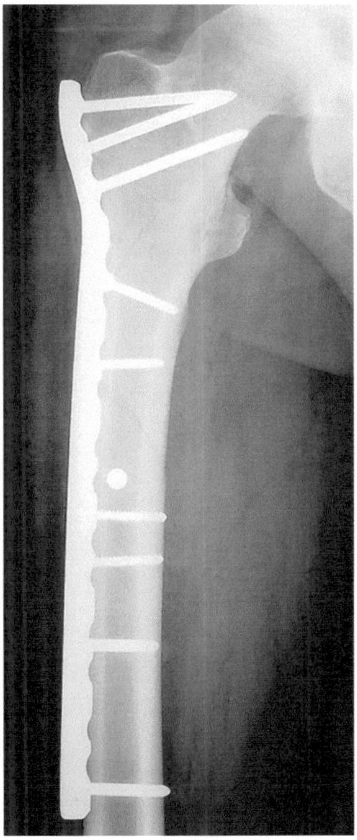

Fig. 33.6 AP right femur radiograph of the same fracture as shown in Fig. 33.1 after open reduction and internal fixation with a proximal femoral locking plate and screws system

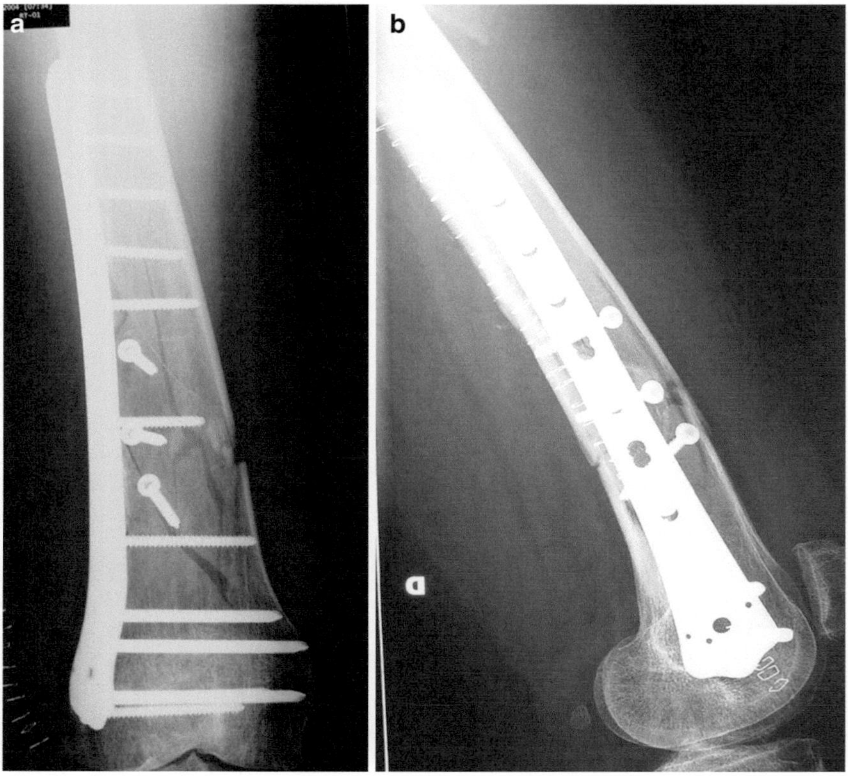

Fig. 33.7 (**a**) AP radiograph of the same fracture depicted in Fig. 33.2a, b after open reduction and internal fixation with a distal femoral locking plate and screws system. (**b**) Lateral X-ray of the same fracture as shown in Fig. 33.2a, b after open reduction and internal fixation with a distal femoral locking plate and screws system

Fractures Around the Knee

34

34.1 Patho-Anatomy

34.1.1 Distal Femur Fractures

They can be distinguished into:

- ***Supra-condylar fractures*** (extra-articular) (Fig. 34.1),
- ***Inter-condylar fractures*** (intra-articular) (Fig. 34.2a, b), which can be,
  - Simple fractures ("V," "T," or "Y" shape),
  - Comminuted (multi-fragmentary) fractures.
- ***Uni-condylar fractures*** (intra-articular): medial or lateral condyle (Fig. 34.3a–d). The fracture line can be either in:
  - the coronal plane (Hoffa fracture),
  - or the sagittal plane.

34.1.2 Fractures of the Proximal Tibia (Tibial Plateau)

They can be distinguished into:

- ***Uni-condylar fractures*** involving one tibial condyle (Fig. 34.4a, b),
  - Medial condyle fracture: usually displaced in split (wedge shape separation).
  - Lateral condyle fracture: displaced in split, depression (impaction), or combined split-depression.

D. Saragaglia, A. Hassan Chamseddine, *Traumatology for the Emergency Doctor*, https://doi.org/10.1007/978-3-031-63196-2_34

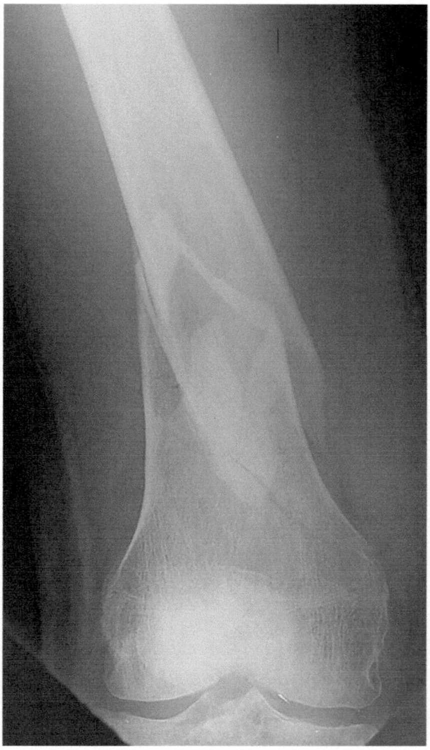

Fig. 34.1 AP X-ray of a distal femur showing a supra-condylar fracture

- ***Bi-condylar fractures*** involving both medial and lateral condyles (Fig. 34.5),
  - Simple fracture pattern,
  - Comminuted fracture pattern.
- ***Partial fractures***
  - *Fracture of the tibial spines*, usually corresponds to avulsion of the distal insertion or footprint of the anterior cruciate ligament (ACL).
  - *Segond fracture*, an extra-articular fleck of bone avulsion from the lateral tibial plateauimmediately below the articular surface, usually associated with ACL rupture.
  - *Fracture of the lateral margin of the lateral tibial* plateau, seen on oblique knee views, and may represent an associated injury with ACL rupture.

34.1.3 Fractures of the Patella

Trauma series of the patella should always include antero-posterior, lateral, and axial tangential views.

Patellar fractures can be distinguished into:

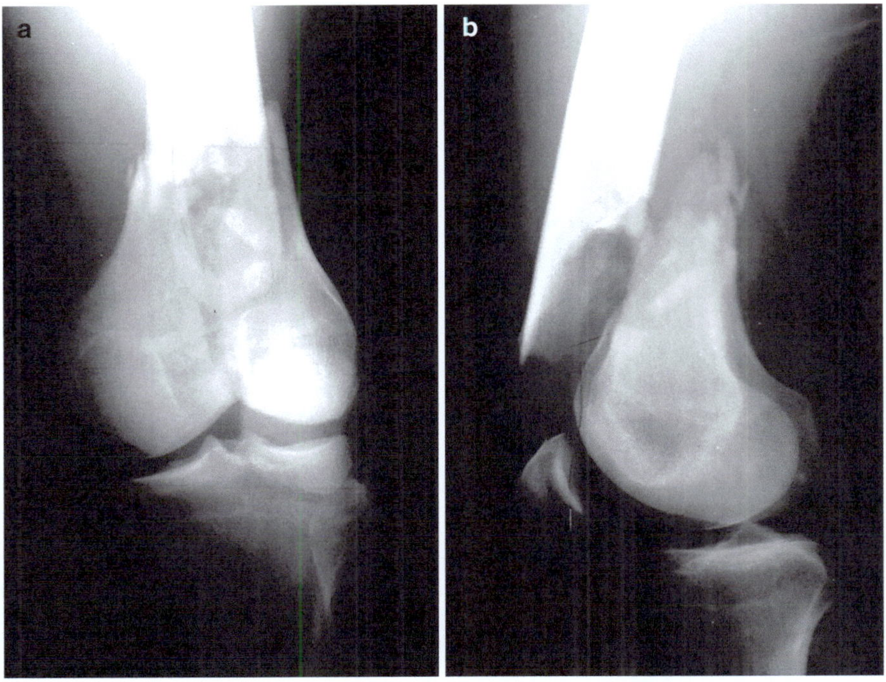

Fig. 34.2 (**a**) AP X-ray of a distal femur showing an inter-condylar fracture. (**b**) Lateral X-ray of the same inter-condylar fracture depicted in Fig. **a**

- ***Transverse fractures*** (Fig. 34.6).
  - These can have simple or complex pattern,
  - They are seen on the lateral knee radiographs,
  - They induce interruption of the extensor mechanism of the knee (with a deficit of active extension of the knee on physical exam).
- ***Sagittal fractures*** (Fig. 34.7a, b).
  - These are often/only seen on the tangential or axial knee views ("sunrise" views).
  - They do not interrupt the knee extensor mechanism (with no impairment of the active knee extension on physical exam).
  - *Bipartite patella* is a differential diagnosis (Fig. 34.8): comparative bilateral radiographs are necessary (bipartite patella is unfused accessory ossification center typically located at the supero-lateral border of the patella and usually corresponds to a bilateral finding).
- ***Marginal bony avulsion*** of the medial femoro-patellar retinaculum at the patellar side (on axial views). This is usually associated with patellar dislocation (refer to chapter "Traumatic dislocations of the patella").

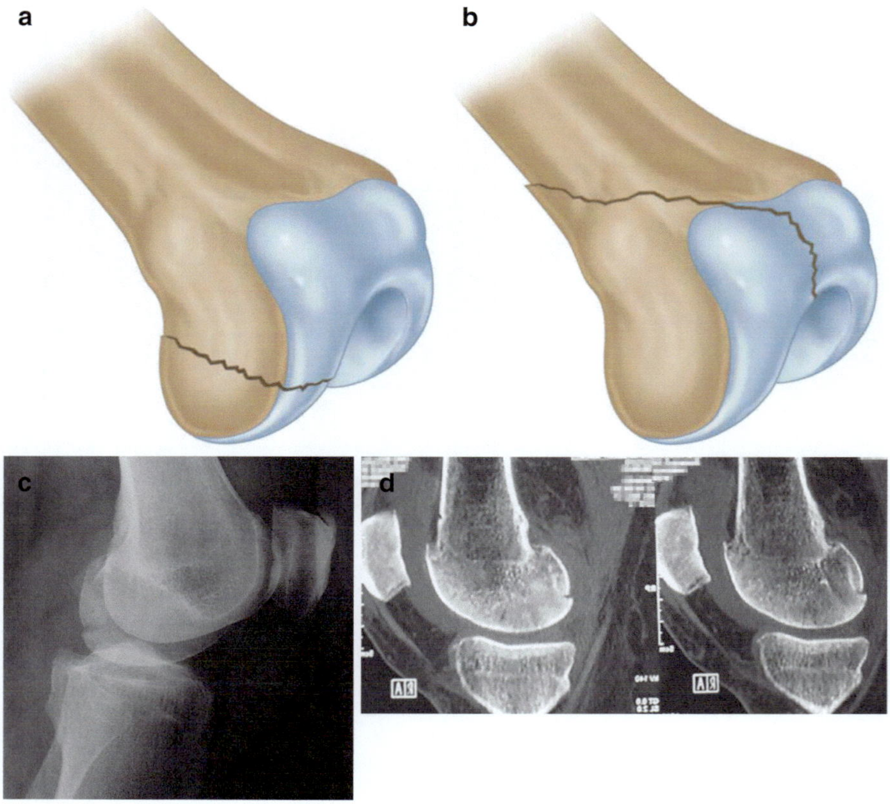

Fig. 34.3 (**a**) Illustration of a uni-condylar distal femur fracture with the fracture line running in the coronal (frontal) plane, consistent with a Hoffa fracture. (**b**) Illustration of a uni-condylar distal femur fracture with the fracture line running in the sagittal plane. (**c**) Lateral distal femur radiograph showing a Hoffa fracture of the medial condyle. (**d**) Sagittal CT scan cuts of the same distal femur as shown in Fig. **c**

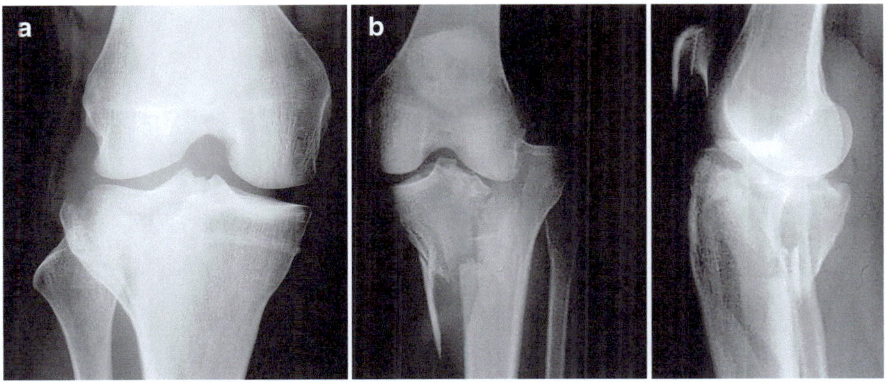

Fig. 34.4 (**a**) AP knee radiograph showing a lateral tibial plateau fracture. (**b**) AP and lateral knee radiographs showing a very displaced medial tibial plateau fracture with a lateral knee sub-luxation

Fig. 34.5 AP knee X-ray showing a bi-condylar tibial plateau fracture

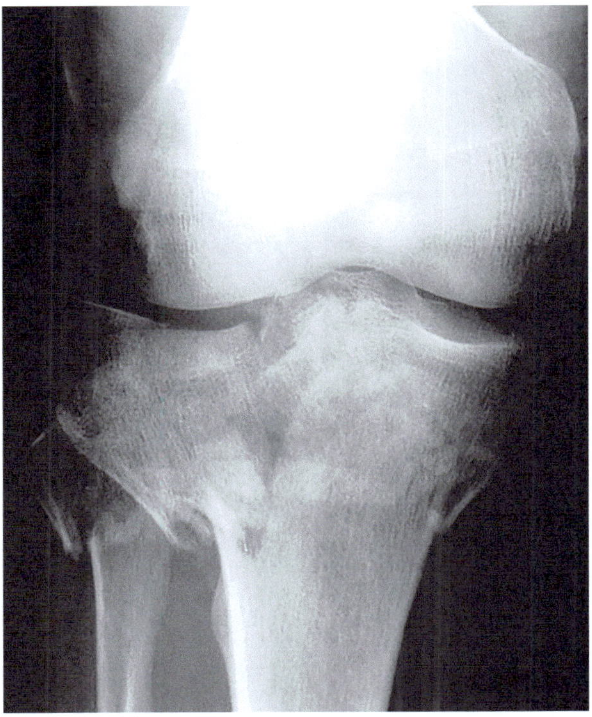

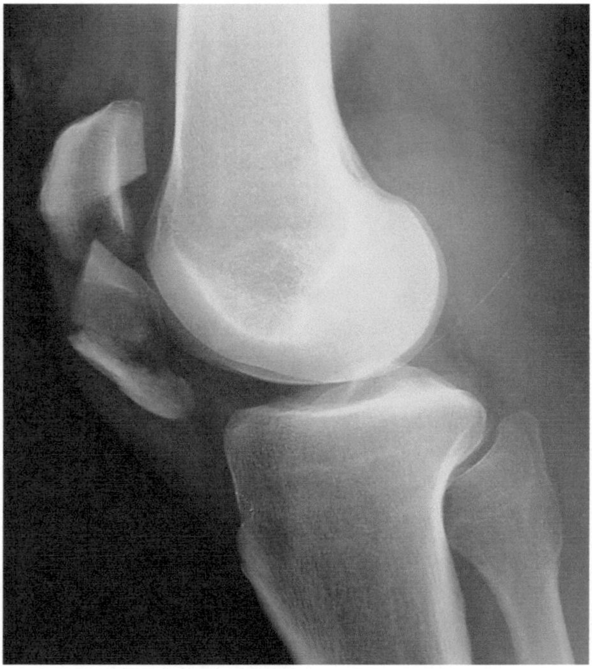

Fig. 34.6 Lateral knee X-ray showing a comminuted fracture of the patella

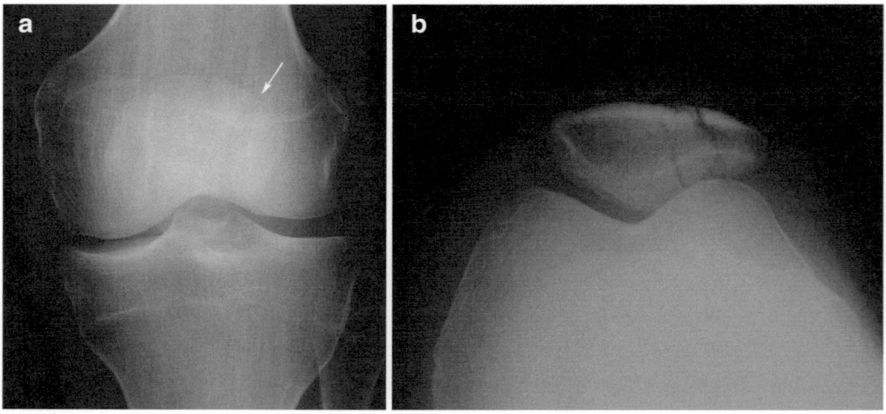

Fig. 34.7 (**a**) AP knee radiograph showing a sagittal fracture of the supero-lateral border of the patella. (**b**) Axial view ("sunrise" view) of the same knee as shown in Fig. **a** clearly showing the sagittal fracture of the lateral patellar edge

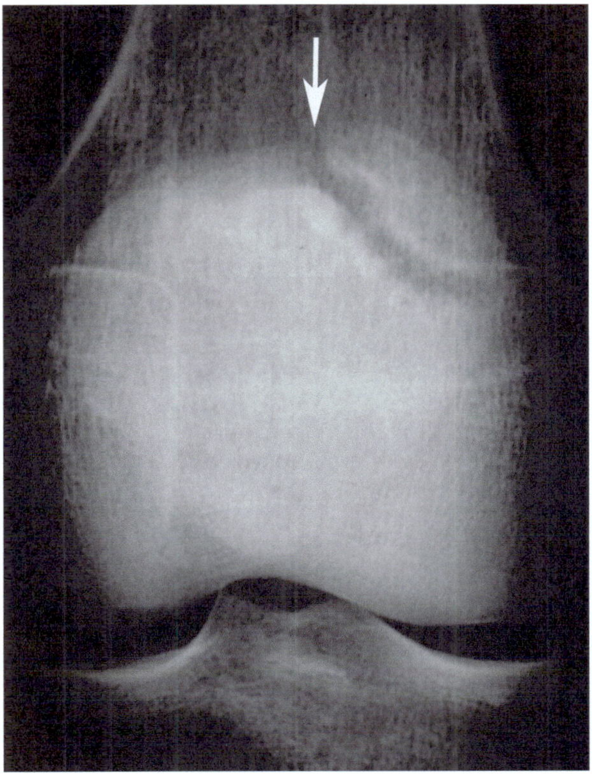

Fig. 34.8 AP knee radiograph with incidental finding of a "bipartite patella"

34.2 Assessment and Management

34.2.1 Distal Femur Fractures

- *Surgical consultation* is always requested regardless of the type of fracture.
- *Pre-operative CT scan (2D and 3D)* is very helpful for surgical planning in articular fractures.
- *Open reduction and internal fixation* is the gold standard treatment (Fig. 34.9).

34.2.2 Fractures of the Proximal Tibia (Tibial Plateau)

- *For displaced fractures* (split, depression, split-depression).
  - Pre-operative CT scan (2D and 3D) is required for surgical planning (Fig. 34.10).
  - Surgical treatment is indicated for reduction and internal fixation (Fig. 34.11a, b).

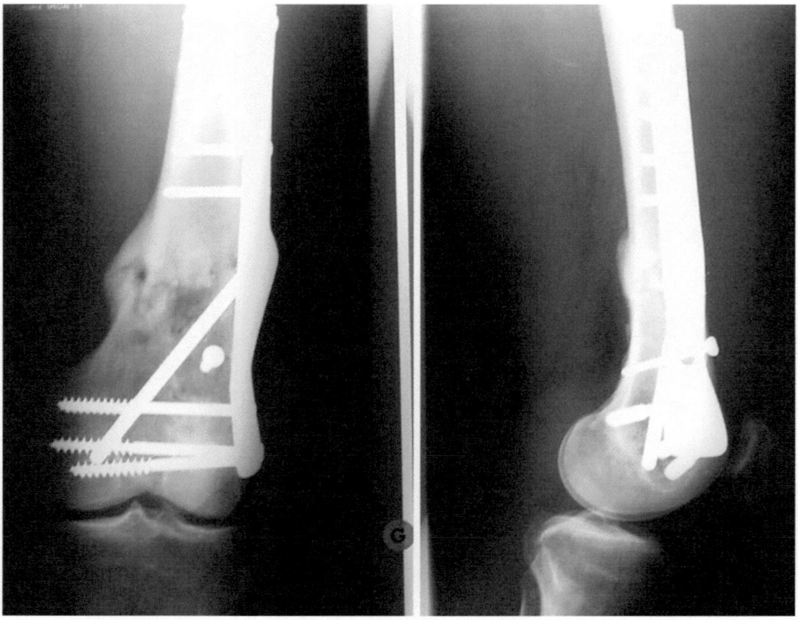

Fig. 34.9 AP and lateral distal femur radiographs of the same patient as shown in Fig. 34.2a, b (inter-condylar fracture) after treatment with open reduction and internal fixation using plate and screws

- *For undisplaced fractures*
  - Orthopedic treatment

    Removable knee brace with non-weight bearing for 45–90 days,

    Early rehabilitation for range of motion and muscular strengthening,

    Weekly radiographic control for the first 3 weeks followed by monthly control until complete fracture healing (usually 3 months).
  - Functional treatment: same scheme of treatment, without bracing.
- *For partial fractures*
  - Fractures of the tibial spines

    Undisplaced fractures: above knee cast or knee brace for 45 days.

    Displaced fractures: surgical reduction with internal fixation.
- Segond fracture (refer to ACL rupture).
- Fracture of the lateral margin of the lateral tibial plateau: orthopedic (cast/Brace) or functional treatment (after elimination of an ACL rupture by MRI).

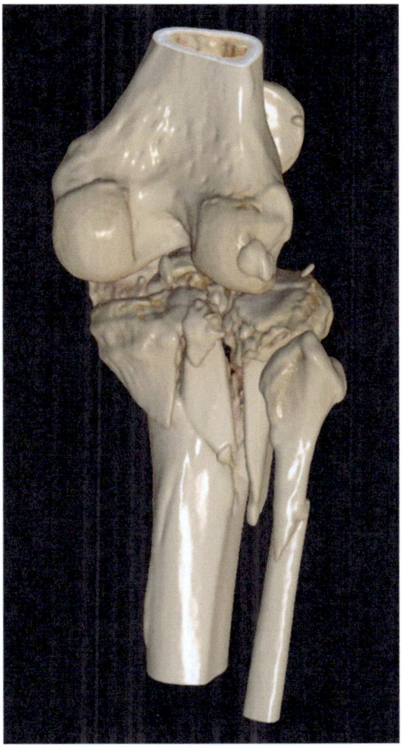

Fig. 34.10 3D CT-Scan of a comminuted bicondylar tibial plateau fracture

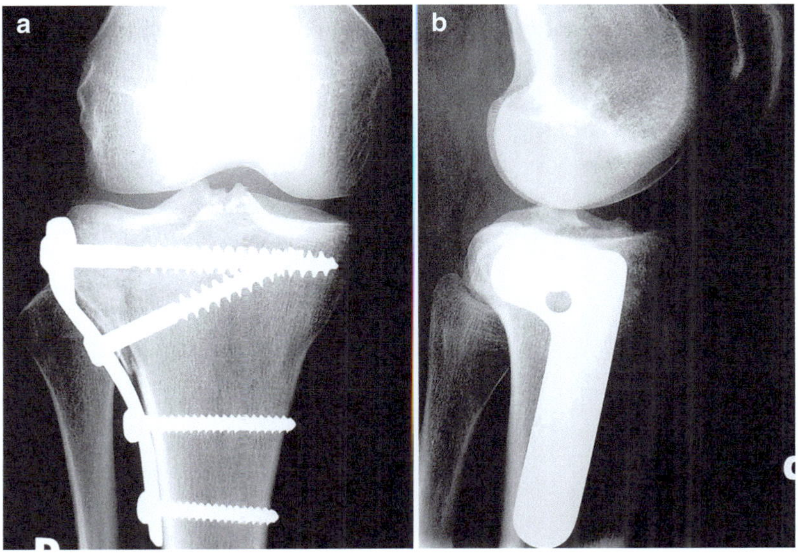

Fig. 34.11 3D CT scan of a comminuted bicondylar tibial plateau fracture. (**a**) AP knee radiograph of a right knee after open reduction and internal fixation of a lateral tibial plateau fracture with plate and screws. (**b**) Lateral knee radiograph of the same patient as shown in Fig. **a**

34.3 Fractures of the Patella

- *Transverse and complex fractures*
  - Displaced fractures: surgical treatment with open reduction and internal fixation (Fig. 34.12a, b).

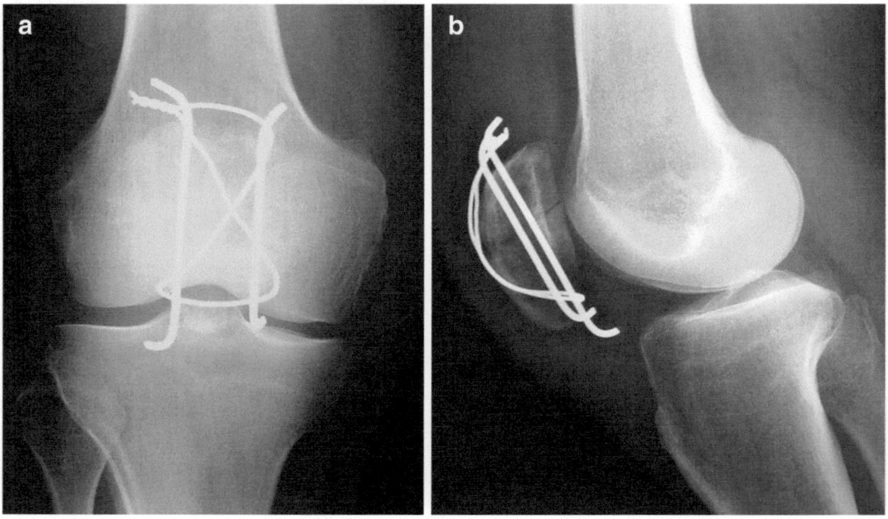

Fig. 34.12 (**a**) AP radiograph of the same knee as shown in Fig. 34.6 after open reduction and internal fixation of a patellar fracture using two pins and metallic wire ("figure of 8" construct). (**b**) Lateral radiograph of the same knee showing a "figure of 8" internal fixation of a patellar fracture

   - Undisplaced fractures: orthopedic treatment with cast immobilization for 45 days followed by rehabilitation (Fig. 34.13a, b).
- *Sagittal fractures*
   - Displaced fractures: surgical treatment with open reduction and internal fixation.
   - Undisplaced fractures: functional treatment (removable knee brace and rehabilitation).

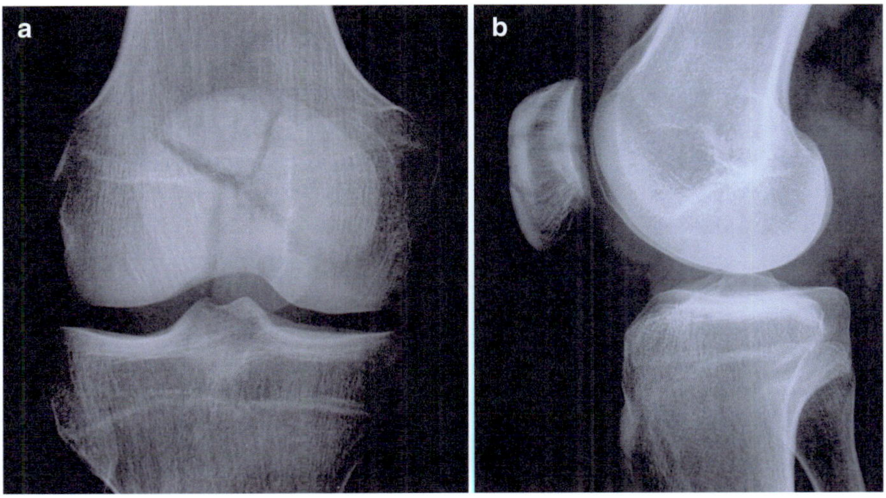

Fig. 34.13 (**a**) AP knee X-ray showing an undisplaced patella fracture. (**b**) Lateral knee X-ray showing an undisplaced patella fracture

35 Assessment of Acute Knee Trauma

Two situations should be distinguished:

- The knee is edematous, painful, with functional disability: radiographic assessment (AP and lateral views) of the knee should be first performed after neurovascular assessment and before any physical examination or testing of the knee joint.
- The knee is mildly painful, with moderate edema and minor functional impairment: the physical assessment and testing of the knee joint can be performed before the radiographic evaluation.

35.1 History

The following notions have to be made clear:

- Type and circumstances of the accident.
  - Road traffic?
  - Sports? Type of sport?
  - Work accident?
  - Domestic accident? etc.
- History of previous injuries to the knee
  - Sprain?
  - Surgery?
- Mechanism of injury
  - Direct impact?
  - Rotational injury?
  - Position of the knee during the accident (flexion, extension, hyperextension, hyperflexion)?

D. Saragaglia, A. Hassan Chamseddine, *Traumatology for the Emergency Doctor*, https://doi.org/10.1007/978-3-031-63196-2_35

- Initial symptoms during, and immediately following the accident
  - Intense, deep, or fainting pain,
  - Popping sound,
  - Immediate swelling,
  - Knee instability and giving way.

35.2 Physical Assessment

35.2.1 Inspection

Look for the presence of:

- Old surgical scar,
- Contusion, skin abrasion, ecchymosis, wound, etc. (Fig. 35.1),
- Knee swelling (effusion),
- Generalized knee edema,
- Posterior sagging of the anterior tibial tubercle when the knee is flexed at 70–80° (Fig. 35.2).
- Spontaneous antalgic flexion position of the knee.

35.2.2 Palpation

- *Patellar rebound* when the patella is pushed against the trochlea (also known as "patellar tap test" or "ballottement patellae": sign of knee joint effusion/hemarthrosis), (Fig. 35.3)
- *Localized tenderness*,
  - Medial collateral ligament (proximal femoral insertion, distal tibial insertion, mid-substance),
  - Lateral collateral ligament (proximal femoral insertion, distal fibular insertion, mid-substance),

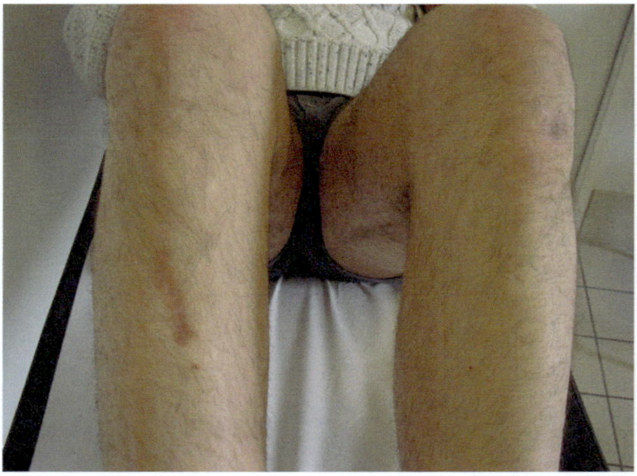

Fig. 35.1 Photo of both knees in a patient presenting with right knee issues. Notably, there is a skin scar on the anterior aspect of the right proximal tibia, likely resulting from direct impact, raising the possibility of a PCL rupture

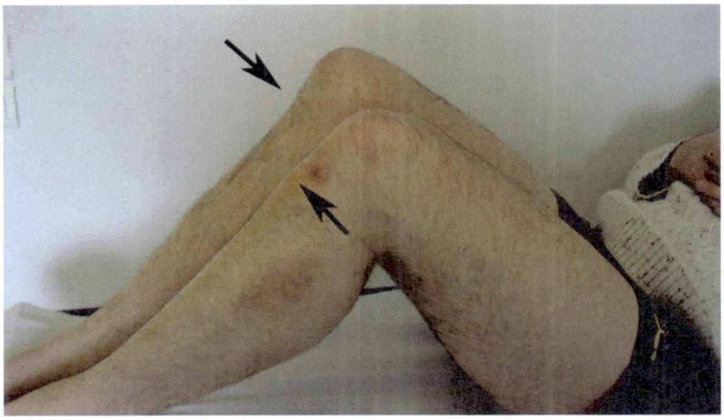

Fig. 35.2 Lateral photographic view of both knees of the same patient, showing the posterior sagging of the right knee's anterior tibial tubercle compared to the left, suggestive of PCL rupture

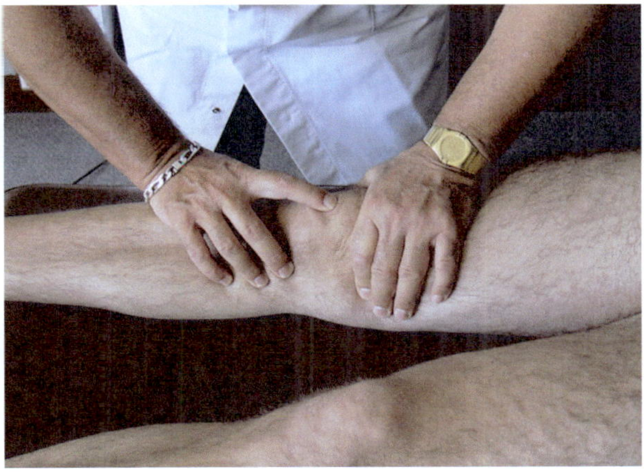

Fig. 35.3 Photo illustrating the technique for assessing patellar rebound or ballottement, in the diagnosis of knee effusion

- Medial and lateral joint line from back to front (Fig. 35.4),
- Medial patellar retinaculum and medial patellar edge,
- Popliteal fossa.

35.2.3 Testing for Knee Laxity (Comparative with the Opposite Side)

- **In knee extension position**
  - ***Testing for laxity in the frontal plane***

    Valgus laxity medial collateral ligament (MCL) and postero-medial corner injuries,

    Varus laxity indicates lateral collateral ligament (LCL) and postero-lateral corner injuries (variable degree involvement of the posterior insertion of the lateral meniscus, biceps femoris tendon, popliteus tendon, ilio-tibial band, lateral head of the Gastrocnemius).
  - ***Testing for laxity in the sagittal plane***

    Anterior drawer test close to the extension position (*Lachman test* at 10–20° knee flexion) (Fig. 35.5) indicates an ACL rupture,

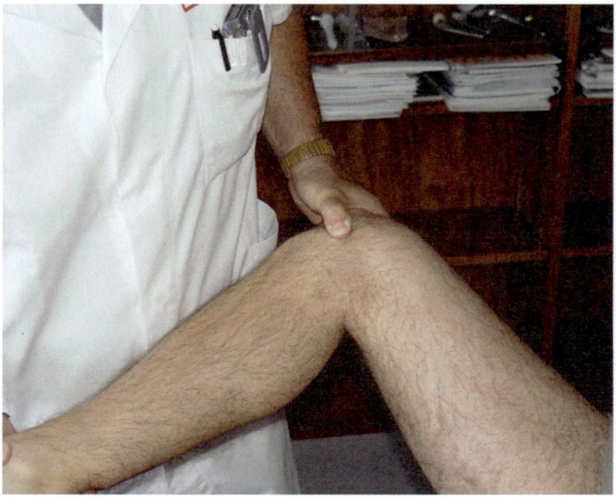

Fig. 35.4 Photo demonstrating palpation of the medial tibio-femoral joint line: painful palpation is highly indicative of a meniscal tear

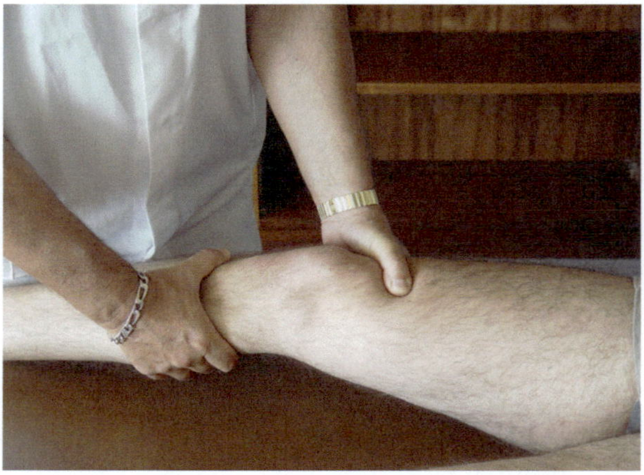

Fig. 35.5 Photo illustrating the technique for performing the Lachman test, which is used to diagnose an ACL rupture

External rotation recurvatum test of Hughston (Fig. 35.6) indicates injury to the postero-lateral corner (LCL + postero-lateral corner +/− biceps femoris tendon and ilio-tibial band).

- **In knee flexion position**
  - ***Testing in the frontal plane at 30° knee flexion***

    Valgus laxity indicates MCL injury (Fig. 35.7),

    Varus laxity indicates LCL injury (Fig. 35.8).
  - ***Testing in the sagittal plane at 70–80° knee flexion***

    Anterior drawer test (Fig. 35.9) in neutral and in external rotation of the foot, indicates ACL rupture associated with medial capsulo-ligamentous injury if the drawer is increased in external rotation position,

    Posterior drawer test indicates PCL rupture (attention not to misinterpret the posterior drawer as an anterior drawer because of pre-existing initial posterior sagging of the anterior tibial tubercle),

    Antero-posterior drawer of large amplitude indicates rupture of both ACL and PCL.

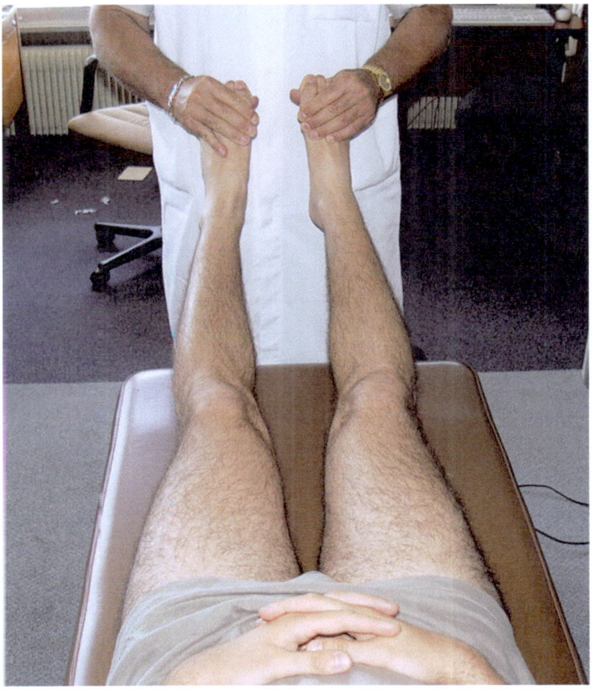

Fig. 35.6 Photo of the Hughston's recurvatum test, showing the left leg in hyperextension and external rotation compared to the right leg

35.2.4 Knee Specific Testing Maneuvers (Comparative with the Opposite Side)

- *Pivot shift test*: pathognomonic of ACL rupture. It can be performed in neutral, external, or internal rotation of the foot (Fig. 35.10).
- *Lelli's lever sign test* (less sensitive than Lachman test in emergency): it corresponds to placing a fulcrum under the proximal third of the patient's calf (in supine position) and applying a vertical force to the distal third of the thigh: When the ACL is intact the force applied over the distal thigh causes the heel to rise; when the ACL is damaged the force applied over the distal thigh causes an anterior translation of the tibia in relation to the femoral condyle, and the heel will not rise (Fig. 35.11).
- *Smilie test* (Fig. 35.12): it is a provocative test designed to identify a lateral patellar instability. The knee in full extension position, the examiner's thumb places a mediolateral force to the patella (pushing it into lateral dislocation) with simultaneous progressive flexion of the knee. A positive test corresponds to oral apprehension by the patient or an apprehensive quadriceps recruitment in response to the provocative maneuver.

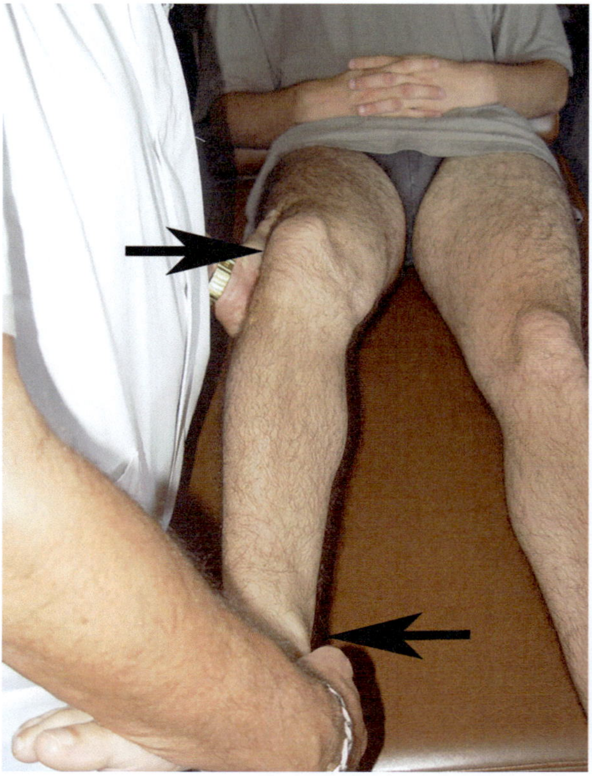

Fig. 35.7 Photo illustrating the test for medial knee laxity in the valgus-flexion position

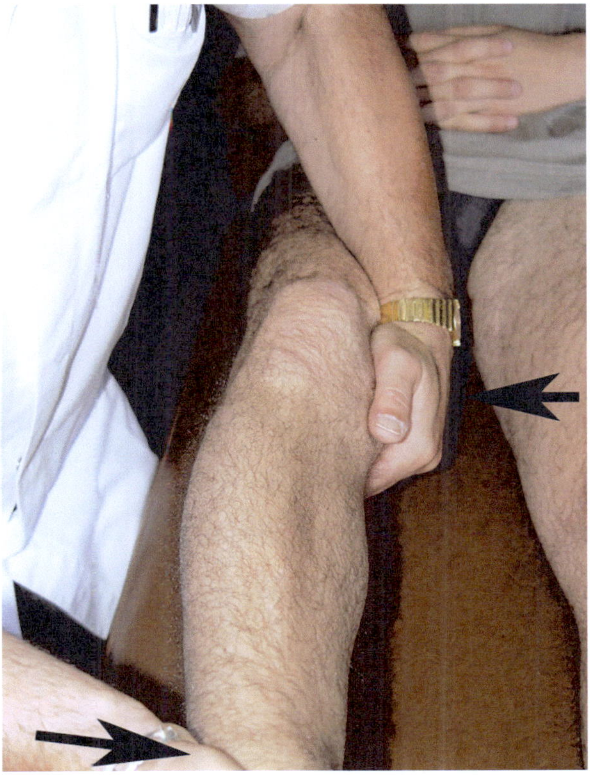

Fig. 35.8 Photo illustrating the test for lateral knee laxity in the varus-flexion position

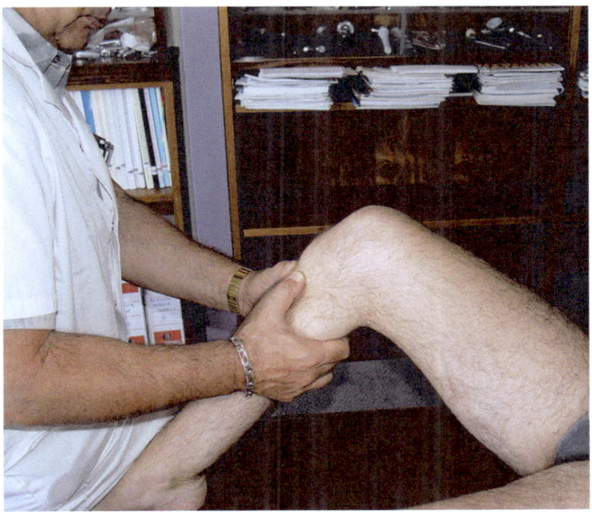

Fig. 35.9 Photo illustrating the anterior drawer test of the knee in the flexion position

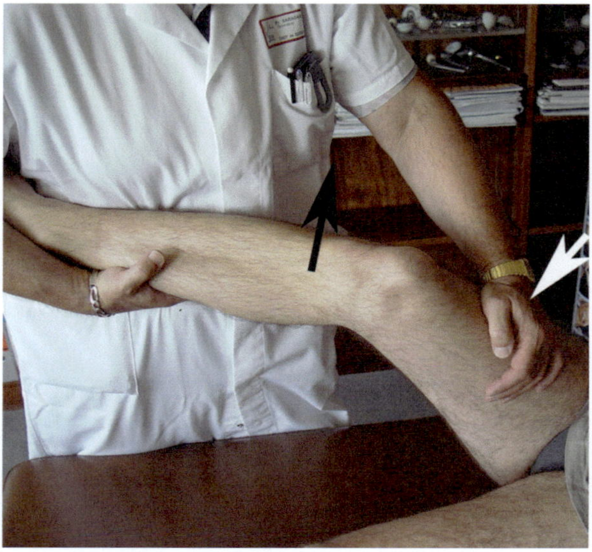

Fig. 35.10 Photo illustrating the technique for performing the Jerk test maneuver, which is used to diagnose an ACL rupture

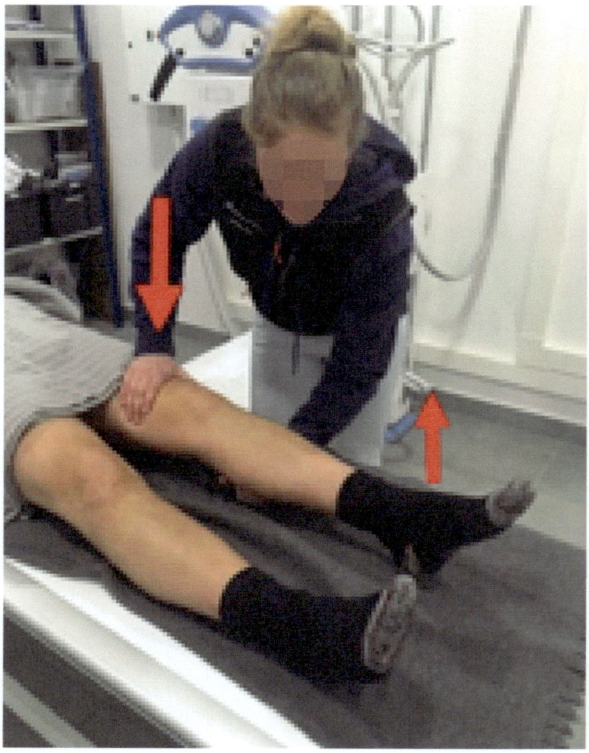

Fig. 35.11 Photo illustrating the technique for performing the Lelli's test, which is used to diagnose an ACL rupture

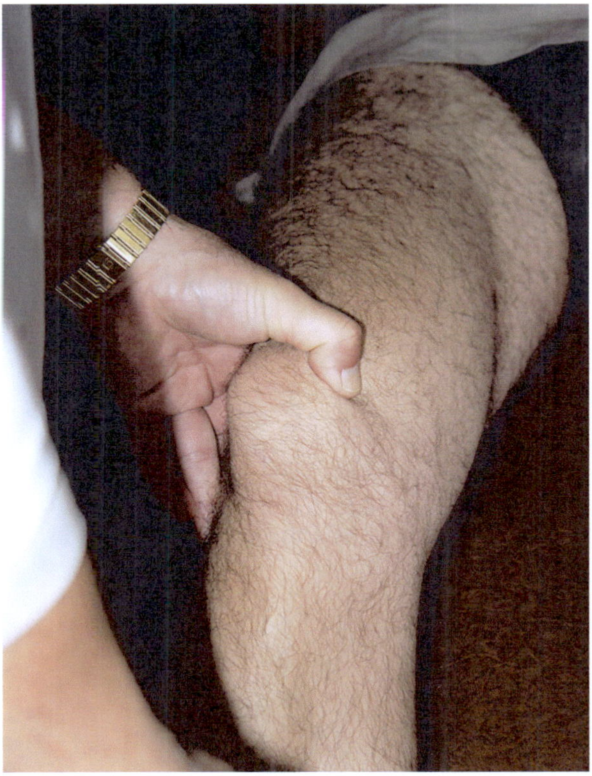

Fig. 35.12 Photo illustrating the technique for performing the Smilie provocative test, which is used to diagnose a lateral patellar instability

35.3 Radiographic Assessment

- Adequate ***standard radiographs of the knee are the primary indispensable*** step in the diagnostic process.
- The following views correspond to the basic trauma series: Antero-posterior, axial (at 30° knee flexion), lateral (at 30° knee flexion), and external and internal oblique.
- The following radiographic images may be seen:
  - Early osteoarthritic changes,
  - Femoro-trochlear dysplasia,
  - Fracture-avulsion of the tibial spines,
  - Segond fracture,
  - Femoral condyle osteochondritis,
  - Tibial plateau fracture (split, compression),
  - Incidental finding of bone tumor.

Traumatic Dislocation of the Patella

36

The large majority of patellar dislocations are secondary to trochlear dysplasia (more than 80% of cases). The injury usually occurs after a valgus-external rotation traumatic mechanism (90% of cases). This entity is different from the injury entitled "knee dislocation" which is discussed separately.

36.1 Diagnosis

Two presentations are possible:

36.1.1 The Patient Presents with the Patella in Dislocated Position

- The diagnosis is obvious with,
  - The patella lying on the lateral aspect of the lateral femoral condyle (Fig. 36.1),
  - The knee is in spontaneous position of 30–45° flexion.
- The ER physician should,
  - Relocate the patella by applying a gentle extension to the knee, with a concomitant direct latero-medial force to the patella,
  - Look for any suspicious radiographic signs after prescribing the appropriate radiographic views (antero-posterior, strict lateral, and axial both at 30° flexion):

    Trochlear dysplasia (Fig. 36.2a, b),

    Avulsion of the medial border of the patella (medial retinaculum) (Fig. 36.3),

    Intra-articular loose body (osteochondral sleeve fracture of the posterior aspect of the patella or the anterior aspect of the lateral condyle) (Fig. 36.4).

D. Saragaglia, A. Hassan Chamseddine, *Traumatology for the Emergency Doctor*, https://doi.org/10.1007/978-3-031-63196-2_36

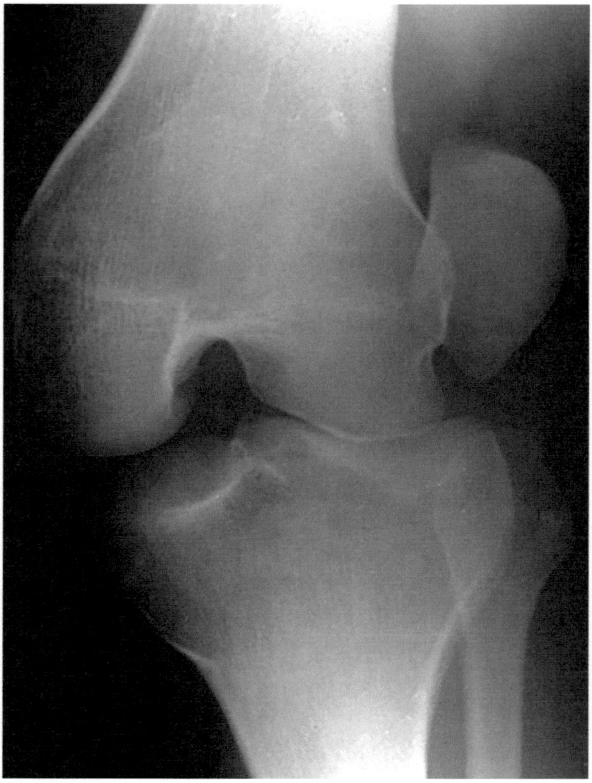

Fig. 36.1 AP knee X-ray demonstrating lateral patellar dislocation with the patella located at the lateral aspect of the lateral femoral condyle

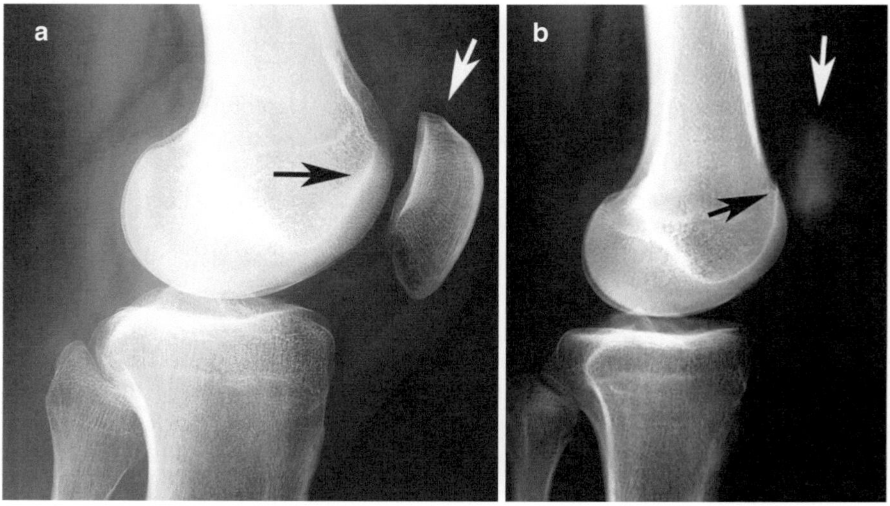

Fig. 36.2 (**a**) Strict lateral knee view showing a normal presentation of the femoro-patellar joint. Note the parallelism between the trochlear groove line and the anterior borders of the lateral and medial femoral condyles, as well as the rectangular shape of the patella. (**b**) Strict lateral knee radiograph revealing a dysplastic proximal pole of the trochlear groove, indicated by a "crossing sign," along with a lateral tilt of the patella, presenting an oval shape

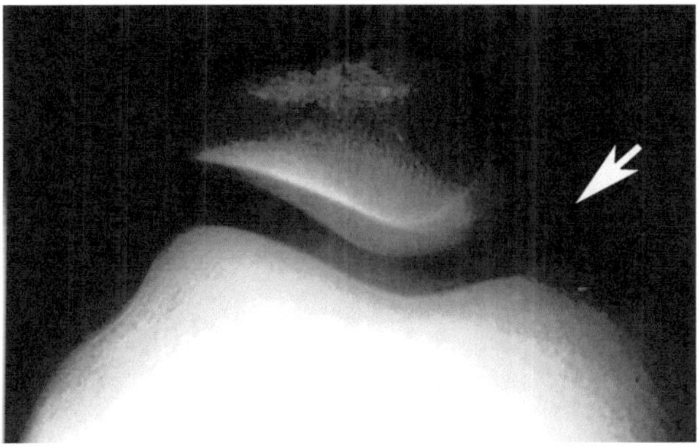

Fig. 36.3 Axial knee X-ray showing a bony avulsion of the medial retinaculum

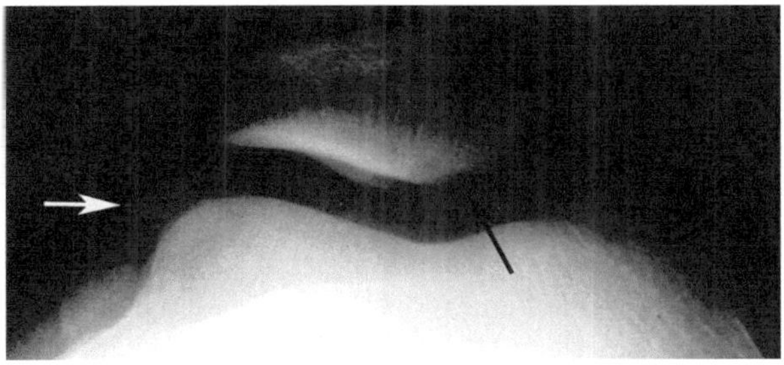

Fig. 36.4 Axial knee X-ray showing an osteochondral fracture of the crest of the patella with a loose fragment located at the anterolateral aspect of the lateral femoral condyle

36.1.2 The Patient Presents after the Patella Has Been Reduced

- The diagnosis is more difficult.
  - The knee joint is edematous,
  - Presence of a *patellar rebound* (sign of knee hemarthrosis),
  - *Presence of an Ecchymosis* of the medial aspect of the knee,
  - *Presence of a Tenderness* of the medial retinaculum and the medial patellar edge,
  - *Negative physical exam* for laxity (varus, valgus, Lachman, anterior drawer, etc.).
- The *radiographic assessment is fundamental* and includes the same radiographic views as in the previous paragraph, with the same radiographic potential findings (Figs. 36.3 and 36.4).

36.2 Assessment and Management

- Ask for the appropriate radiographic views (as previous) in order not to miss the right diagnosis.
- ***Ask for an MRI***
  - It serves in confirming the diagnosis.

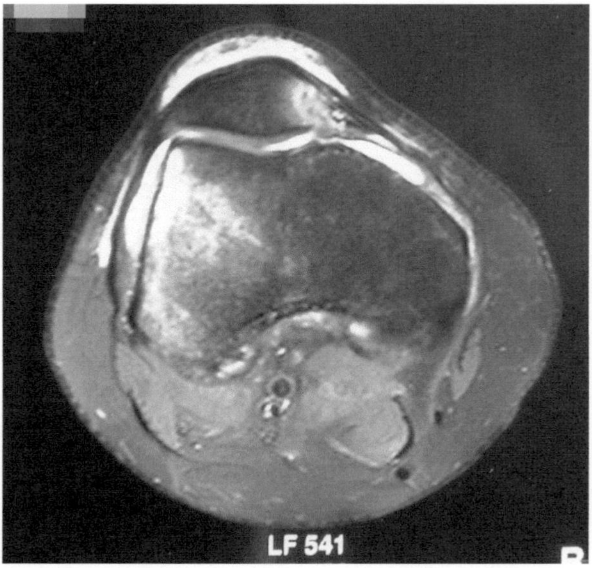

Fig. 36.5 Axial cut of knee MRI revealing an osteochondral bruise of the medial aspect of the articular patellar surface

- It may show the subtle signs of patellar dislocation:
  Sub-chondral intra-osseous edema (contusion) of the medial patellar facet and border (Fig. 36.5) and the anterior aspect of the lateral condyle (Fig. 36.6),
  Intra-articular osteochondral loose fragment (Figs. 36.7 and 36.8).

- A few days period of knee immobilization using a removable knee brace is prescribed (strict and long-term knee immobilization in extension may be harmful: fibrous scar healing of the medial retinaculum, atrophy of the quadriceps muscle).
- ***Early rehabilitation is preferred*** (8 days after the accident), with the use of a patellar brace (Fig. 36.9), analgesics, and NSAIDs:
  - Quadriceps muscle strengthening,
  - Proprioceptive rehabilitation,
  - Early full weight bearing as tolerated with the use of two crutches for the first 10–15 days.
- Early surgical treatment is only discussed to remove or to fix an incarcerated intra-articular osteochondral fragment that may bother or disturb the progression of the rehabilitation program (Fig. 36.8).
- *In case of recurrent instability*, an elaborated radiographic assessment (CT scan) is requested (with evaluation of the trochlear dysplasia and measurement of the distance anterior tibial tubercle-trochlear groove) in order to consider a potential surgical treatment.

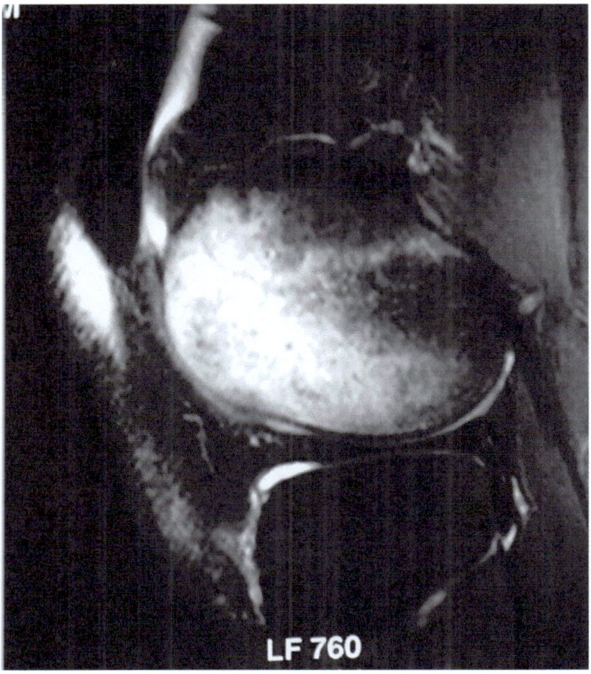

Fig. 36.6 Sagittal cut of knee MRI revealing an osteochondral post-traumatic bruise of the lateral femoral condyle

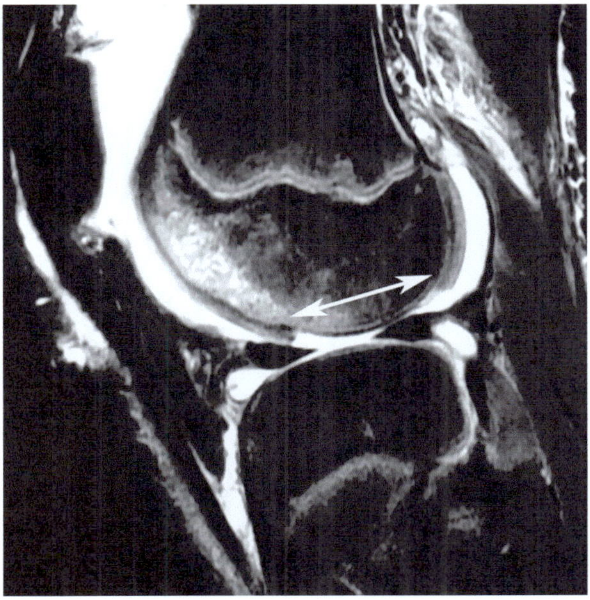

Fig. 36.7 Sagittal cut of knee MRI revealing a significant osteochondral post-traumatic defect of the lateral femoral condyle

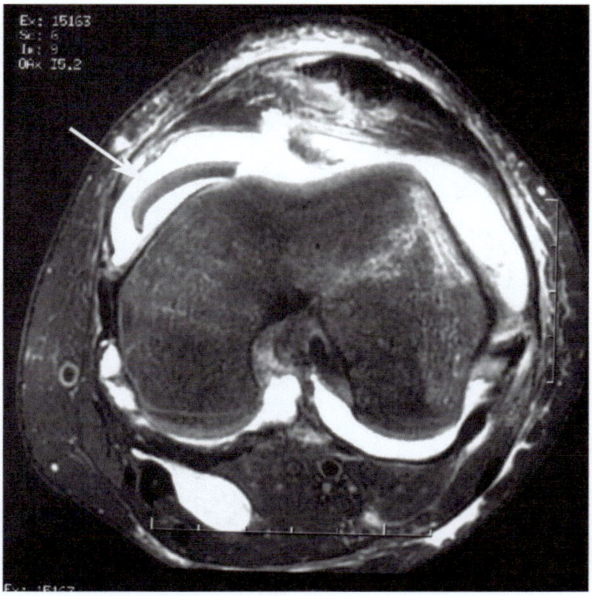

Fig. 36.8 Axial cut of knee MRI revealing an intra-articular osteochondral loose fragment (same patient as in Fig. 36.7)

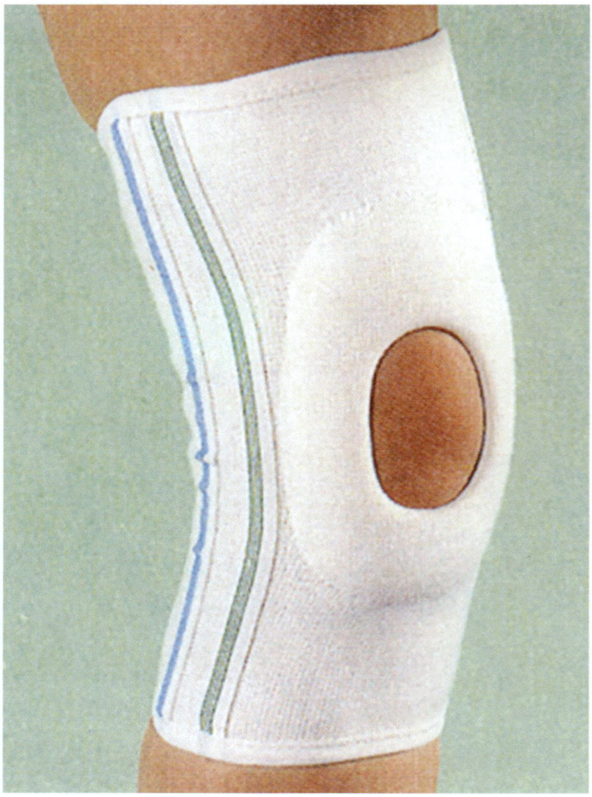

Fig. 36.9 Photo of a patellar knee brace (with an anterior patellar window)

37 Knee Dislocations

37.1 Patho-Anatomy

Knee dislocations are described and named according to the direction of displacement of the tibia in relation to the femur.

37.1.1 Anterior Dislocations (Fig. 37.1)

- Frequent: 30–40%.
- Associated vascular injuries are common (up to 40%).
- Rupture of both the ACL and the PCL is common; the PCL remains rarely intact.
- Mechanism
  - Knee hyperextension.
  - Direct postero-anterior trauma to the posterior aspect of the proximal tibia (less common).

37.1.2 Posterior Dislocations

- As common as the anterior dislocations.
- Popliteal artery injuries are frequent (up to 40%).
- Rupture of both the ACL and the PCL is common; the ACL remains rarely intact.
- Mechanism: direct antero-posterior trauma to the anterior aspect of the proximal tibia (tibial tubercle).

37.1.3 Lateral and Medial Dislocations (Figs. 37.2a, b and 37.3a, b)

- Less common than the anterior and posterior types, except in skiing accidents.

D. Saragaglia, A. Hassan Chamseddine, *Traumatology for the Emergency Doctor*, https://doi.org/10.1007/978-3-031-63196-2_37

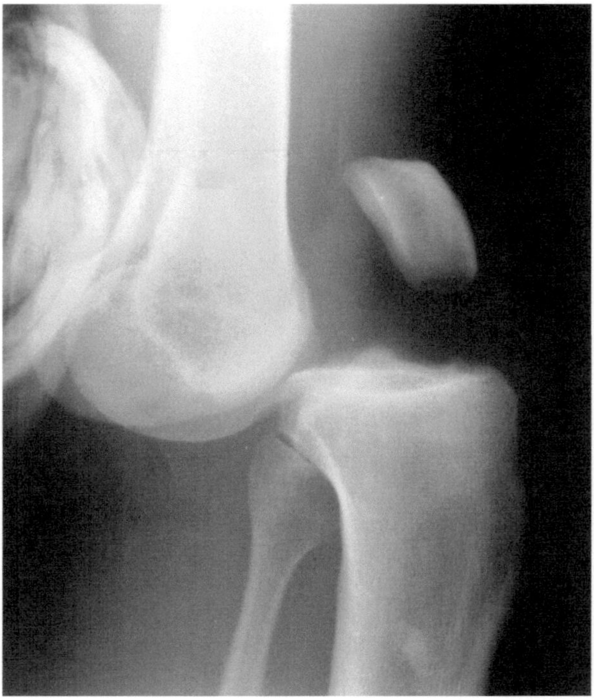

Fig. 37.1 Lateral knee X-ray demonstrating an anterior knee dislocation

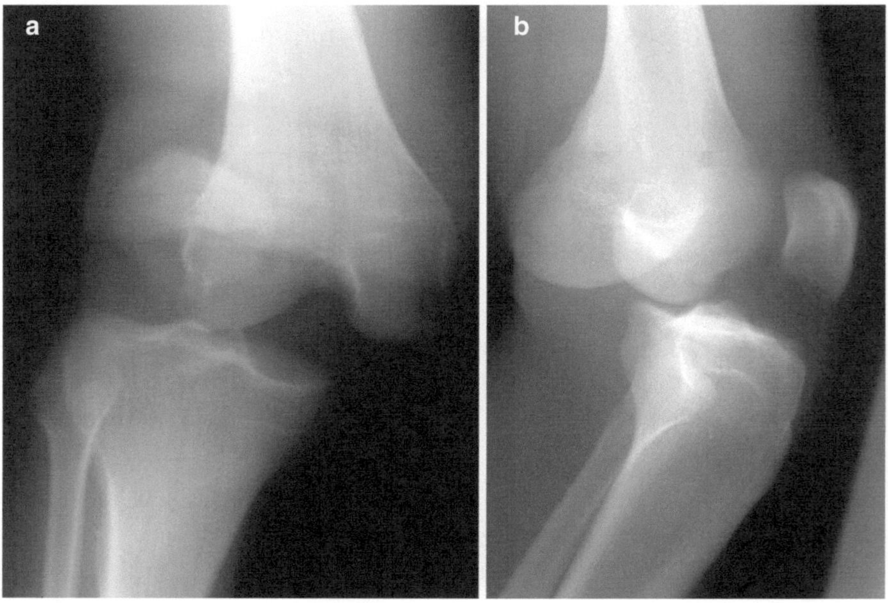

Fig. 37.2 (**a**) AP knee X-ray demonstrating an anterolateral knee dislocation. (**b**) Lateral knee X-ray demonstrating an anterolateral knee dislocation

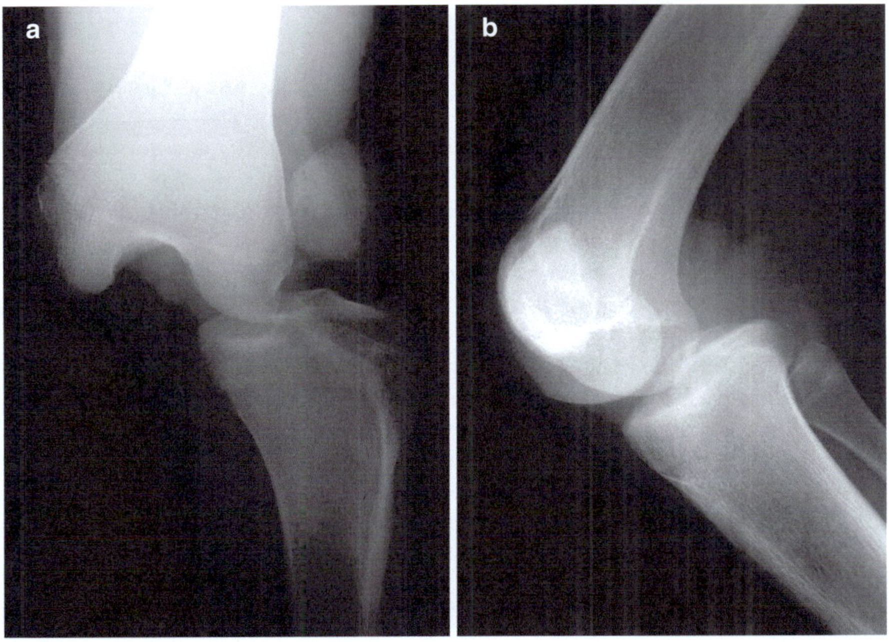

Fig. 37.3 (**a**) AP knee radiograph demonstrating a posterolateral knee dislocation. (**b**) Lateral knee radiograph demonstrating a posterolateral knee dislocation

- Vascular injuries are rare (5–20%) especially in low-energy trauma, in opposition to high energy trauma.
- They encompass ruptures of the ACL, PCL, and the peripheral medial or lateral capsulo-ligamentous structures.
- The mechanism of injury is usually a direct choc applied to the medial or lateral aspect of the knee.

37.1.4 Rotatory Dislocations

- These are rare (5% of all knee dislocations).
- They involve multidirectional laxity.
- Mechanism
  - Valgus-external rotation: anterolateral and posterolateral dislocations,
  - Varus-internal rotation: anteromedial and posteromedial dislocations.
- Associated vascular injuries are less common than in medial and lateral dislocations.
- They involve ruptures of the ACL, PCL, and the peripheral medial and lateral capsulo-ligamentous injuries.

37.2 Assessment and Management

- Relocate and realign the lower limb (general anesthesia is necessary for anterior and posterior dislocations).
- Assess the vascularity of the lower limb: posterior tibialis and dorsalis pedius pulses, capillary refill, venous return.
- Assess the neurologic condition of the lower limb (common fibular nerve).
- ***Ask for an orthopedic surgery opinion***
- ***If associated vascular injuries: ask for a vascular surgery opinion***
  - Urgent arteriography (after closed reduction of the dislocation),
  - Vascular repair in emergency (first 6 h),
  - The repair of the ligamentous injuries is delayed (not urgent).
- ***In the absence of initial vascular injuries*** (Fig. 37.4).
  - Assess for any latent ongoing vascular injury: arterial Doppler, *angio-scan.*
  - *MRI* for a more precise diagnosis of the capsulo-ligamentous injuries,
  - Delayed ligamentous reconstructive surgery after full assessment.
  - In some cases, orthopedic treatment may lead to good functional results.

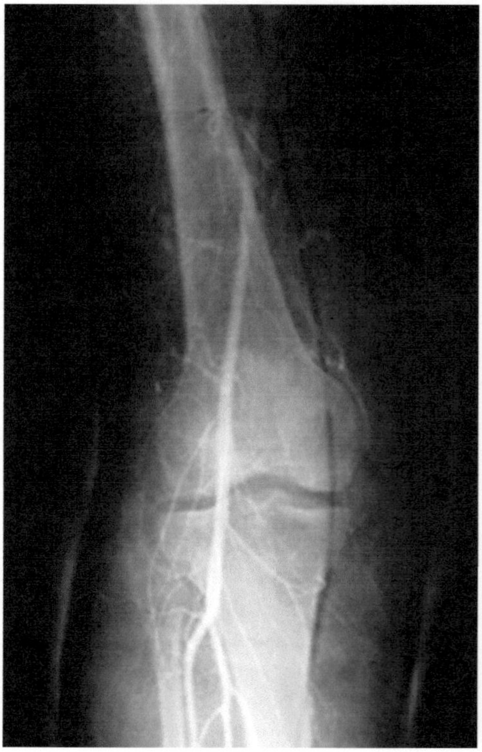

Fig. 37.4 Lower limb arteriogram labeled as "normal," performed urgently after closed reduction and prior to the final surgical treatment of a knee dislocation

Knee Trauma with "Normal" Radiographs 38

We only find what we look for, and we only look for what we know

This chapter intends to give an overview of knee assessment after a traumatic injury with a normal radiographic presentation. The traumatic injury may be secondary to either direct impact or indirect mechanism, i.e., sprain. The aim is to provide a clinical diagnostic orientation with a therapeutic guidance.

An "apparently" simple knee trauma may result in serious injuries to the ligaments and menisci, according to different isolated patterns and variable associated modes.

38.1 Ligamentous Injuries

Ligamentous injuries are the direct anatomo-clinical manifestations of "knee sprains." They are frequent in some sports such as football, basketball, rugby, and skiing, to name a few. They are usually secondary to an indirect trauma which associates variable combinations of varus/valgus and external/internal rotation or twist. Direct trauma to the medial, lateral, anterior, or posterior aspect of the knee may also result in ligamentous injuries. The lesion may affect one or more ligaments, with or without meniscal tear, according to the mechanism and severity of the accident. The diagnosis of these injuries should be made at early stage to avoid secondary progression into chronic instability with more severe and complicated prognosis.

38.1.1 Isolated Medial Collateral Ligament (MCL) Injury

- ***Mechanism***
  - Forced knee valgus in mild flexion and external rotation,
  - Direct trauma to the lateral aspect of the knee in fixed valgus position.

D. Saragaglia, A. Hassan Chamseddine, *Traumatology for the Emergency Doctor*, https://doi.org/10.1007/978-3-031-63196-2_38

- ***Diagnosis***
  - Presentation
    Pain at the medial aspect of the knee,
    Painful and difficult walk with weight bearing.
  - Physical exam
    Tenderness of the medial aspect of the knee joint (along the course of the MCL, especially at the proximal femoral insertion),
    Medial joint line laxity (valgus laxity) as compared to the opposite side, with more important laxity for more severe injury (superficial and deep MCL).
    Negative anterior drawer and Lachman test,
    Negative Jerk test.
- ***Imaging***
  - *Radiographs*: Normal.
  - *MRI*
    Is the best diagnostic tool,
    It identifies the site of injury (usually proximal),
    It discloses other potential associated injuries (meniscus, ACL, etc.).
- ***Differential diagnosis***
  - Medial meniscus tear,
  - Patellar dislocation with spontaneous reduction,
  - Knee contusion.
- ***Management***
  - Knee brace for 4–6 weeks associated with early rehabilitation to *avoid knee flessum* and stiffness and to restore the range of motion,
  - Avoid knee strapping: risk of irreducible antalgic knee flessum position.
  - Surgical treatment is rarely indicated.

38.1.2 Central Pivot Injuries Involving at Least the ACL (Anterior Cruciate Ligament)

38.1.2.1 Isolated ACL Tear

The term isolated ACL tear corresponds to an ACL injury without associated "peripheral" ligamentous injuries, such as injury to the MCL, or the LCL. The injury pattern can be either a "pure" ACL injury or associated with meniscal tear.

1. ***History***
   (a) Audible pop with severe pain at the moment of accident,
   (b) Immediate inability to continue the ongoing activity,
   (c) "Giving way" or sensation of knee instability when walking with weight bearing,
   (d) Immediate or rapid knee swelling,
   (e) Possible early limitation of knee range of motion.
2. ***Physical examination*** (for more details refer to Chap. 35 "assessment of acute knee trauma")

(a) Tenderness on knee palpation (usual posterolateral point of maximal tenderness),
(b) Patellar rebound or ballottement (sign of knee joint effusion/hemarthrosis),
(c) Absence of any peripheral laxities in varus–valgus stress,
(d) Negative anterior drawer test at 70–80° of knee flexion,
(e) Positive signs for ACL tear:
   - *Lachman test* (anterior drawer test close to extension position, at 10–20° knee flexion),
   - *Lelli test*,
   - *Jerk test* or pivot shift test.

3. ***Differential diagnosis includes***
   (a) LCL sprain: very rare isolated injury pattern,
   (b) Medial and or lateral meniscal tears: these can occur as isolated injuries or associated to an ACL rupture (see paragraph "meniscal injuries" below). Tenderness of the medial or lateral joint line is the most sensitive sign especially when it is associated with a painful deficit of complete active extension, and lack of the final degrees of passive extension, with feeling of "elastic" resistance (meniscal flap interposition, bucket handle tear, meniscal extrusion, etc.).
   (c) Traumatic patellar dislocation (see Chap. 36 "Traumatic dislocation of the patella").
   (d) Knee contusion: painful knee with negative physical exam findings.
4. ***Imaging***
   (a) ***Radiographic assessment*** includes AP, lateral, axial, and oblique views.
   - It is usually normal.
   - It may demonstrate,
     - A "*Segond fracture*" (Fig. 38.1) in 5–10% of cases, usually associated to ACL rupture (small extra-articular bone avulsion at the lateral aspect of the lateral tibial plateau),
     - A *fracture-avulsion of the tibial spines* (Fig. 38.2) in 5–10% of cases (distal ACL footprint insertion),
     - An *Image of notch in the lateral condyle* on the lateral view. When it is more than 5 mm deep, it indicates an ACL rupture (Fig. 38.3).
   - It serves to eliminate other pathologies such as tibial plateau fractures, trochlear dysplasia (usually associated to femoro-patellar dislocation), etc.

   (b) ***MRI assessment***
   - It confirms the presence of the ACL tear, (Fig. 38.4)
   - It discloses the presence of potential associated injuries (menisci, bone bruise, etc.),
   - It is not requested in emergency, as the ACL surgical reconstruction is not an urgent procedure.
5. ***Early management***
   (a) Knee brace for 7–10 days,
   (b) Painkillers, with or without NSAIDs,

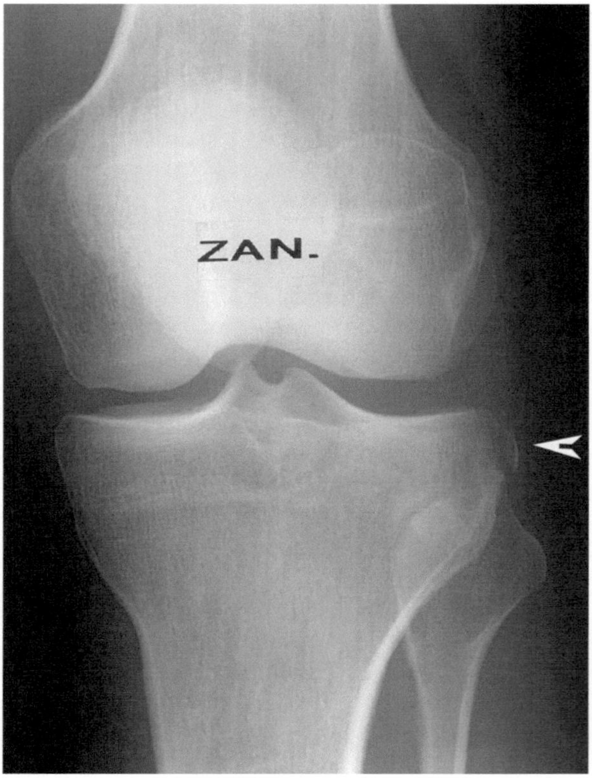

Fig. 38.1 AP knee radiograph revealing a "Segond fracture"

(c) DVT prevention according to the patient's individual risk factors,
(d) Early rehabilitation program for restoration of the range of motion and strengthening of the quadriceps and hamstrings,
(e) Knee reassessment after 10 days (after decrease of the knee effusion and pain). This may involve radiographic views in stress using a Telos^{R} stress device with measurement of the anterior translation of the proximal tibia under the distal femur on the lateral knee view, compared to the opposite side (Fig. 38.5).

6. ***Treatment***
   (a) The treatment is almost always surgical in young and active patients.
   (b) The timing of repair is usually delayed for 2–3 months in order to restore the range of motion and to strengthen the quadriceps and the hamstrings, as well as to decrease the risk of post-operative potential complications (stiffness, algodystrophy, and arthrofibrosis). This period can be shortened for professional or high-level athletes or in case of meniscal tear (bucket handle).
   (c) Fracture-avulsion of the tibial spines may benefit from an urgent surgical treatment (especially when there is a displaced large fragment). Early specialized opinion is therefore required.

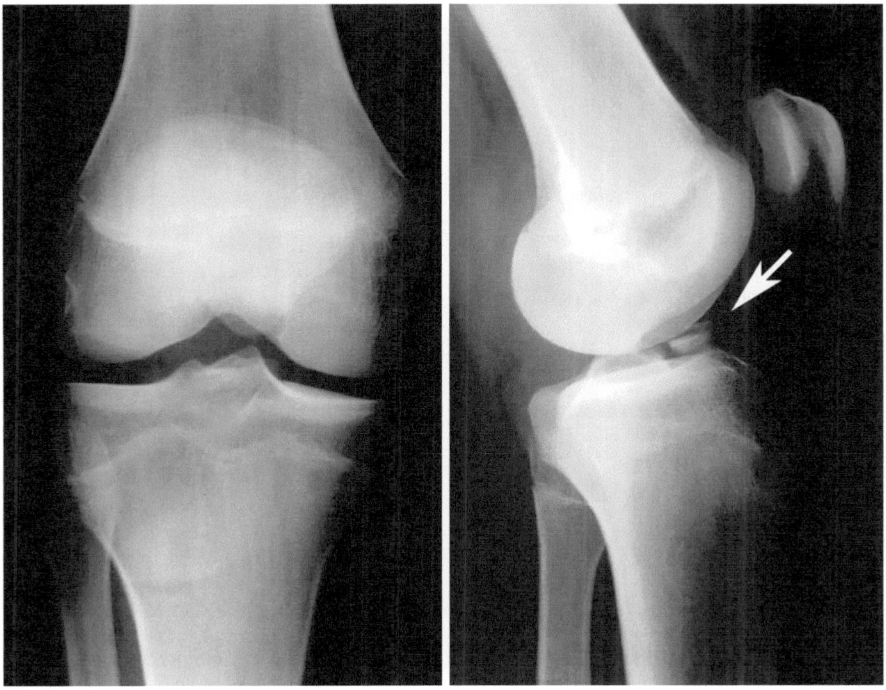

Fig. 38.2 AP and lateral knee views revealing a fracture-avulsion of the tibial spines

38.1.2.2 Associated ACL and "Peripheral" Ligamentous Injuries

Different types of ACL sprains are distinguished by the clinical evaluation and by the associated injuries, with several degrees of increasing severity. In many situations, the elaboration of the final appropriate diagnosis is based on the MRI findings and the physical examination performed under anesthesia. These injuries should be managed in collaboration with an orthopedic surgeon who is competent in sports and knee surgery.

- ***Antero-medial sprains***
  - These involve associated injuries to the ACL and the medial capsulo-ligamentous structures.
  - The clinical presentation corresponds to:

    Medial laxity in knee valgus-flexion and or valgus-extension stress (according to the involvement of the posteromedial corner),

    Positive Lachman test,

    Positive Lelli test,

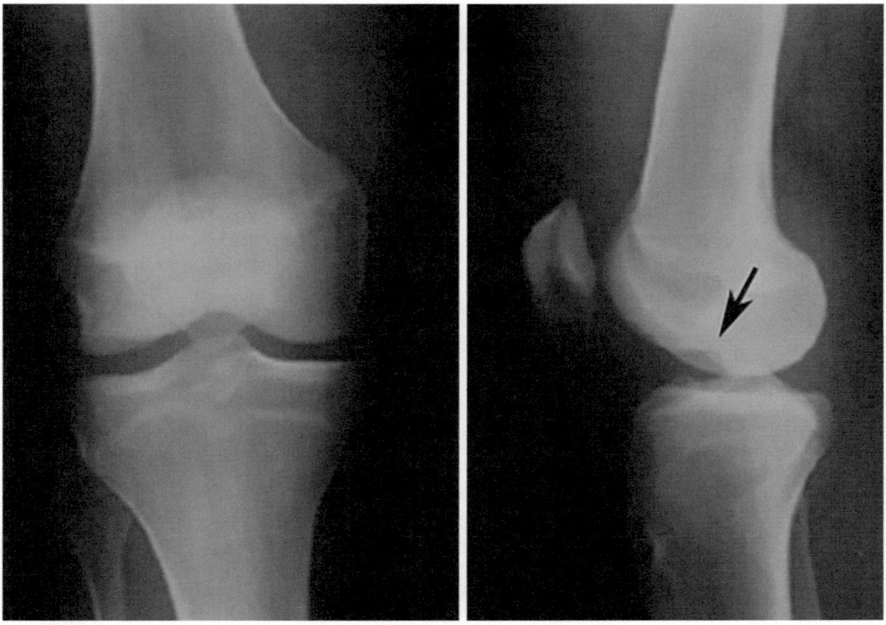

Fig. 38.3 AP and lateral knee views revealing an impaction of the lateral condyle (notching), indicative of an ACL rupture

Fig. 38.4 Sagittal cut of knee MRI showing an ACL rupture

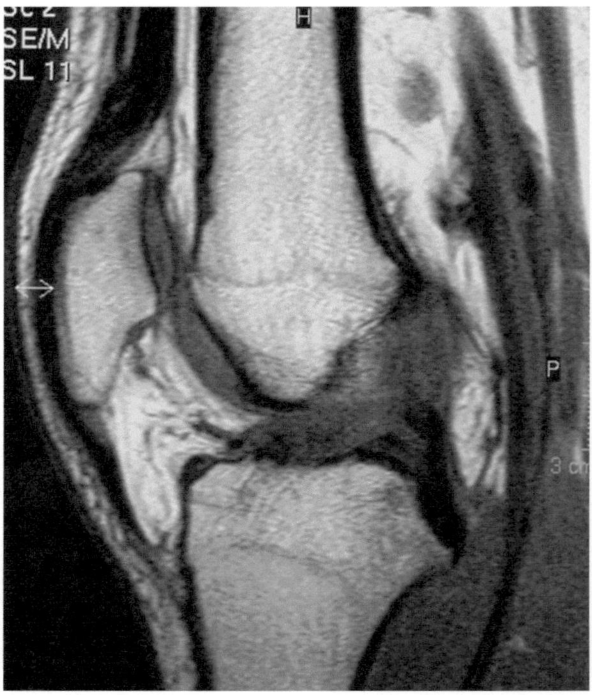

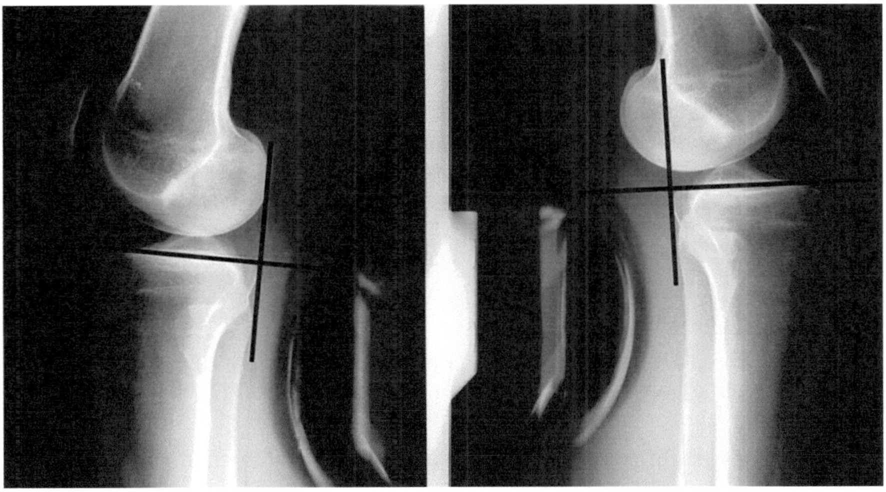

Fig. 38.5 Bilateral comparative lateral knee stress radiographs using the Telos^R stress device showing a significant anterior shift of the proximal tibia beneath the distal femur on the right knee compared to the left side

Positive anterior drawer test (70–80° of knee flexion), increased in external rotation position of the foot.
Positive Jerk test (may be lessened by the occurrence of a medial laxity—-medial joint line opening—during the test).

- ***Antero-lateral sprains***
  - These involve associated injuries to the ACL and the lateral capsulo-ligamentous structures.
  - The clinical presentation corresponds to:
    Lateral laxity in knee varus-flexion and or varus-extension stress (according to the involvement of the posterolateral capsulo-ligamentous structures—LCL, popliteal tendon, biceps femori tendon, postero-lateral corner, etc.),
    Positive Hughston recurvatum test,
    Positive anterior drawer test (70–80° of knee flexion), increased in internal rotation position of the foot,
    Positive Lachman test,
    Positive Lelli test,
    Positive Jerk test.

38.1.2.3 Combined ACL–PCL Tears

These involve rupture of both the ACL and the PCL, associated with injury to either the medial or lateral capsulo-ligamentous structures, or both. They should be considered as "aborted" or incomplete knee dislocations, and should be managed as such (refer to Chap. 37 "Knee dislocations").

38.1.2.4 General Guidelines for the Management of Associated ACL and "Peripheral" Ligamentous Injuries

These injuries commonly lead to serious knee disability, imposing a substantial burden on the daily living activities, especially for young, active, and athletic patients. Since associated "peripheral" injuries are often difficult to manage at a late stage, early diagnosis and prompt treatment of these injuries are of primary importance.

The author's preferred diagnostic scheme is as follows:

- *Adequate radiographic assessment* is a must for elimination of any potential fractures,
- *An MRI* should be considered a virtually urgent exam, in contrast to other situations with "isolated ACL tear".

The author's preferred algorithm of treatment is the following:

- Urgent surgical repair in case of "peripheral" mediolateral laxity that occurs in knee extension position,
- Conservative orthopedic treatment (cast for 45 days) in case of "peripheral" mediolateral laxity that occurs in knee flexion position and disappears in extension position. Secondary ACL reconstruction is performed depending on the patient's situation, such as the extent of knee instability or the additional knee injuries.
- Urgent surgical repair for combined ACL–PCL ruptures (refer to Chap. 37).

38.1.3 Posterior Cruciate Ligament (PCL) Tears

They can be categorized as isolated PCL tears, and PCL tears associated with peripheral injuries (MCL, LCL). These types of injuries are relatively rare, especially in sports practice, and can be easily overlooked in an emergency setting. Misdiagnosing a PCL injury is unfortunate, as this lesion may heal with a simple well conducted conservative orthopedic treatment when diagnosed early.

38.1.3.1 Isolated PCL Tears

- ***Elements of positive diagnosis***
  - Common history of *antero-posterior impact* applied to the anterior aspect of the proximal tibia, e.g., the anterior tibial tubercle (50%),
  - Pain in the popliteal fossa,
  - Positive patellar ballottement or patella tap sign (Knee effusion, i.e., hemarthrosis),
  - Negative varus–valgus stress laxity,

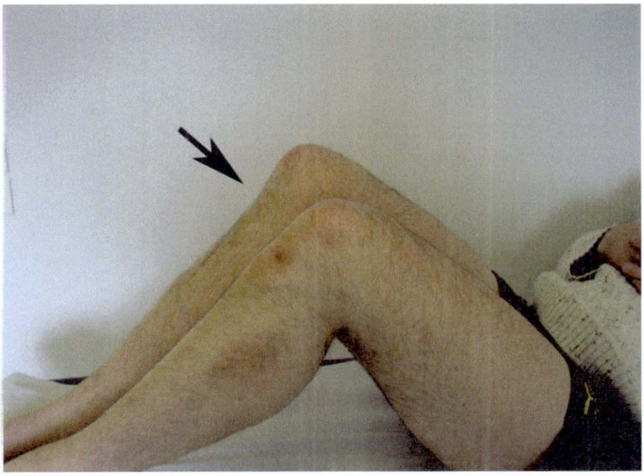

Fig. 38.6 Photograph showing posterior sagging of the anterior tibial tubercle on the right knee compared to the left, indicative of a PCL rupture

  - *Spontaneous posterior sagging* of the anterior tibial tubercle at 70–80° knee flexion position (Fig. 38.6): this appearance is the clinical manifestation of the posterior "drop back" of the proximal tibia under the distal femur in the abovementioned knee flexion position.
  - *False positive anterior drawer test*: When the examiner performs an anterior drawer maneuver starting from the position of "drop back" in knee flexion, the anterior shift or displacement of the proximal tibia gives a false impression of positive anterior drawer test.
  - *False positive Lachman test*: the "false" impression of anterior tibial translation during the test is in fact related to the manual correction of the spontaneous posterior sagging of the proximal tibia under the distal femur.
  - Negative Jerk test.
- ***Radiographic assessment***
  - Usually normal.
  - The lateral view may demonstrate a *bony fracture-avulsion* of the retro-spinal surface of the proximal tibia (footprint of the distal PCL insertion, also called PCL facet).
  - May show a spontaneous posterior displacement of the proximal tibia under the distal femur on lateral radiograph (posterior sagging).
  - A lateral view, with the application of a *forced posterior drawer at 90° knee flexion*, is helpful in quantifying the amount of posterior tibial displacement (Fig. 38.7).
- ***Management***
  - *MRI is essential* for the confirmation of the diagnosis, identification of the site of rupture and disclosure of any associated potential lesions (Fig. 38.8).
  - Knee brace is used for temporary immobilization.
  - Specialized orthopedic opinion is requested within a few days after the accident.
  - Treatment is controversial between partisans of conservative orthopedic management and partisans of surgical treatment.

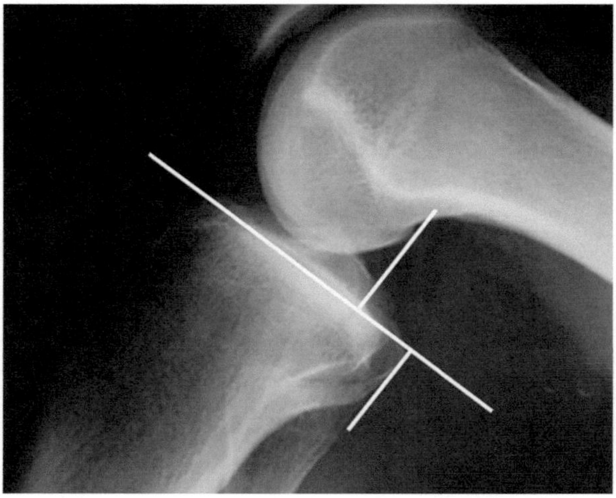

Fig. 38.7 Lateral knee stress view at 90° knee flexion showing a posterior drawer sign, with the proximal tibia shifted posteriorly beneath the distal femur by more than 10 mm, indicative of a PCL rupture

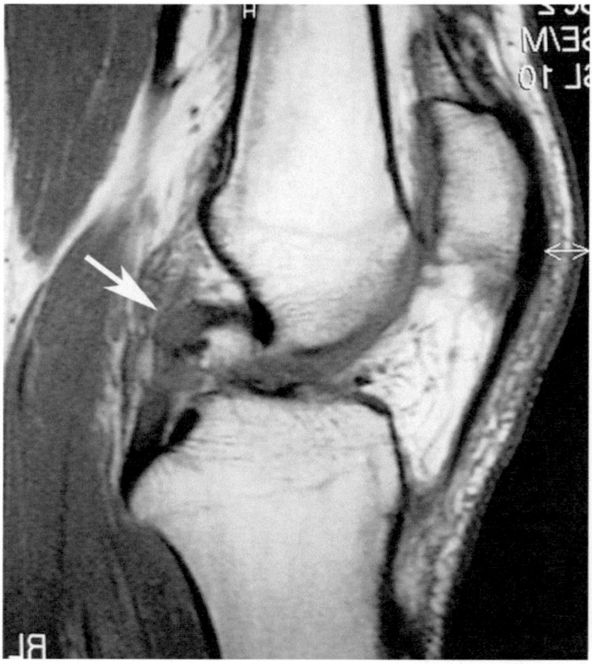

Fig. 38.8 Sagittal cut of a knee MRI showing a PCL rupture

– Authors' preferred method:

PCL tear without bony avulsion: cast immobilization in knee extension for 45 days (position of reduction of the posterior sagging), followed by rehabilitation.

Bony avulsion-fracture of the PCL tibial insertion: early surgical repair.

38.1.3.2 Associated PCL and "Peripheral" Ligamentous Injuries

- These correspond to the so-called *postero-postero-lateral and postero-postero-medial sprains* (PCL rupture with injury to the posterolateral and posteromedial capsulo-ligamentous structures, respectively).
- The clinical presentation combines signs of PCL rupture (posterior sagging, negative Jerk test) and signs of peripheral medial or lateral injury (laxity in valgus–varus stress as detailed above for ACL sprains).
- *MRI is indispensable* to refine the diagnosis, particularly when the result is analyzed in light of the knee examination performed under anesthesia.
- *A specialized orthopedic opinion* is essential, as surgical treatment is often indicated.

38.2 Meniscal Injuries

38.2.1 Medial Meniscus

Medial meniscus tears are more common than lateral meniscus (except for acute ACL injury where the lateral meniscus tears are more common).

A patient with a medial meniscal tear may clinically present in one of the following two circumstances:

1. ***Acute knee locking***
   (a) Relatively rare presentation,
   (b) Usually in young patients,
   (c) Secondary to a twisting-flexion mechanism in a weight-loaded knee,
   (d) May be associated with an ACL tear.
   (e) Clinical presentation with,
      - Medial joint line pain and tenderness,
      - Knee flexion limited to 100–110°,
      - Patient unable to extend their knee: *extension deficit of 20–30°*,
      - Moderate knee effusion.
2. ***Post-traumatic medial joint line pain***
   (a) More common presentation.
   (b) The patient may complain of intermittent knee locking and or giving way.
   (c) Clinical exam:
      - Tenderness of the medial joint line (most simple and reliable physical sign of meniscal tear).
      - Always assess for any associated laxities (antero-posterior and medio-lateral).
      - Always evaluate the knee alignment (normal axis, genu varum, genu valgum).
3. ***Differential diagnosis*** of medial meniscal injury includes:
   (a) MCL sprain, especially when the MCL tear is located in the mid-substance (relatively rare situation),

   (b) Tendinitis or bursitis of the "pes anserinus" (even rarer).
4. ***Management***
   (a) *For acute knee locking*
      - Standard knee radiographs are first requested for elimination of any intra-articular loose bodies (usually seen in the cases of osteochondritis of the femoral condyles) (Fig. 38.9a, b)
      - If an orthopedic surgeon is available: Arthroscopy is indicated as early as possible for the removal of "loose body" (Fig. 38.10), partial meniscectomy, or meniscal repair according to the findings.
      - If an orthopedic surgeon is not available: Attempt unlocking the knee with alternation of valgus-internal and valgus-external rotation movements, pushing on the medial joint line.
         – If unlocking is successful: ask for an MRI and refer the patient for an orthopedic consultation within a few days.
         – If unlocking is not successful: prescribe painkillers, NSAIDs, and muscle relaxant. The knee will then frequently unlock spontaneously in 2–3 days.
      - A specialized orthopedic opinion is a must in all cases and should be arranged within the following few days.
   (b) *Post-traumatic medial joint line pain*
      - Medical treatment is started: NSAIDs, painkillers, rest.
      - *For patients of >45 years age*: Ask for a complete radiographic knee assessment for evaluation of medial femoro-tibial potential early

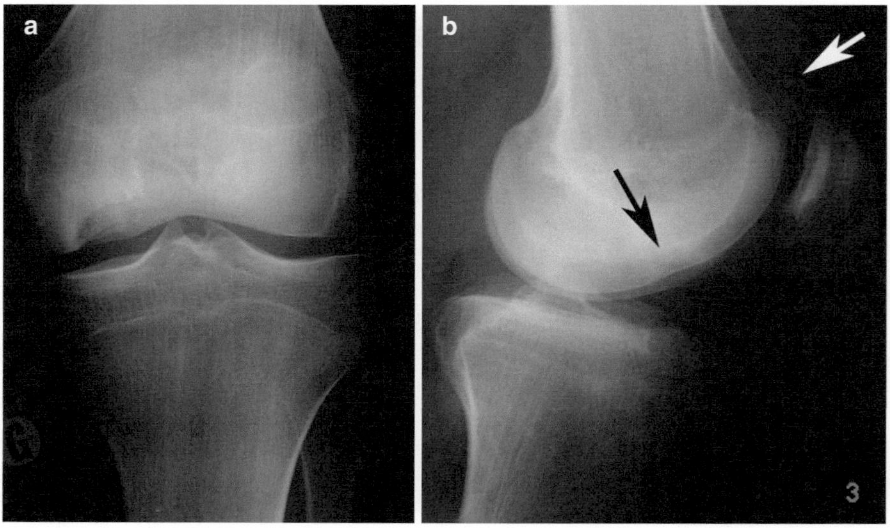

Fig. 38.9 (**a**) AP view of the left knee showing an "osteochondral defect" of the distal aspect of the medial femoral condyle. (**b**) Lateral view of the left knee showing a large "osteochondral defect" of the distal aspect of the medial femoral condyle. Note the presence of a loose body proximal to the trochlea

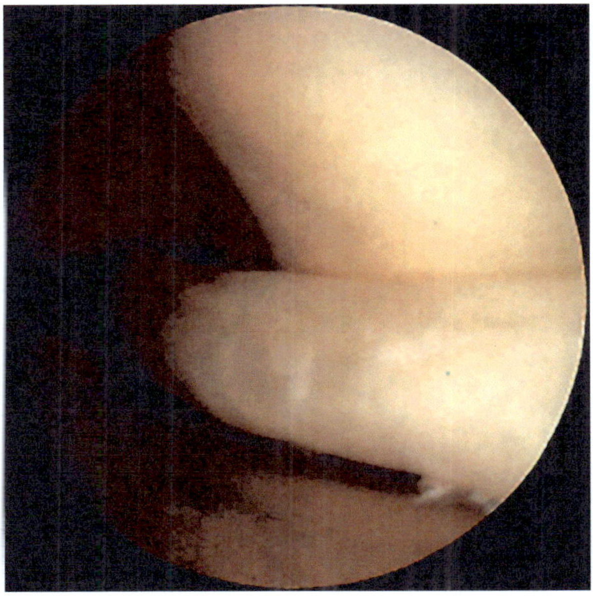

Fig. 38.10 Arthroscopic view of a bucket handle injury of the medial meniscus

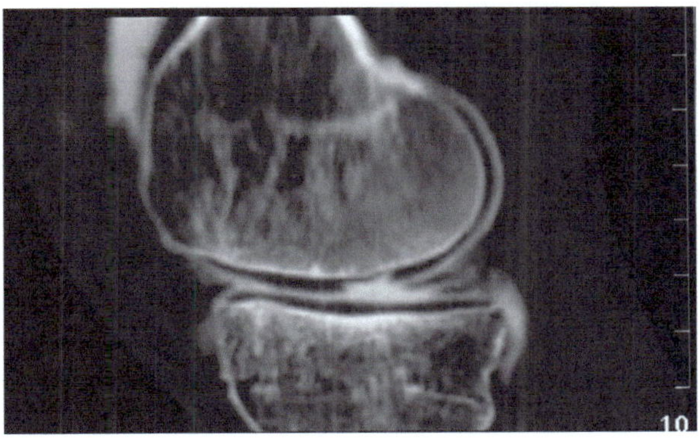

Fig. 38.11 Sagittal cut of a knee arthro-CT scan in an adult patient over 50 years old, showing a medial meniscus injury. Note also the cartilage lesion on the medial femoral condyle

osteoarthritis (the medial meniscal tear is a common consequent association, especially in the presence of genu varum malalignment).

- AP view with knee extension position and weight bearing,
- postero-anterior view with 30° knee flexion position and weight bearing ("schuss" view),
- A full length radiograph of both lower limbs in standing position (Scanogram) is helpful for the assessment of knee alignment (normal axis, varus, or valgus).
- If the radiographic assessment is normal: evaluation of the knee articular cartilage using arthro-CT scan rather than MRI (Fig. 38.11).

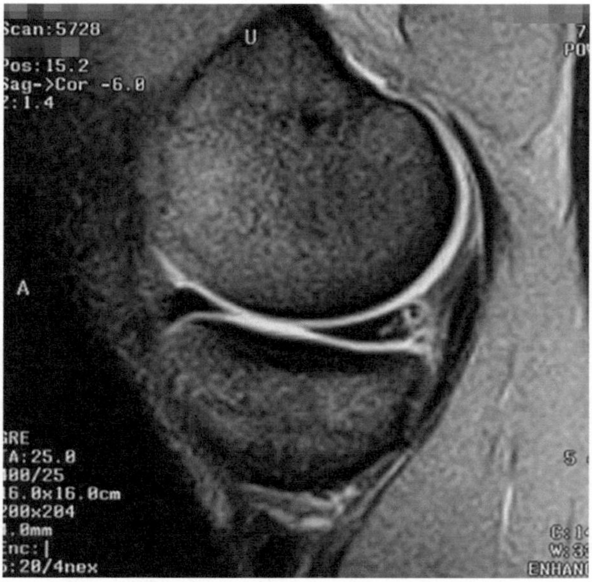

Fig. 38.12 Sagittal cut of a knee MRI showing a medial meniscus injury in a young adult patient

- *For patients of* <*45 years age*: if the standard radiographic assessment is normal, an MRI is requested to confirm the diagnosis of meniscal tear (Fig. 38.12).

38.2.2 Lateral Meniscus

- Lateral meniscus tears are 5–10 times less common than medial meniscus tears.
- Symptoms are similar for both menisci, with the understanding that symptoms of the lateral meniscus are located at the lateral side of the knee.
- Management is similar for both menisci, although it is known that lateral meniscectomy yields less satisfactory results than medial meniscectomy (75% vs. 90% satisfactory rates).

38.3 Ruptures of the Extensor Mechanism of the Knee

These correspond to ruptures of the quadriceps tendon and patellar tendon. These injuries are discussed in Chap. 44 "Tendino-muscular injuries of the lower limb."

38.4 Knee Contusion

- Knee contusion is almost always associated with a cutaneous footmark of the traumatic impact.

- Knee contusion may be accompanied with one or more of the following intra-articular injuries:
  - PCL rupture (antero-posterior impact to the anterior aspect of the proximal tibia),
  - ACL rupture (postero-anterior impact to the posterior aspect of the proximal tibia),
  - MCL rupture (impact to the lateral aspect of knee),
  - Patellar dislocation,
  - Meniscal tear,
- Any patient with knee contusion should undergo a complete clinical evaluation and a well-guided radiographic assessment.
- Initial radiographs can be valuable for the differential diagnosis in many situations.
- Initial radiographs may be labeled "normal," as many bony injuries are subtle and easily missed by an undiscerning or an inexperienced eye (Fig. 38.13a, b).
- Some situations may remain confusing as the history, the primary clinical evaluation, and the initial radiographic assessment are deceiving and not conclusive.
- ***Management***
  - When the clinical evaluation is smooth and the radiographic presentation is irrefutable, the diagnosis is almost always conclusive and the treatment is consequently diagnosis-guided.
  - When the clinical evaluation is dull and/or the radiographic presentation is not conclusive:
    - Prescribe the use of a knee brace,
    - Allow walking with no weight bearing,
    - Prescribe NSAIDs and local ice application,

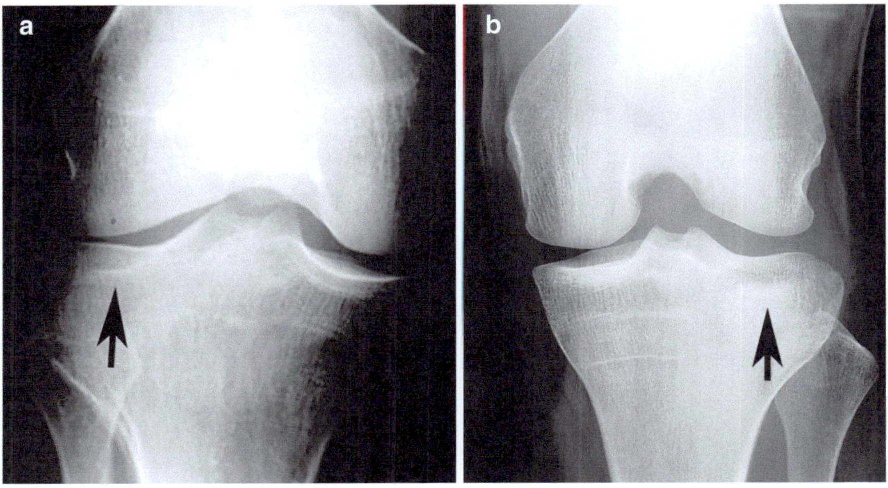

Fig. 38.13 (**a**) AP knee X-ray revealing a localized impaction-fracture of the lateral tibial plateau, initially overlooked in the ER. (**b**) AP knee X-ray showing the same findings as depicted in Fig. **a**

Reassess after 1 week for either the confirmation of the initial diagnosis of "simple knee contusion" or redirection for a new final more serious diagnosis that has been initially missed. A simple contusion usually recovers in 10–15 days.

Fractures of the Tibia and Fibula

39

39.1 Patho-Anatomy

Fractures of the tibia and fibula may occur in isolation or in combination. They are fractures located in the area extending from just below the anterior tibial tubercle to 4 cm proximal to the tibial plafond. Fractures of the fibula are often considered secondary, especially if they occur along the shaft.

39.1.1 Anatomic Varieties

- Simple fractures: transverse and short oblique fractures (Fig. 39.1a, b), and spiral fractures.
- Wedge fractures (frequent in skiing accidents).
- Fragmentary or comminuted fractures (Fig. 39.2).
- Segmental fractures (simple and fragmentary).
- *Red flag*: spiral diaphyseal fractures of the tibia may involve the tibial plafond, especially the posterior margin or "posterior malleolus" of the distal tibia (knee and ankle joints should always be included in the radiographic views).

39.1.2 Associated Injuries

1. **Open fractures**
   (a) They are frequent especially in high-energy trauma, as the medial aspect of the tibia is "subcutaneous."
   (b) *The Gustilo classification* for open fractures is widely used and categorizes fractures into three grades of increasing severity. These grades are based on the amount of energy involved, the degree of soft tissue damage, and the level of contamination. The progression from grade I to III indicates a

D. Saragaglia, A. Hassan Chamseddine, *Traumatology for the Emergency Doctor*, https://doi.org/10.1007/978-3-031-63196-2_39

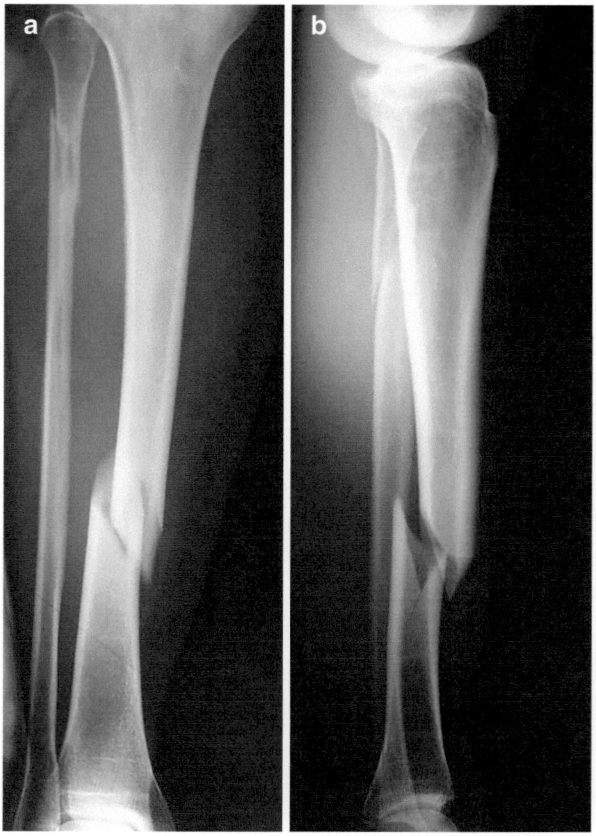

Fig. 39.1 (**a**) AP leg radiograph showing an oblique fracture pattern of the tibial shaft. (**b**) lateral leg radiograph showing the same oblique fracture pattern of the tibial shaft

greater amount of traumatic energy, more soft tissue and bone damage, and a higher potential risk for complications.

- Grade I: clean wound <1 cm in length,
- Grade II: wound size >1 cm but <10 cm without extensive soft tissue damage (no avulsion, detachment, or flaps),
- Grade III: indicates either an open fracture with segmental component or an extensive soft tissue damage, and is divided into three sub-groups:
  - IIIA: adequate soft tissue coverage despite the size and the extent of the laceration,
  - IIIB: extensive soft tissue defect or loss with periosteal stripping, bone damage, and important contamination. It usually requires bone coverage with flap,
  - IIIC: arterial injury requiring surgical repair regardless of the amount of soft tissue damage, mangled extremity, and open fractures with traumatic amputation.

2. **Neurovascular injuries**
   (a) Rare in closed fractures.

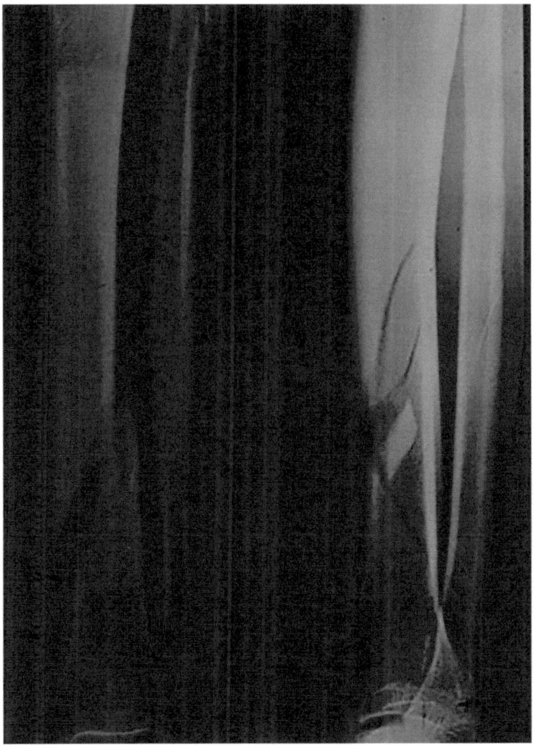

Fig. 39.2 AP and lateral leg radiographs showing a spiral wedge fracture pattern of the tibial shaft, resulting from a ski accident

   (b) More common in high-energy open fractures with soft tissue and muscular damage.
3. **Compartment syndrome**
   (a) Should be suspected:
      - In transverse fractures induced by important contusion or direct impact to the anterolateral aspect of the leg,
      - In case of significant displacement of associated fibular fracture.
   (b) Measurement of compartment pressures is mandatory in case of any doubt.

39.2 Clinical Presentation

39.2.1 Diagnosis

- The clinical diagnosis is obvious in the presence of deformity (shortening, angulation, rotation), pain, and functional disability.
- The diagnosis is suspected in the presence of partial functional disability (undisplaced hairline "sub-periosteal" fracture).

39.2.2 Physical Examination for Associated or Complicated Injuries

- Open fracture (Gustilo's classification),
- Vascular complication (distal pulses, capillary refill, venous return),
- Neurologic impairment (motor and sensory),
- Compartment syndrome (the pain is intense and exaggerated by passive dorsal flexion of the ankle and foot, presence of tense anterolateral compartment of the leg, and distal paresthesia).

39.2.3 Radiographic Assessment

- Final diagnosis is based on the radiographic assessment of the leg,
- A minimum of two orthogonal radiographic views are required, including the adjacent proximal and distal joints (knee and ankle).

39.3 Management

39.3.1 For Open Fractures

- Inform the orthopedic surgeon,
- Install tetanus prevention schedule,
- Start intra-venous preventive antibiotics (usually amoxicillin or Amoxicillin/Clavulanic acid),
- Pre-operative assessment (Blood workup, cardio-vascular, and general).
- Active abundant irrigation of the open fracture site using high pressure lavage (normal saline, Betadine solution),
- Cover the leg with sterile draping,
- Temporary immobilization of the leg with rigid splint,
- Transfer the patient to the operative theater.

39.3.2 For Closed Displaced Fractures

- Displaced fractures are usually surgically treated in adult patients.
- Early surgical treatment may be done based on the availability of the surgeon and the operating theater and provided that the patient is fit and prepared for surgery (a temporary rigid splint of the leg is applied while awaiting surgery).
- If surgery must be postponed for any reason, skeletal trans-calcaneal traction weighing 6–8 kg is installed and the leg is elevated.
- Surgical fixation is performed using intra-medullary nail (Fig. 39.3) or plate and screws (Fig. 39.4) according to the fracture type and surgeon preferences.

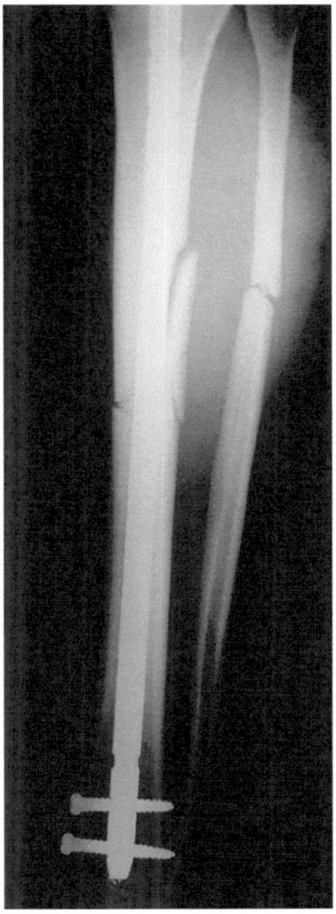

Fig. 39.3 AP leg X-ray showing an intra-medullary interlocking nail fixation for a wedge fracture of the proximal tibial shaft

39.3.3 For Closed Non-displaced Fractures

- Non-displaced fractures may be treated non-surgically (conservative orthopedic treatment).
- *Long leg above knee cast* is applied:
  - it should be well molded to prevent secondary displacement,
  - the use of "plaster of Paris" is recommended for better molding of the cast.
- *Weekly radiographic control* is mandatory for the first 3 weeks for early detection of secondary displacement of the fracture site that will be treated with cast re-adjustment when possible ("gypsotomy") (Fig. 39.5) or with open reduction and internal fixation.
- Duration of healing is 3 months for non-displaced fractures in adult patients.
- If the fracture is stable (transverse fracture), a weight bearing cast with rocker bottom sole can be used.
- Thrombo-embolic prevention is recommended in adult patients.

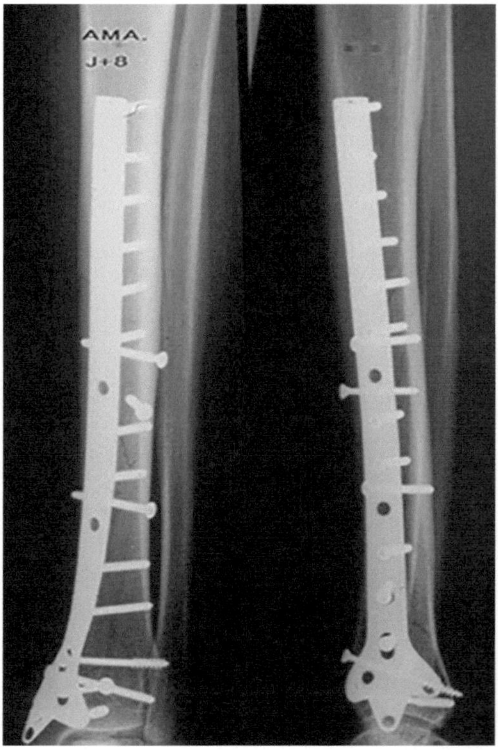

Fig. 39.4 AP and lateral leg X-rays after open reduction and internal fixation of the same fracture depicted in Fig. 39.2

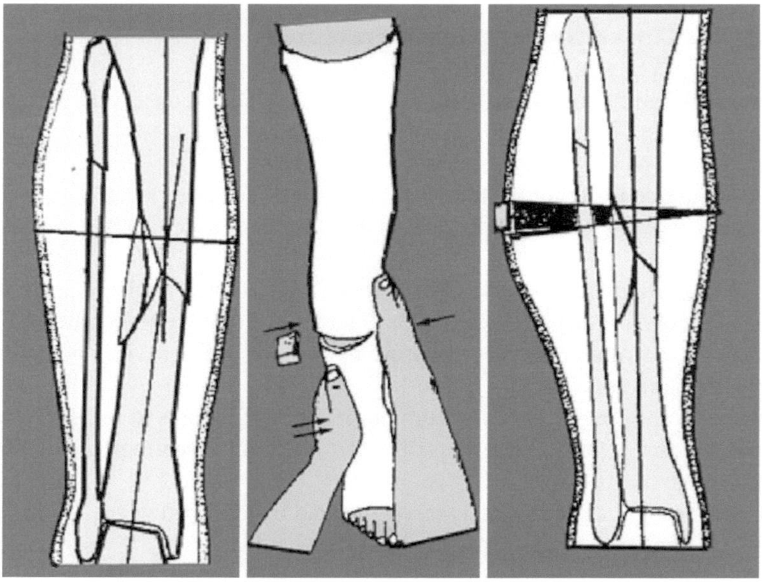

Fig. 39.5 Illustration of a lateral open wedge "gypsotomy" at the site of a tibial fracture, performed for the correction of valgus displacement in the cast

39.3.4 Isolated Fractures of the Fibular Shaft

- Usually benefit from functional treatment without immobilization.
- Pain disappears after 4–6 weeks.

39.4 Conclusion

Undisplaced tibial shaft fractures may be conservatively treated by the ER physician in collaboration with the orthopedic surgeon.

However, regular radiographic controls are mandatory to detect any secondary displacement, which should be handled by the orthopedic team.

Ankle Fractures

40

Ankle fractures are one of the most common injuries seen in the ER. They are usually secondary to twisting mechanism.

40.1 Patho-Anatomy

They are categorized as:

40.1.1 Malleolar Fractures

40.1.1.1 Isolated Malleolus Fractures

They correspond to:

- Fractures of the ***medial malleolus***,
- Fractures of the ***lateral malleolus***.
- Fractures of the ***posterior malleolus*** ("Volkmann" or "curbstone" fracture).

40.1.1.2 Bimalleolar Fractures

They involve fractures of both medial and lateral malleoli and are described according to the location of the fibular fracture in relation to the distal tibio-fibular syndesmosis (distal tibio-fibular ligaments):

- ***Supra-syndesmotic fractures*** (Fig. 40.1)
  - The fibular fracture is located proximal to the inferior tibio-fibular ligaments,
  - They involve injury to the distal tibio-fibular syndesmosis.
- ***Infra-syndesmotic fractures*** (Fig. 40.2)
  - The fibular fracture is located distal to the inferior tibio-fibular ligaments,
  - The distal tibio-fibular syndesmosis is respected.

D. Saragaglia, A. Hassan Chamseddine, *Traumatology for the Emergency Doctor*, https://doi.org/10.1007/978-3-031-63196-2_40

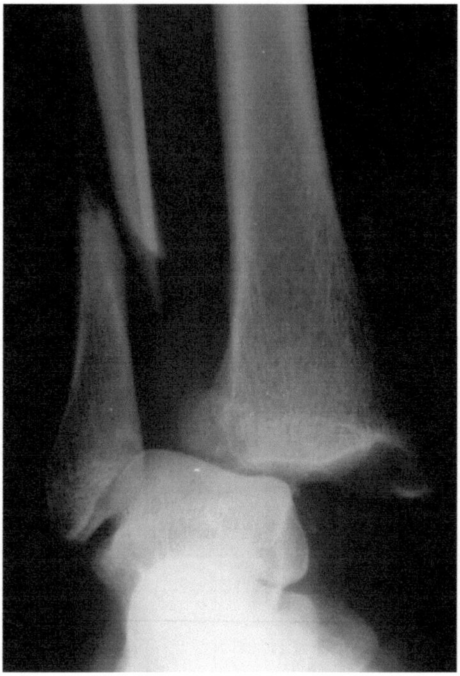

Fig. 40.1 AP right ankle X-ray revealing a bi-malleolar supra-syndesmotic fracture

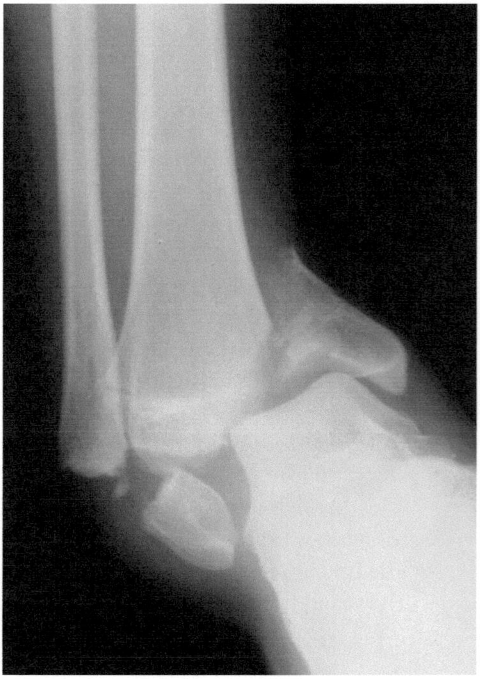

Fig. 40.2 AP right ankle X-ray revealing a bi-malleolar infra-syndesmotic fracture

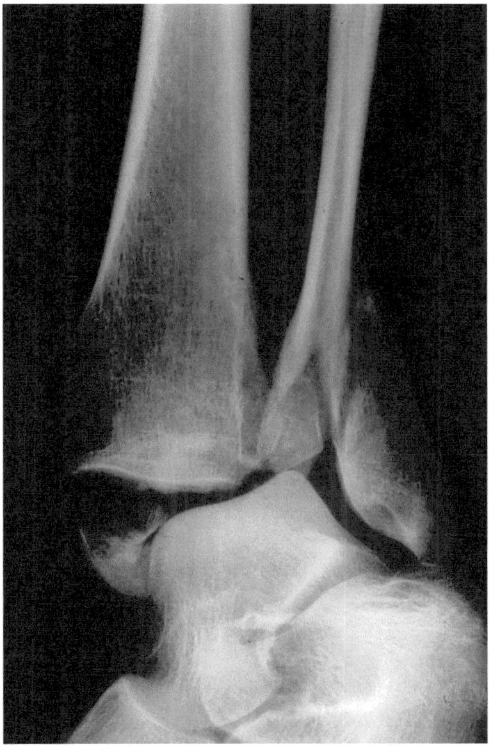

Fig. 40.3 AP left ankle X-ray revealing a bi-malleolar trans-syndesmotic fracture

- ***Trans-syndesmotic fractures*** (Fig. 40.3)
  - The fibular fracture is located at the site of the inferior tibio-fibular ligament,
  - The distal tibio-fibular syndesmosis may either be involved or intact.
- ***Maisonneuve's fracture***
  - Is a particular fracture type.
  - It involves fracture of the fibular shaft or neck associated with fracture of the medial malleolus or rupture of the deltoid ligament of the ankle (Medial Collateral Ligament) (Fig. 40.4).
- ***Bimalleolar-equivalent fractures***: they involve fracture of the lateral malleolus associated with rupture of the deltoid ligament (Fig. 40.5).
- ***Trimalleolar fractures and equivalents***
  - They involve associated fractures of the medial, lateral, and posterior malleoli (Fig. 40.6a, b).
  - An equivalent to trimalleolar fractures is represented by an association of a rupture of the deltoid ligament with fractures of the lateral and posterior malleoli.
- **Tillaux–Chaput fracture**
  - Is a particular partial fracture type,
  - It corresponds to the fracture of the anterolateral tibial margin,
  - It relates an avulsion of the antero-inferior tibio-fibular ligament (AITFL).

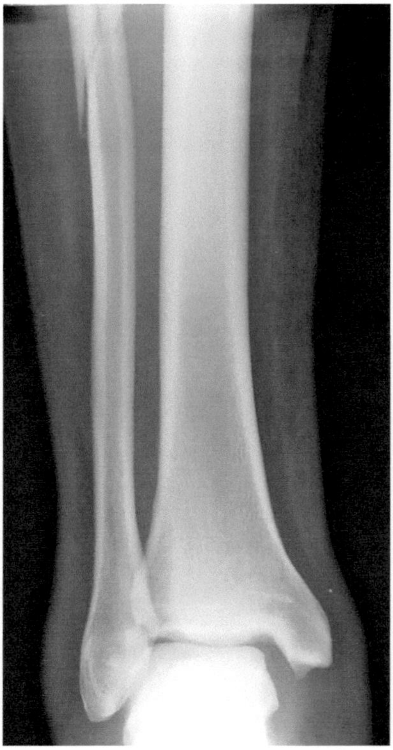

Fig. 40.4 Equivalent to a Maisonneuve fracture: a fibular shaft fracture with associated injury to the MCL, resulting in widening of the medial tibio-talar space

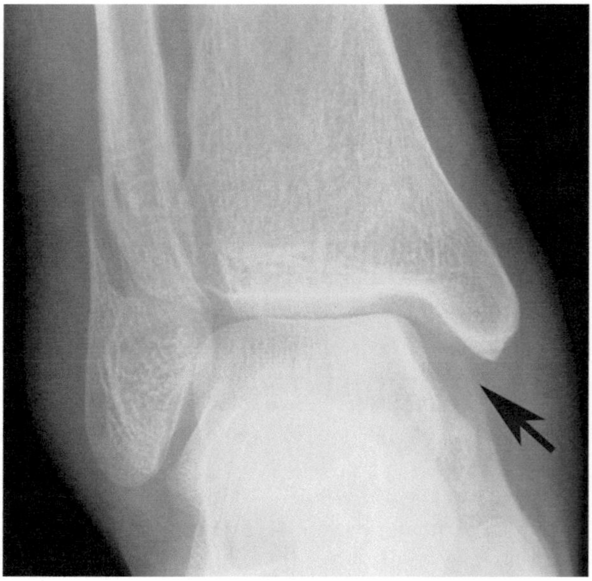

Fig. 40.5 Equivalent to a bi-malleolar fracture: fracture of the lateral malleolus with associated injury to the MCL, resulting in widening of the medial tibio-talar space

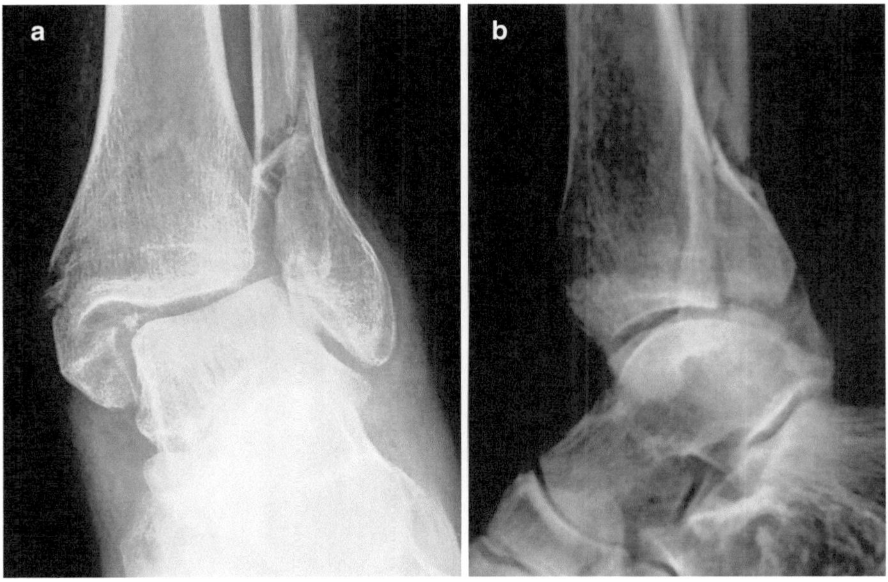

Fig. 40.6 (**a**) AP ankle X-ray of a patient with a trimalleolar fracture. Note that the fracture of the posterior malleolus is ill-defined on the AP view. (**b**) Lateral radiograph of the same trimalleolar fracture depicted in Fig. **a**. Note that the posterior malleolus fracture is well identified on the lateral view

40.1.2 Fractures of the Tibial Pilon or Plafond

- Tibial pilon (or plafond) fractures correspond to distal tibial fractures with intra-articular involvement.
- Associated metaphyseal and/or articular comminution is common.
- Associated soft tissue damage is frequent (contusion, abrasion, bullae, blisters, open wound, etc.).
- They may be categorized as:
  - ***Partial articular fractures*** involving
    The *posterior or the anterior tibial margin* (Fig. 40.7a, b).
    The *medial malleolus and the anterior or the posterior tibial margin* (Fig. 40.8a, b).
  - ***Complete articular fractures*** involving *both tibial margins without or with fracture of the medial malleolus* (Fig. 40.9a, b).
- They frequently present an impaction of the articular surface.
- They are frequently associated with fracture of the lateral malleolus.

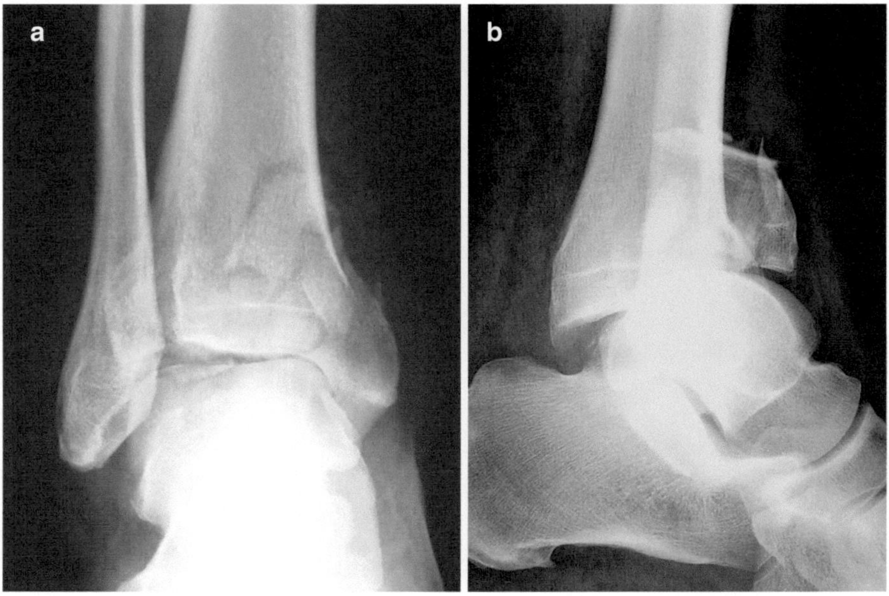

Fig. 40.7 (**a**) AP ankle X-ray of a patient with a tibial pilon fracture involving an ill-defined anterior tibial margin fracture. (**b**) Lateral ankle radiograph of the same patient depicted in Fig. **a**. Note that the anterior tibial margin fracture is now well identified

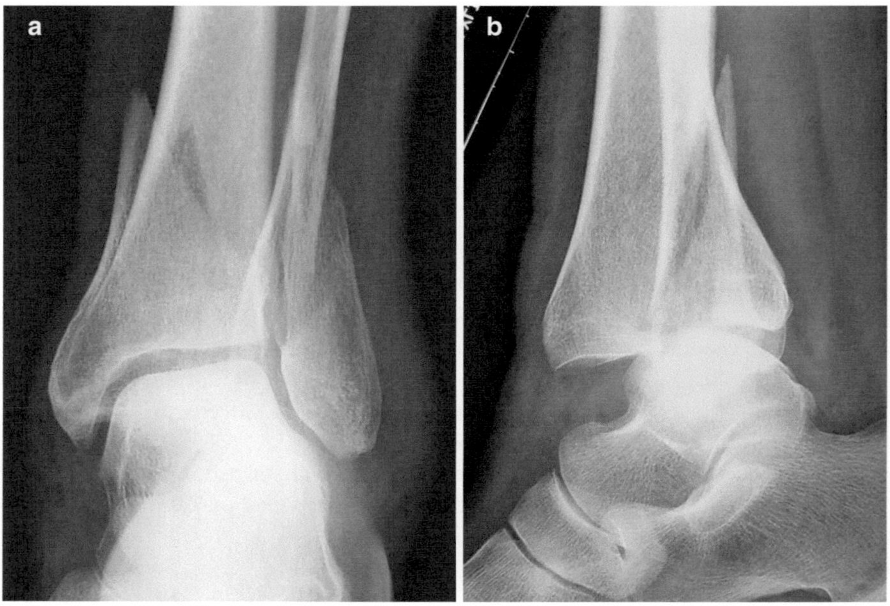

Fig. 40.8 (**a**) AP ankle radiograph of a patient with a tibial pilon fracture involving an ill-defined posterior tibial margin fracture. (**b**) Lateral ankle radiograph of the same patient as shown in Fig. **a**. Note that the posterior tibial margin fracture is now well identified

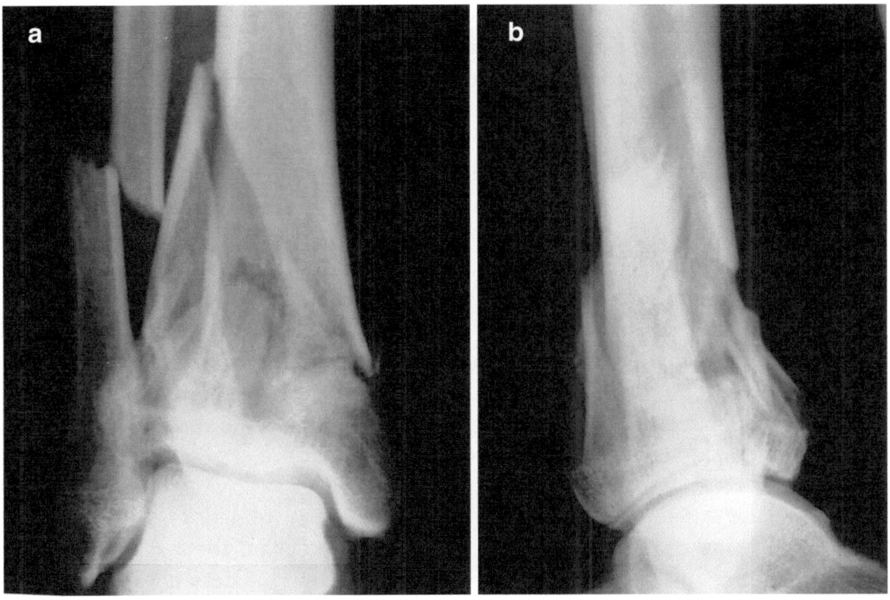

Fig. 40.9 (**a**) AP ankle radiograph showing a tibial pilon fracture with a complete articular involvement. (**b**) Lateral radiograph of the same ankle as shown in Fig. **a** showing a tibial pilon fracture with a complete articular involvement (anterior and posterior margins)

40.2 Clinical Presentation

- The clinical diagnosis of "displaced" ankle fracture is evident when the patient presents to the ER with deformity, edema, and functional disability.
- The radiographic assessment (AP, lateral, and mortise views) confirms the preliminary diagnosis and usually shows the type of fracture.
- The clinical diagnosis may easily be missed if the fracture is undisplaced and the patient presents with minimal disability, making the ER physician confident not to ask for radiographic assessment (as the injury is misdiagnosed for an "ankle sprain" according to the "Ottawa ankle rules").
- An apparently "isolated" fracture of the medial malleolus should always be assessed for an associated fracture of the fibular shaft by appropriate palpation and radiographic views (Maisonneuve's fracture).
- **A CT scan with 2D and 3D reconstruction** is usually requested in pre-operative, especially for tibial pilon fractures.

40.3 Management

- An orthopedic specialized consultation is always recommended, as ankle fractures involve the joint itself ("articular fractures"). Their reduction should be "perfect" in order to minimize the risk of secondary post-traumatic osteo-arthritis.

- The fixation of these fractures should be stable enough to facilitate early rehabilitation, as soon as the skin has healed.
- The following schematic management is proposed for the ER physician:

40.3.1 Non-surgical Management

- *Non-displaced fractures ("hairline" and "sub-periosteal" fractures)*
  - Below knee cast immobilization, ankle at 90°:
    45 days for Lateral malleolus,
    75 days for pilon fractures.
  - For isolated malleolus fractures (lateral, medial, or small posterior fragment) a weight bearing cast with a rocker bottom sole can be applied.
  - For pilon fractures, weight bearing is not allowed (risk of fracture impaction).
  - Radiographic control should be done after 8 days of starting bearing weight and at the time of cast removal.
  - For lateral malleolus fractures, "radiographic consolidation" with complete obliteration of the fracture line is frequently delayed for 3–6 months. The absence of fracture line obliteration in the early period does not indicate non-union, especially if it is asymptomatic.
- *For isolated lateral malleolus fractures*
  - Make sure not to miss a bimalleolar-equivalent fracture (with associated rupture of the deltoid ligament) (Fig. 40.10).
  - Carefully assess for any potential syndesmotic injury on the radiographic views and ask for orthopedic surgical opinion when there is an increased medial clear space (normal medial tibio-talar space ≤4 mm on mortise view) (Fig. 40.10).

40.3.2 Surgical Management Is Indicated for

- All displaced fractures (Figs. 40.11a, b and 40.12a, b),
- Fractures at risk for secondary displacement (e.g., bimalleolar-equivalent fractures),
- Open fractures.

40.3.3 Management of Fracture-Dislocations

- Fracture-dislocations and very displaced fractures (Fig. 40.13a, b) should be urgently relocated by the ER physician, especially if the orthopedic surgeon is not immediately available. These injuries encompass an important risk of complications if they are not early reduced (soft tissue and neuro-vascular threats).

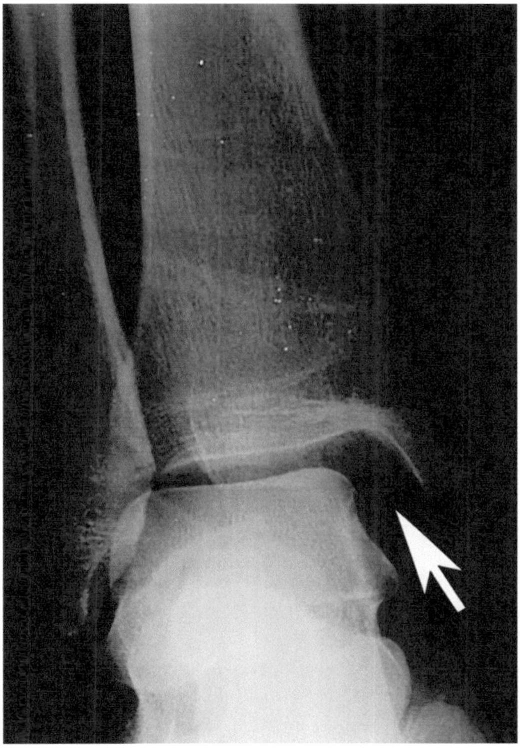

Fig. 40.10 AP ankle X-ray showing an abnormal widening of the medial tibio-talar space

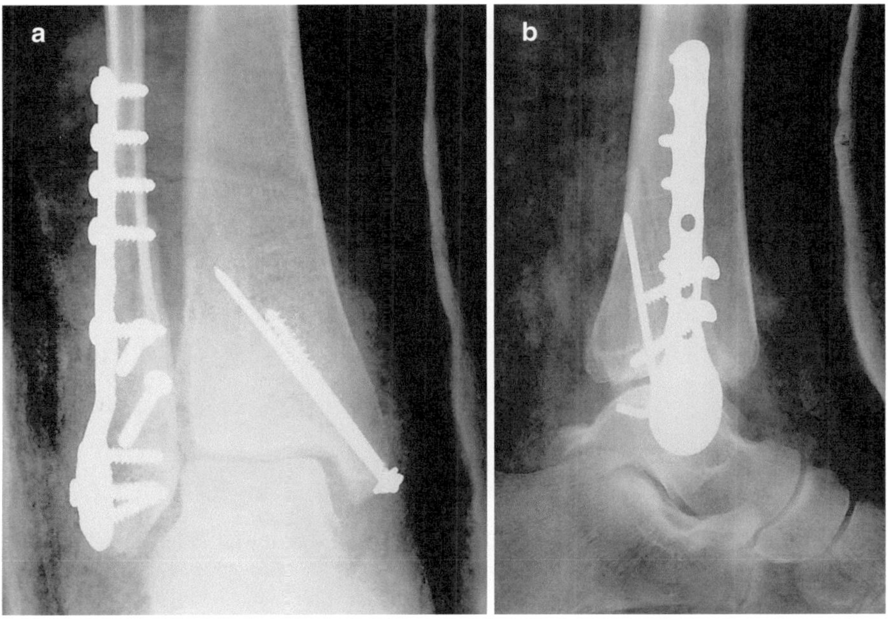

Fig. 40.11 (**a**) AP ankle X-ray after open reduction and internal fixation of a bi-malleolar fracture. (**b**) Lateral radiograph of the same ankle as shown in Fig. **a**

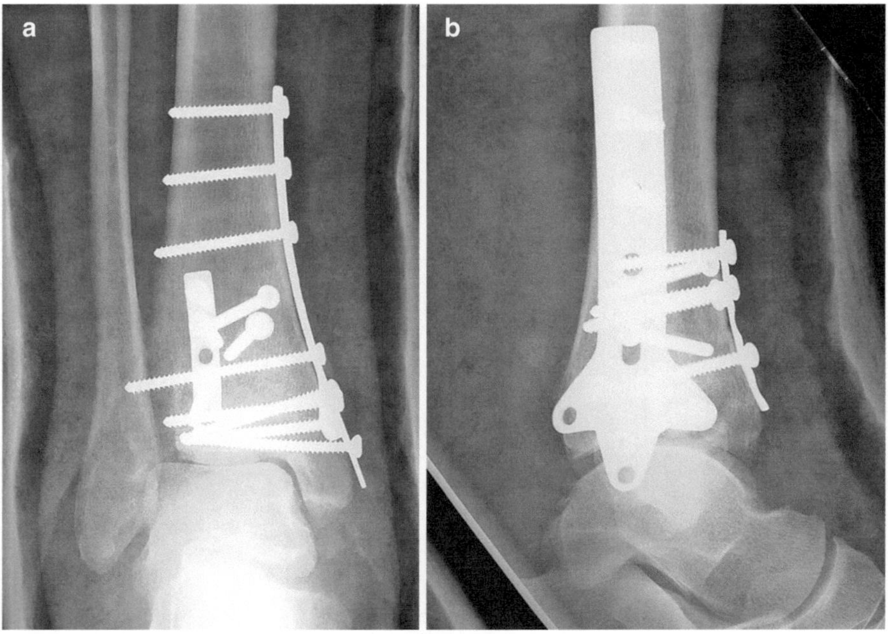

Fig. 40.12 (**a**) AP post-operative ankle X-ray showing the radiographic result of open reduction and internal fixation of a tibial pilon fracture. (**b**) Lateral radiograph of the same ankle as shown in Fig. **a**

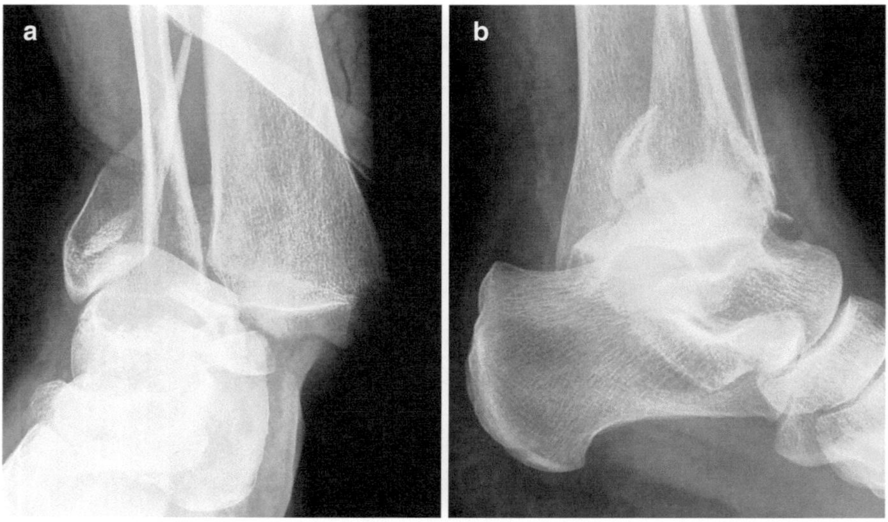

Fig. 40.13 (**a**) AP ankle X-ray of a bi-malleolar fracture associated with a tibio-talar dislocation (ankle fracture-dislocation). (**b**) Lateral radiographic view of the same ankle as shown in Fig. **a**

- The reduction is usually performed using a maneuver that imitates the "*boot pulling-out*" *maneuver* to relocate and put back the ankle in place; reduction is followed by cast immobilization (below knee plaster of Paris cast).
- For tibial pilon fractures, skeletal trans-calcaneal traction (6–8 kg) is recommended while awaiting the final treatment (if delayed).
- Radiographic control and CT scans are performed after reduction and immobilization or traction. This allows for a more detailed analysis of the fracture to facilitate better therapeutic planning.
- The lower limb is elevated in the bed (anti-edema) while awaiting the final treatment.
- For patients with peripheral artery disease, the lower limb should be positioned straight and aligned with the plane of the bed (Red flag: ischemia).
- Intra-venous NSAID's may be prescribed if no contraindications.

Ankle Trauma with "Normal" Radiographs

41

Normal radiographs are a common finding after ankle trauma. Consequently, many authors have defined the "Ottawa ankle rules" to restrict the prescription of ankle radiographs in the ER. However, we believe that this approach may lead to misinterpretation:

- Even a comprehensive physical exam is not 100% reliable, as pain perception or threshold is subjective and may vary from one patient to another.
- The cost of radiographs is modest compared to the expense and burden of an initial misdiagnosis, which could be induced by the absence of an initial radiographic assessment.
- The waiting time for performing non-urgent ankle radiographs in a busy ER department can be reduced if the radiographs are conducted at an outside facility either the same day or the next day.
- The medico-legal value of initial radiographs is irreplaceable, especially in circumstances such as differentiating between an osteochondral fracture and osteochondritis of the talar dome or between an os trigonum and a fracture of the posterior tubercle of the talus.
- Diagnostic errors can be minimized if the radiographic request and analysis are clinically guided.

41.1 Lateral Ankle Sprains

- They are very common and represent 10–15% of the overall limbs' injuries.
- The majority are benign injuries (80–85%).
- The mechanism of injury is commonly an inversion of the ankle with plantar flexion of the foot.
- They frequently present in the form of recurrent sprain with chronic ankle instability.
- They affect the lateral collateral ligament (LCL) formed by three components:

D. Saragaglia, A. Hassan Chamseddine, *Traumatology for the Emergency Doctor*, https://doi.org/10.1007/978-3-031-63196-2_41

  - The anterior talo-fibular ligament (ATFL),
  - The calcaneo-fibular ligament (CFL),
  - The posterior talo-fibular ligament (PTFL).
- They are typically categorized into three grades of severity based on the clinical presentation, involvement of the various components of the LCL, and the degree of laxity observed during the physical exam.
- The assessment of the degree of laxity during the physical exam is a crucial indicator for guiding appropriate treatment.

41.1.1 Diagnosis of the Degree of Severity

- **The clinical presentation** (signs and symptoms) is not pathognomonic for the diagnosis:
  - Popping,
  - Swelling,
  - Ecchymosis,
  - Functional disability and inability to bear weight,
  - Peri-malleolar tenderness.
- There are theoretically three *degrees of sprain* severity based on the extent of injury to the LCL:
  - Grade I (mild): No LCL disruption (only stretch),
  - Grade II (moderate): Rupture of the ATFL,
  - Grade III (severe): Complete tear of the LCL (rupture of the ATFL and CFL with or without PTFL involvement).
- **Bilateral comparative ankle radiographs with stress** in AP and lateral views are very helpful in determining the degree of severity of the sprain and the extent of the ligamentous injury (Fig. 41.1a, b):
  - *In an AP view with varus stress*, a lateral tilt of the talus and an opening of the lateral tibio-talar joint space greater than 12° indicate a combined injury of both the ATFL and the CFL (grade III) (Fig. 41.1a),
  - *In a Lateral view with anterior drawer* and 20° plantar flexion position, an opening of the posterior tibio-talar joint space greater than 8 mm indicates a rupture of the ATFL (Fig. 41.1b).
- **Ultrasound imaging of the ankle**, in both static and dynamic modes, is helpful for visualizing the extent of ligamentous injury; however, it requires a skilled radiologist.

41.1.2 Management

The initial phase of management, known as **RICE** (Rest, Ice application, Compression, Elevation), is followed by the definitive treatment based on the severity of the injury.

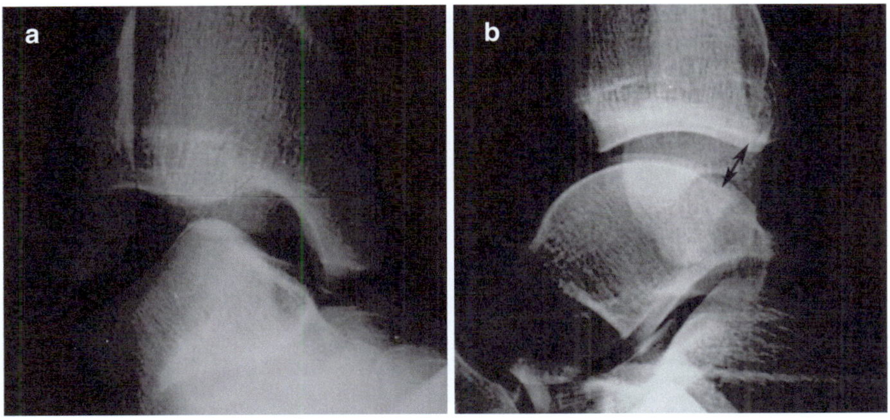

Fig. 41.1 (**a**) AP varus stress ankle X-ray using the Telos^{R} stress device. Note the significant lateral tilt of the talus associated with an important lateral tibio-talar joint space opening, indicative of a complete LCL tear. (**b**) Lateral X-ray of the same ankle as shown in Fig. **a**. Note the anterior drawer of the talus beneath the distal tibia, resulting in widening of the posterior tibio-talar joint space

- **Mild and moderate sprains** (Grade I and II)
  - They are defined based on,
    - The presence of a mild functional disability (the patient can walk on the affected limb),
    - The presence of a moderate swelling or edema,
    - The absence of ecchymosis.
    - The following radiographic findings: a varus stress laxity <12° with an anterior drawer <8 mm if the ATFL is intact and >8 mm if the ATFL is injured,
    - The following ultrasound findings: absence of LCL rupture or only rupture of the anterior LCL component (ATFL).
  - Ankle stabilization using either,
    - Ankle strapping (usually changed several times during the treatment),
    - Or removable ankle brace.
  - Functional treatment using a specific rehabilitation program with,
    - Restoration of the range of motion (ROM),
    - Physiotherapy,
    - And proprioceptive rehabilitation.
- **Severe sprain (Grade III)**
  - They are defined based on,
    - The presence of a severe functional disability (while patients often cannot bear weight on the affected limb, this is not always the case),
    - The presence of a significant swelling and edema,
    - The presence of ecchymosis,

The following radiographic findings: a Varus stress laxity >12° with an anterior drawer >8 mm,

The following ultrasound findings: rupture of the ATFL and CFL.

- Treatment:

  It is usually conservative, using a below-knee cast immobilization for 6 weeks, followed by a specific rehabilitation program as previously mentioned.

  The surgical treatment for LCL repair is a rare indication.

- **Recurrent sprain** and chronic lateral instability of the ankle
  - Cast immobilization is not considered a viable option, as the healing of ligaments is often ineffective,
  - The initial phase of management involves functional treatment, similar to the protocols detailed for mild and moderate sprains,
  - A consultation with a specialized orthopedic surgeon is recommended to discuss the possibility of surgical intervention, taking into account factors such as the patient's response to the specific rehabilitation program, the frequency of recurrent instability episodes, and the patient's activity level, needs, and expectations.

41.2 Other Ankle Sprains

41.2.1 Distal Tibio-Fibular Sprain (or High Ankle Sprain)

1. It corresponds to an injury of the tibio-fibular syndesmosis (distal tibio-fibular ligaments).
2. The injury typically occurs due to a forced external rotation or dorsal hyperflexion of the ankle.
3. The patient presents with painful weight-bearing ambulation.
4. The physical exam commonly reveals pain and tenderness at the distal tibio-fibular joint upon palpation, during anteroposterior movements to the distal fibula, with manual compression of the fibula toward the tibia, and when external rotation and dorsi-flexion of the ankle are provoked.
5. Radiographic assessment
   (a) Conventional AP, mortise, and lateral views,
   - Usually show normal findings,
   - May reveal,
     - A fracture-avulsion of the distal anterolateral tibial tubercle (Tillaux-Chaput).
     - More rarely a widening of the distal tibio-fibular clear space on both AP and mortise views (Fig. 41.2).

   (b) The AP view with stress applied through forced external rotation and dorsiflexion of the ankle is optional but may aid in the diagnosis.

   (c) The CT scan and Ultrasound or MRI are useful when there is a clinical suspicion of "high ankle sprain" with normal radiographic findings.

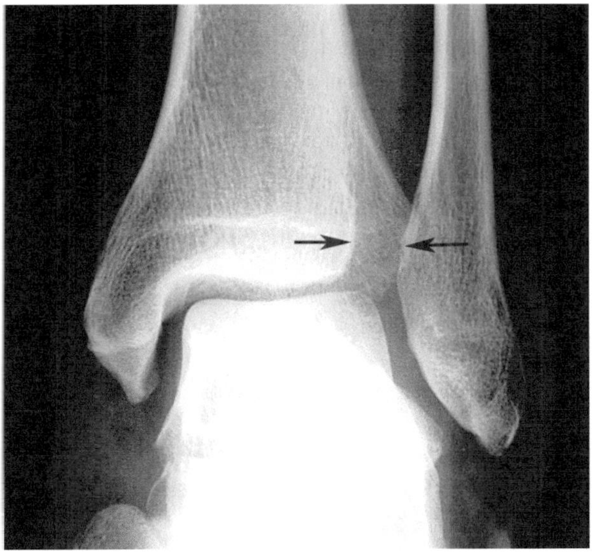

Fig. 41.2 AP ankle X-ray showing widening of the distal tibio-fibular joint space, indicative of a distal tibio-fibular or high ankle sprain

6. Treatment
   (a) Orthopedic treatment with below-knee cast immobilization for 6 weeks is indicated when the radiographs are normal or in the presence of small avulsion of the anterolateral distal tibial tubercle.
   (b) A specialized orthopedic consultation is recommended for potential surgical intervention in cases of widening of the distal tibio-fibular clear space or the presence of a large anterolateral distal tubercle avulsion fracture.

41.2.2 Anterior Ankle Sprain

- It refers to an injury of the anterior capsulo-ligamentous structures of the tibio-talar joint.
- The usual mechanism is plantar hyperflexion of the ankle.
- It clinically presents with anterior ankle pain, swelling, and tenderness.
- Radiographic assessment typically appears normal.
- Functional treatment, such as strapping and rehabilitation, is generally indicated.

41.2.3 Medial Ankle Sprain

- A sprain of the medial collateral ligament (deltoid Ligament) is a rare injury.
- The injury is typically caused by a forced valgus stress on the ankle.
- Clinically, it presents with pain and tenderness below the medial malleolus.
- It is important to consider a possible injury or dislocation of the *posterior tibialis tendon*, which can mimic a medial ankle sprain and is confirmable by ultrasound.

- Functional treatment, including strapping and rehabilitation, is commonly used. Below-knee cast immobilization may be necessary if the pain is severe and impedes weight-bearing.

41.2.4 Mid-Tarsal Sprain

- It is a common presentation.
- The injury is typically caused by a plantar forced hyperflexion of the foot.
- The pain and tenderness are located at the dorsal aspect of the tarsal bones.
- The radiographic assessment may reveal a small bony avulsion at the dorsal aspect of the talo-navicular joint or the calcaneo-cuboid joint.
- Functional treatment, including strapping and rehabilitation, is usually indicated for mild and moderate pain.
- A below-knee cast immobilization is applied for 4–6 weeks if the pain is severe and impedes walking.

41.3 Dislocation of the Peroneal Tendons

- It is an uncommon injury.
- It often goes undiagnosed in the emergency setting.
- The mechanism of injury typically resembles that of a lateral ankle sprain.
- The clinical presentation and examination typically include:
  - *Lateral retro-malleolar* pain and tenderness, which is different from lateral ankle sprains where the pain is usually located pre and sub-malleolar
  - Palpation of the peroneal tendons in an anteriorly dislocated position in relation to the lateral malleolus,
  - Provocative maneuvers to induce tendon dislocation are generally not feasible in the emergency setting due to the significant pain they cause.
- Radiographic ankle assessment
  - Usually normal findings.
  - May reveal a small chip of bone located posterior to the lateral malleolus (in the AP or oblique view).
- *Ultrasound*, both in static and dynamic modes, is helpful for initial diagnostic orientation. It can visualize the tendons and any abnormal movement or position.
- *CT scans and/or MRI* are more definitive imaging techniques that can confirm the diagnosis by clearly showing the position of the peroneal tendons whether there is a complete dislocation or sub-luxation.
- The treatment is surgical.

41.4 "Hidden" or "Unrevealed" Fractures

The radiographic assessment and interpretation should always be clinically guided in order to disclose any "hidden" or "unrevealed" fractures and to reduce the risk of undiagnosed injuries.

41.4.1 Calcaneal Fractures

- Undisplaced extra-articular fracture (posterior tuberosity).
- Undisplaced articular fracture.
- ***Fracture of the sustentaculum tali*** (misdiagnosed as medial ankle sprain):
  - Pain and tenderness located inferior to the medial malleolus,
  - The fracture line is commonly unrevealed on the conventional radiographic ankle views,
  - *Retro-tibial calcaneal view* may disclose the fracture line,
  - *The CT scan* is mandatory in case of doubt.
  - Undisplaced fractures of the sustentaculum tali are treated with below-knee cast immobilization without weight-bearing for 8 weeks,
  - Displaced fractures of the sustentaculum tali are surgically treated with open reduction and internal fixation

41.4.2 Talar Fractures

- **Undisplaced fractures of the body and the neck of the talus** (Fig. 41.3a, b):
  - Fractures of the talar body may easily be missed, as the fracture line is commonly located in the sagittal plane.

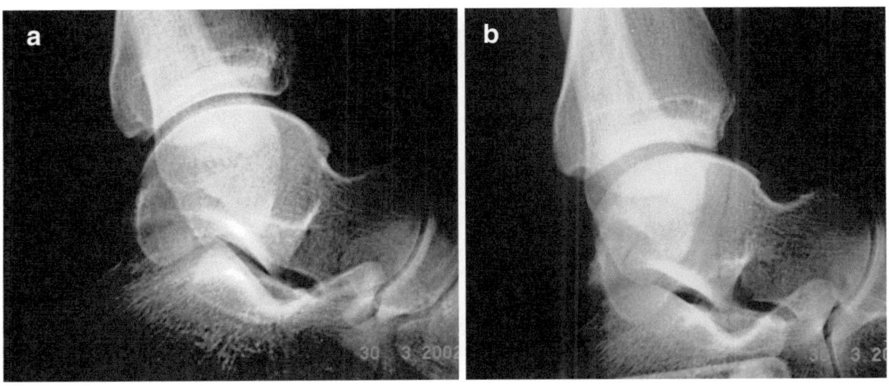

Fig. 41.3 (**a**) Post-traumatic lateral ankle X-ray labeled "Normal." (**b**) Slightly Lateral oblique ankle radiograph of the same patient as shown in Fig. **a** showing a subtle hairline fracture of the talar body

- Oblique views are helpful, and *CT scan* is mandatory to confirm the diagnosis (especially in case of any doubt).

- **Osteochondral lesions of the talar dome**
  - They are usually visible on the initial radiographic evaluation in the ER, presenting as osteochondral hairline fracture located at either the medial, or more commonly, the lateral talar dome, without any radiographic signs of surrounding bone condensation (Fig. 41.4a).
  - The diagnosis becomes more subtle in case of chronic ankle pain unrelated to recent sprains, where it is difficult to differentiate between pre-existing conditions such as osteochondritis of the talus and injuries to the talar dome resulting from the sprain itself (Fig. 41.4b).
  - The *post-traumatic initial radiographic assessment* of the ankle is important for early detection of any associated "occult" bony or osteochondral lesions, especially when the diagnosis of sprain is evoked (the talus tilts in varus into the tibio-peroneal mortise and the talus angles tend to impact against the lateral malleolus or the tibial pilon).
- **Fractures of the posterolateral tubercle of the talus (Shepherd fracture)**
  - The fracture is visible on the lateral ankle view (Fig. 41.5).
  - It may be misinterpreted for an accessory bone, so-called os trigonum, or for an unfused posterolateral tubercle of the talus.
  - The clinical presentation corresponds to:

    Posterior ankle pain in plantar hyperflexion,

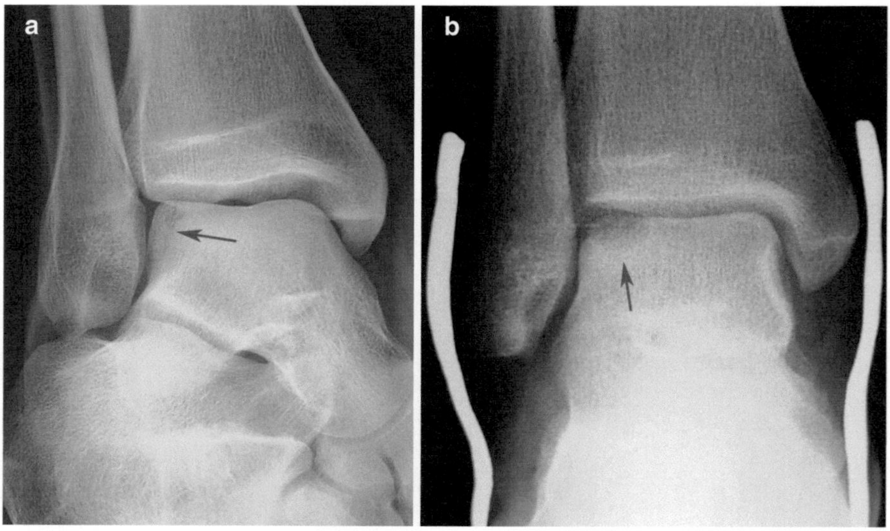

Fig. 41.4 (**a**) Ankle mortise view showing an osteochondral fracture of the supero-lateral talar dome, despite the patient presented initially with negative Ottawa criteria for radiographic imaging. (**b**) AP ankle X-ray of a late presentation of an osteochondral lesion of the supero-lateral talar dome

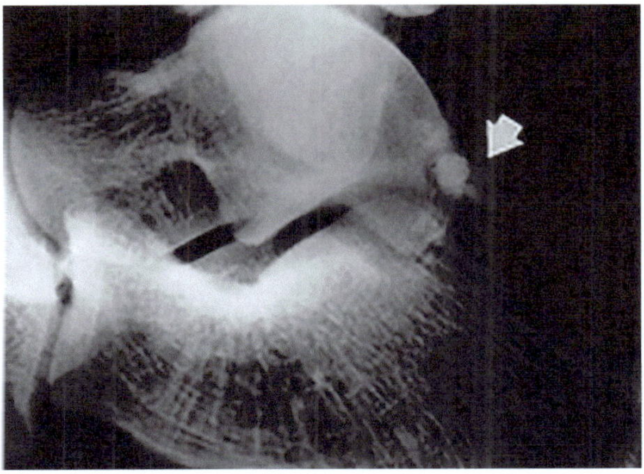

Fig. 41.5 Lateral ankle radiograph showing a fracture of the posterolateral talar tubercle (the so-called Shepherd fracture) which may be misinterpreted for normal accessory bone ("os trigonum")

Medial retro-malleolar pain during plantar flexion of the big toe with manual resistance (the flexor hallucis Longus tendon runs just in contact with the tubercle).

- Comparative radiographic assessment of both ankles is useful for guiding the diagnosis.
- Both *CT scan and MRI* are outstanding for diagnosis. MRI is particularly useful in the early post-traumatic period as it can reveal bony contusions and edematous changes in the posterolateral talar tubercle.
- In later stages, bone scintigraphy may be indicated to distinguish between an os trigonum and a nonunion of a posterolateral tubercle fracture, as indicated by hyperfixation or "hot spot" (Fig. 41.6).

• **Fractures of the lateral process of the talus**
  - Are frequent, yet they are commonly undiagnosed in the early post-traumatic stage.
  - The clinical presentation can be misleading, often resembling a lateral ankle sprain, as the pain and tenderness are localized just below the tip of the lateral malleolus.
  - The initial ankle radiographs in the ER are commonly interpreted as "normal" (Fig. 41.7).
  - The AP ankle view with internal rotation is useful to reveal the fracture (Fig. 41.8).
  - *The CT scan* is mandatory to confirm the diagnosis as well as to indicate the most appropriate treatment plan (Fig. 41.9).
  - Treatment

    Undisplaced fracture: below-knee cast immobilization for 6–8 weeks.

    Displaced fracture: open reduction and internal fixation.

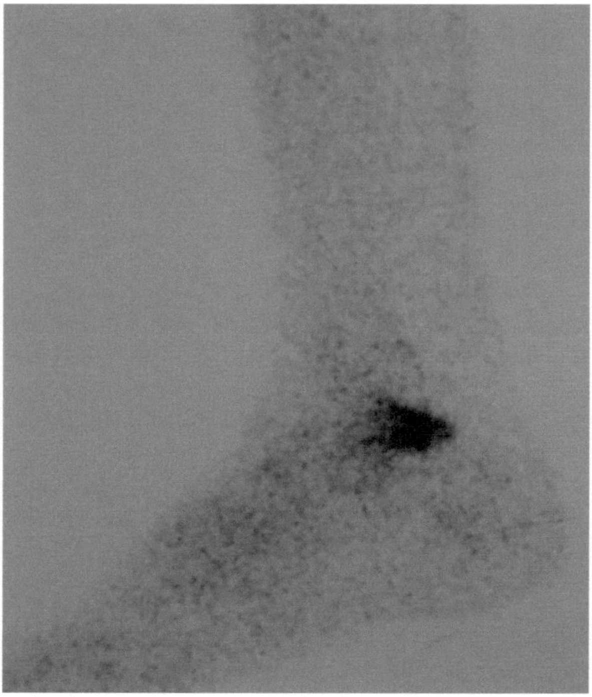

Fig. 41.6 Bone scintigraphy image showing an increased uptake (hotspot) at the posterior aspect of the talus, indicative of nonunion of a fracture of the posterolateral talar tubercle

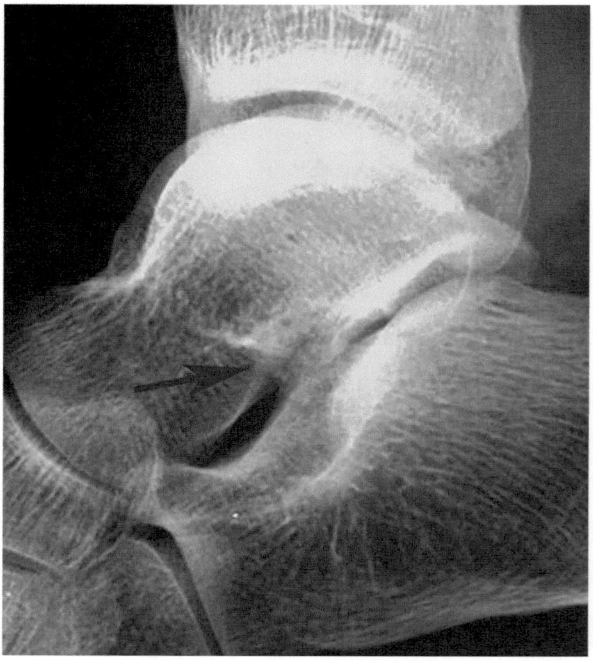

Fig. 41.7 Lateral ankle X-ray showing a very subtle radiographic presentation of a fracture of the lateral talar tubercle

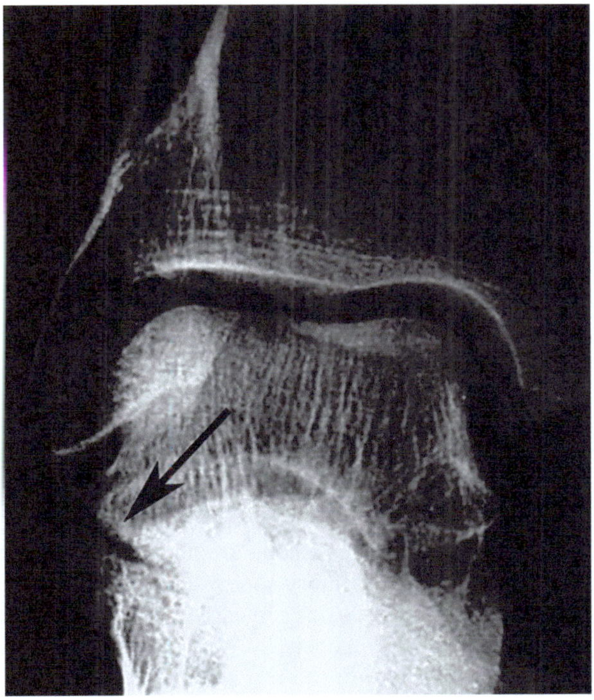

Fig. 41.8 AP X-ray of the same ankle as shown in Fig. 41.7 revealing a more evident radiographic image of the fracture of the lateral talar tubercle

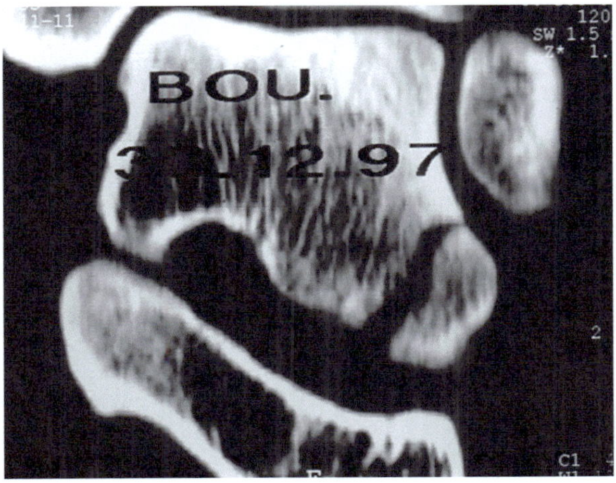

Fig. 41.9 Coronal cut of ankle CT scan revealing an evident image of fracture of the lateral talar tubercle

41.4.3 Navicular Bone Fracture

Undiagnosed fractures of the tarsal navicular bone are usually represented by the stress fractures and fractures of the navicular medial tuberosity.

- **Stress fractures**
  - Uncommon injuries,
  - May induce secondary serious complications such as avascular necrosis and nonunion,
  - The clinical presentation commonly mimics ankle sprain in runners who have increased or modified their training or technique of practice (e.g., running on hard surface),
  - The patient complains of pain at the lateral edge of the navicular bone, just proximal to the sinus tarsi,
  - The pain is reproduced and increases when the *patient stands or walks on tiptoe.*
  - Radiographs are often interpreted as "normal" because special AP views targeting the navicular bone are not typically performed in the ER, and radiographic signs of injury appear late.
  - *MRI is highly sensitive* in early stage: it shows increased signal intensity and confirms the diagnosis.
  - *Bone scintigraphy (bone scan)* could be helpful in case of unexplained chronic ankle pain during sports activities (sprint, jump).
  - *CT scan* is more sensitive than conventional radiographs in late stage.
  - Treatment

    Below-knee cast without weight-bearing for 8 weeks is recommended for patients seen in the early stage, before the occurrence of radiographic "widening" of the fracture line (local bone resorption).

    Surgical treatment, usually with a bone graft (or without), is recommended for patients seen at a late stage.
- **Fractures of the medial tuberosity**
  - Fractures of the medial tuberosity of the tarsal navicular bone may not be a straightforward diagnosis.
  - The clinical exam usually demonstrates a "hypertrophic" medial tuberosity, with tenderness on palpation.
  - The radiographs rarely conclude for the diagnosis of "acute" or "recent" fracture (Fig. 41.10).
  - The *CT scan* may reveal the presence of an accessory navicular bone (os navicularis or os tibiale externum) without being able to conclude whether it is pathological or not (Fig. 41.11).
  - In case of doubt, *bone scintigraphy* is helpful (Fig. 41.12). A "hot spot" at the navicular bone site suggests a "fracture" or rupture of the fibrous connection

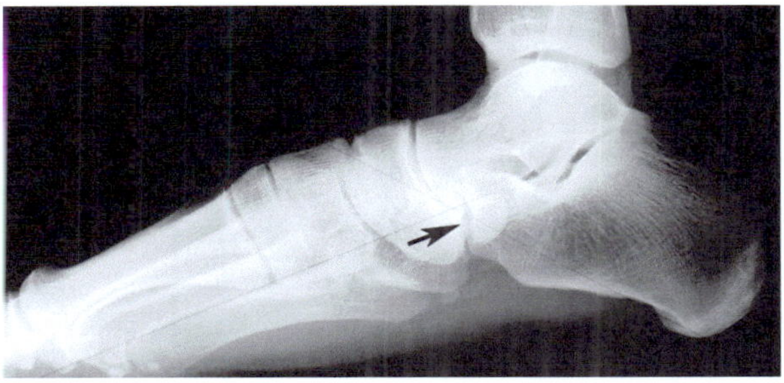

Fig. 41.10 Lateral foot radiograph with an image that shows a suspected fracture of the medial tubercle of the tarsal navicular bone

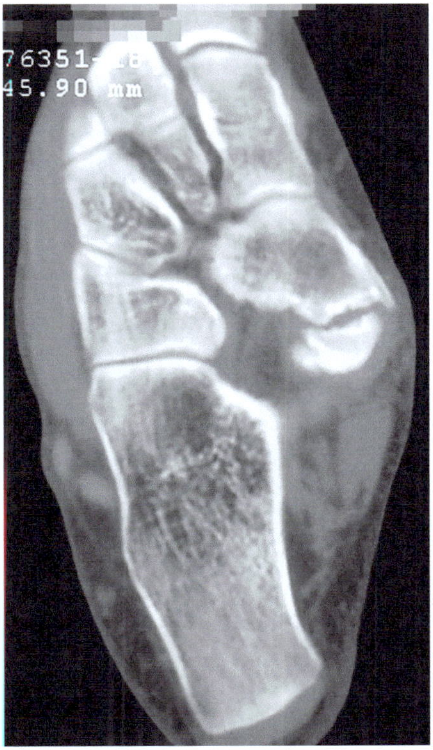

Fig. 41.11 Axial cut of a foot CT scan showing fracture of the medial tubercle of the tarsal navicular bone (difficult to differentiate between recent and old fracture)

between the navicular bone and the os navicularis, indicating the need for surgical treatment (excision of the os navicularis, or internal fixation of the navicular fragment).

- A below-knee cast immobilization for 6 weeks may be used as a trial treatment before scintigraphy or if scintigraphy results are negative (no "hot spot").

Fig. 41.12 Bone scintigraphic image of increased uptake (hotspot) at the site of the tarsal navicular bone, indicative of a recent traumatic injury

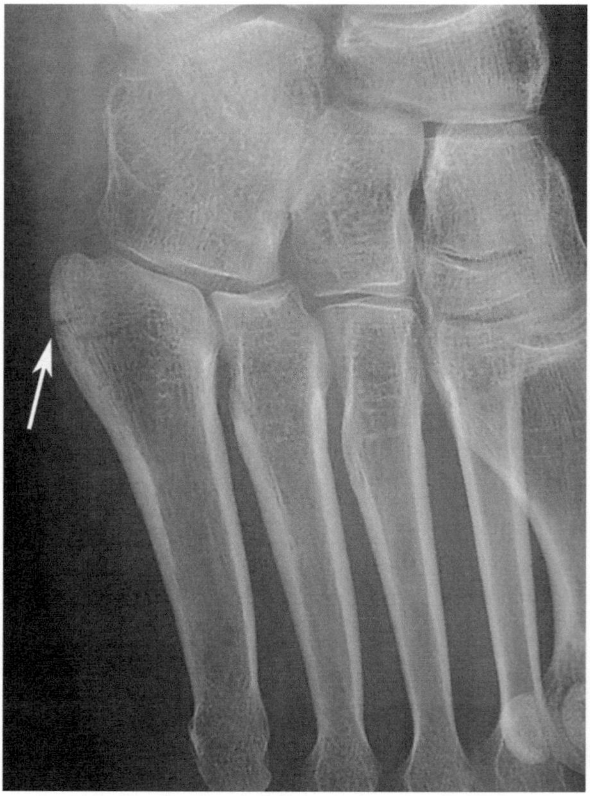

Fig. 41.13 Foot radiograph showing an undisplaced fracture of the base of the fifth metatarsal bone (type 1)

41.4.4 Fractures of the Other Tarsal and Metatarsal Bones of the Foot (Cuboid, Cuneiform, Base of the Fifth Metatarsal, etc.)

The clinical examination and radiographs guided by this examination and including views of the entire foot should enable the diagnosis of these lesions (Fig. 41.13). It is important to avoid indiscriminately requesting a CT scan or MRI, as these may complicate the diagnostic process unnecessarily.

41.5 In Summary

- Any post-traumatic "swollen ankle" for which well-done, well-oriented, and well-interpreted radiographs have found no bone damage should be immobilized in a rigid boot (plaster cast or splint) for at least 1 month.
- Functional treatment should be avoided, as it may lead to equinus stiffness of the ankle, dragging and tedious pain, algodystrophy, pseudarthrosis of an undiagnosed occult fracture.
- The ER physician should not just ask for an MRI at random, without knowing what he is looking for.
- When the cast is removed, and after 1–2 months of rehabilitation, if disabling pain persists, it is preferable to ask for a *bone scan*, which will enable the diagnosis to be made of either an undetected fracture (localized hyperfixation +++) or algodystrophy (global hyperfixation of the foot).

42 Fractures of the Foot

42.1 Fractures of the Talus

42.1.1 Patho-Anatomy

Fractures of the talar bone are often the result of high-energy trauma in forced dorsi-flexion of the ankle and foot, with a variable association of eversion, inversion, supination, pronation, internal or external rotation.

They may affect,

- **The talar neck** (Fig. 42 1),
  - Secondary to high-energy trauma in forced dorsi-flexion of the ankle and foot.
  - Involves the risk of avascular necrosis.
  - May be,
    Undisplaced,
    Displaced,
    Comminuted, fragmentary.
  - May be associated with dislocation of one or more of the following joints:
    Subtalar,
    Tibiotalar,
    Talonavicular.
- **The talar body**, including, sagittal (Fig. 42.2), frontal (Fig. 42.3), partial (dome) (Fig. 42.4), and comminuted fractures.
- **The talar posterior process or Shepherd fracture** (Fig. 42.5): care should be taken not to mistake an os trigonum for a fracture of the posterior process of the talus.
- **The talar lateral process** (Fig. 42.6),
- **The talar head**, with possible involvement of the talonavicular joint.

D. Saragaglia, A. Hassan Chamseddine, *Traumatology for the Emergency Doctor*, https://doi.org/10.1007/978-3-031-63196-2_42

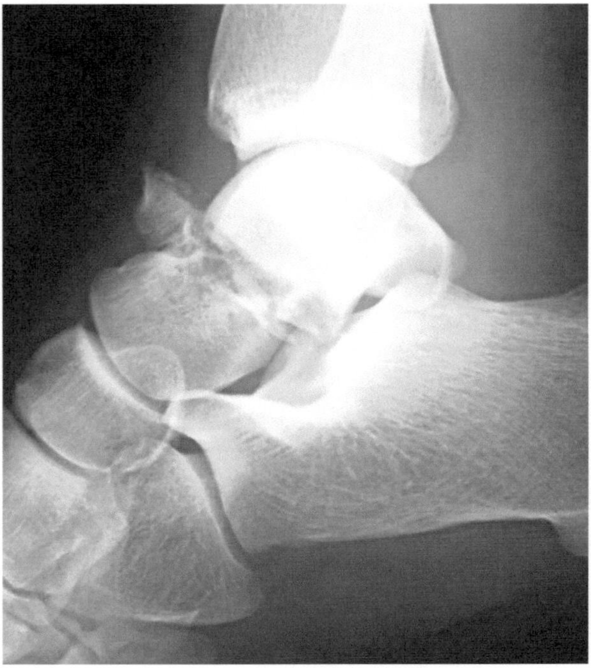

Fig. 42.1 Lateral ankle radiograph showing a comminuted fracture of the talar neck

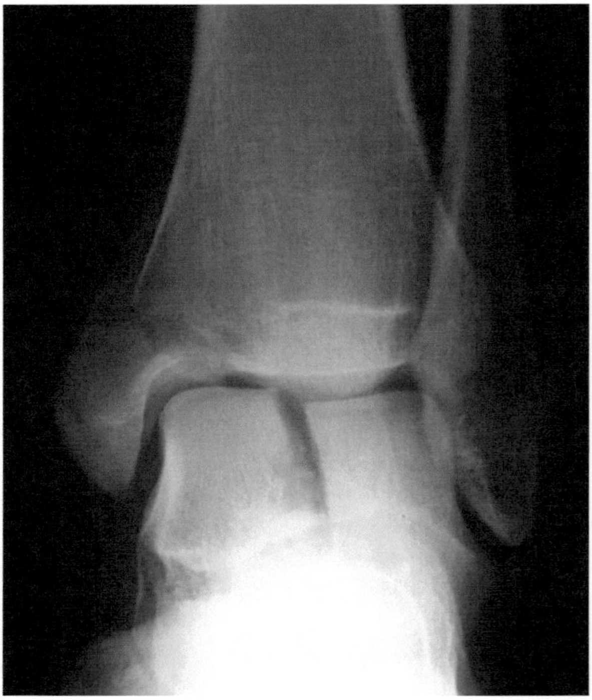

Fig. 42.2 AP ankle radiograph showing a sagittal fracture of the talus with a fracture of the medial malleolus

Fig. 42.3 Lateral ankle radiograph revealing a subtle hairline frontal fracture of the talar body

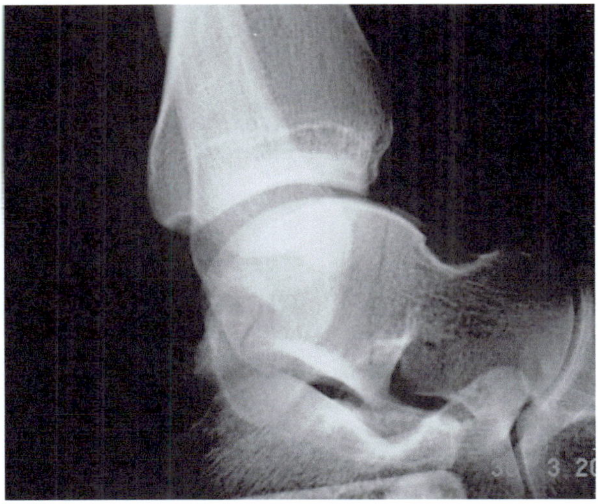

Fig. 42.4 AP ankle X-ray revealing a fracture of the supero-lateral talar dome

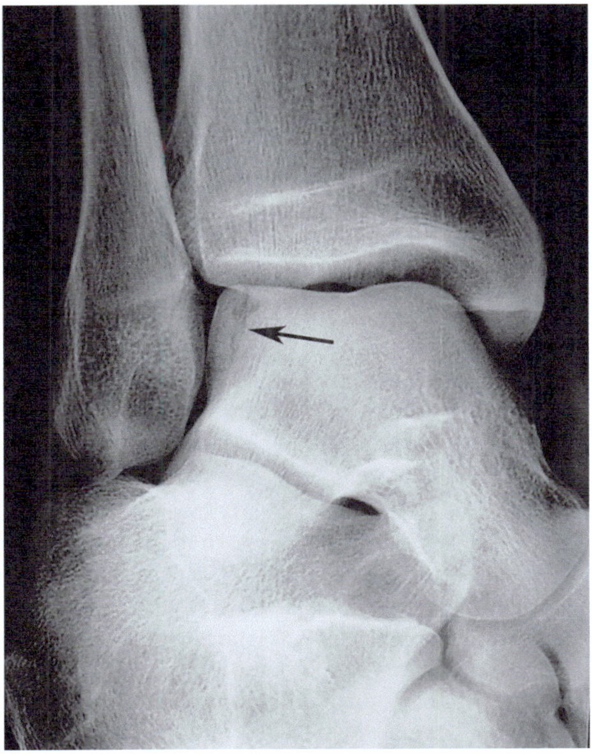

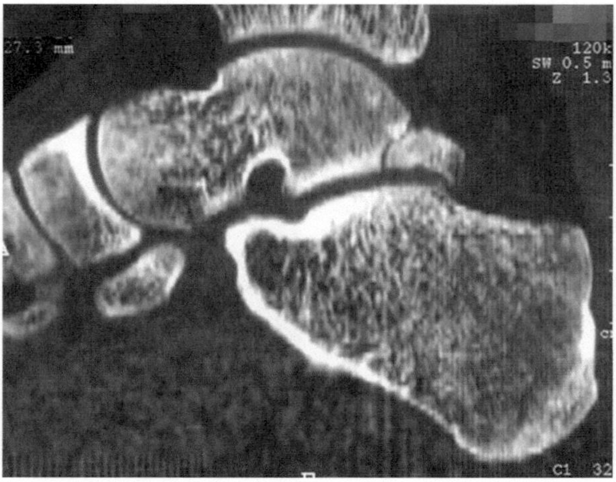

Fig. 42.5 Sagittal cut of ankle CT scan showing a confirmed fracture of the postero-lateral talar tubercle (Shepherd fracture)

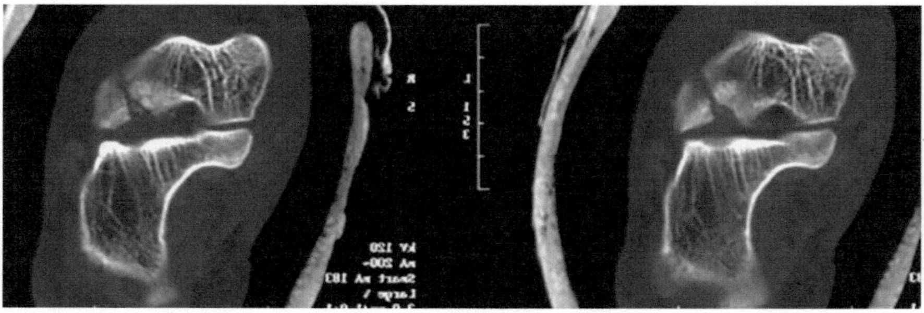

Fig. 42.6 Coronal cuts of ankle CT scan showing a fracture of the lateral talar tubercle

42.1.2 Diagnosis

- The diagnosis is essentially based on the radiographic assessment: AP, lateral.
- Special views may be requested for better visualization of the talar neck:
  - oblique views (internal and external),
  - Canale view for talar neck (full equinus position with 15° ankle pronation, and X-ray beam directed 75° cephalad from the horizontal plane),
  - Pre-tibial dorso-plantar view (to visualize the long axis of the talus).
- Some fractures (such as fractures of the lateral process, posterior process, and sagittal fractures of the body) can be easily missed in the emergency settings because of bad or inappropriate radiographic views.
- *CT scan* is a must in any doubtful situation; it also helps for therapeutic decision.

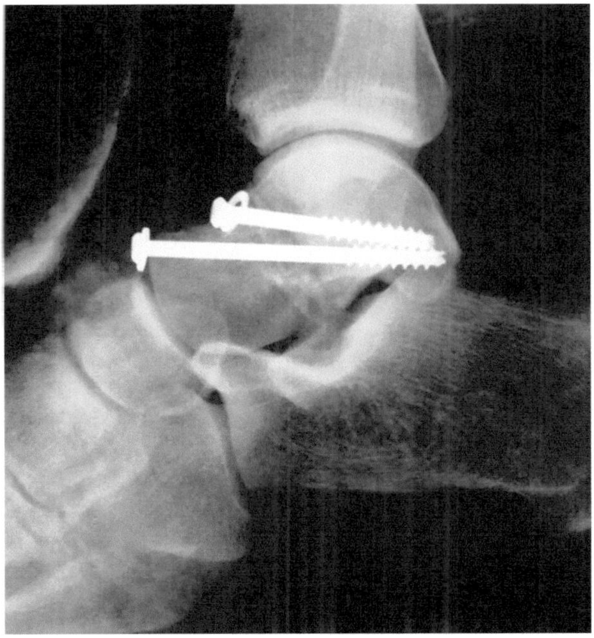

Fig. 42.7 Lateral ankle X-ray showing a post-operative control of open reduction and internal fixation of a talar fracture using two screws

42.1.3 Management

- Undisplaced fractures: below-knee non-weight bearing cast for 8–12 weeks.
- Displaced fractures of the body, neck, and lateral process: open reduction with internal fixation (Fig. 42.7).
- Fractures of the posterior process:
  - They are usually initially treated conservatively,
  - They commonly progress to nonunion,
  - Secondary surgical treatment may be needed with excision of the fragment if it becomes source of pain and functional disability.

42.2 Fractures of the Calcaneus

Calcaneal fractures are the most frequent fractures of the foot.

42.2.1 Patho-Anatomy

1. Fractures of the calcaneus are categorized into:
   (a) ***Extra-articular fractures*** involving,
      - The anterior process,
      - The sustentaculum tali,
      - The posterior tuberosity (site of Achilles tendon insertion).

(b) ***Intra-articular fractures*** involving the posterior articular facet and the subtalar joint.
- The posterior facet may be completely separated from the rest of the calcaneus and displaced into the body of the calcaneus in a "vertical" or "horizontal" depression,
- The posterior facet may,
  - present two or more separate fragments,
  - remain attached to the posterior calcaneal tuberosity and displaced with it (the so-called tongue-type fracture).

2. *Sanders classification* is widely used.
   (a) It is based on the coronal CT images.
   (b) It is divided into four types according to the number of the posterior facet fragments:
   - Type I: Undisplaced fractures, regardless of the number of the fracture lines and fragments,
   - Type II: one fracture line separating the posterior facet in two fragments,
   - Type III: two fracture lines separating the posterior facet in three fragments (Fig. 42.8).
   - Type IV: three or more fracture lines inducing a comminution of the posterior facet in four or more fragments (Figs. 42.9a, b and 42.10).

42.2.2 Clinical Presentation and Diagnosis

- ***Red Flags***
  - Patients with calcaneal fracture should always be assessed for associated injuries (25 to 50%): bilateral calcaneal fractures, lumbar spine fractures, pelvic fractures, etc.
  - Ask for history of peripheral artery disease or insufficiency, diabetes, cigarettes consumption, alcohol abuse.

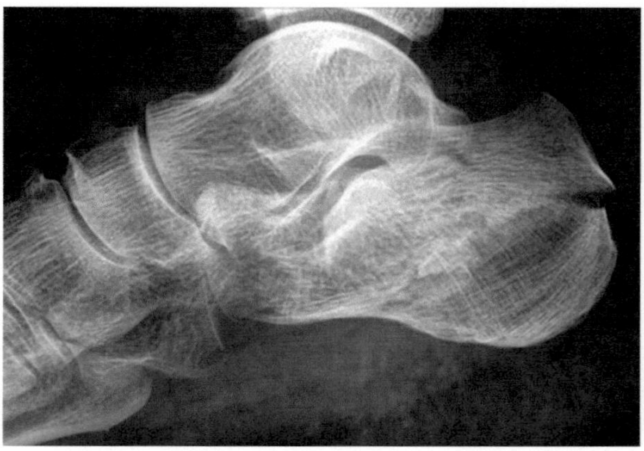

Fig. 42.8 Lateral calcaneal X-ray showing a calcaneal fracture of type 3 resulting in a depression-split

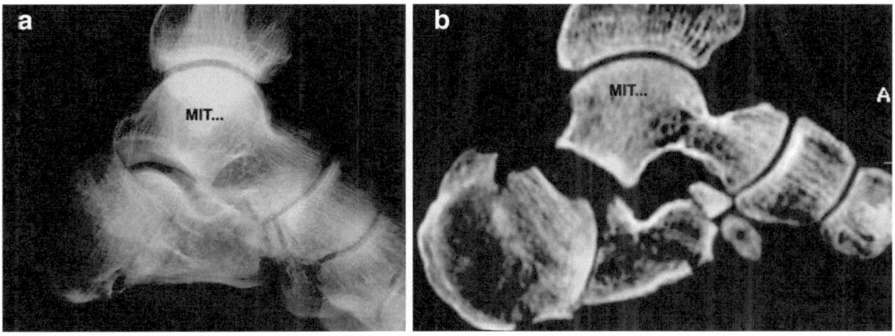

Fig. 42.9 (**a**) Lateral calcaneal X-ray showing a calcaneal fracture of type 4 resulting in a depression-split fracture. (**b**) Sagittal CT scan cut of the same fracture as shown in Fig. **a**

Fig. 42.10 Lateral calcaneal X-ray showing a calcaneal fracture of type 4 resulting in a depression-split fracture (comminuted fracture)

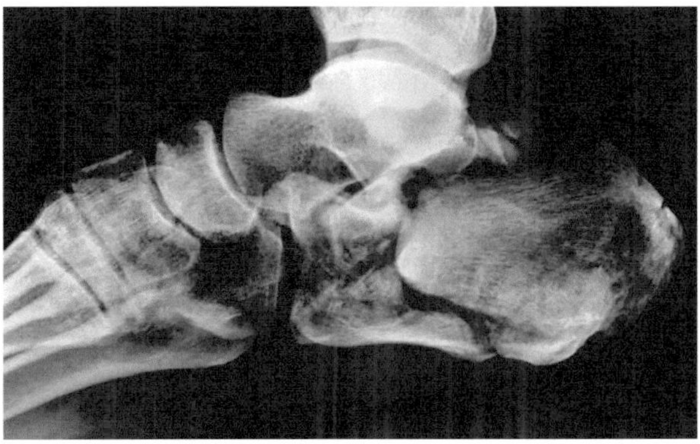

- ***The clinical diagnosis*** is easily evoked when the fracture is displaced and secondary to high-energy trauma:
  - Swelling and ecchymosis of the posterior heel, involving the medial and lateral aspects (medial and lateral infra-malleolar areas),
  - The heel appears widened and shortened with varus deformity.
  - Complete functional disability and inability to bear weight.
- ***The clinical presentation*** may be more subtle when the fracture is undisplaced.
- For late presentation (hours after the accident),
  - Carefully inspect for any impairment of the skin of the posterior heel: open fracture, pale appearance, threatened skin, bullae and blisters (hemorrhagic "red" blisters indicate more severe injury than clear "yellowish" blisters).
  - Carefully assess for the presence of compartment syndrome of the foot: severe pain, exacerbated with passive stretch of the toes, tense swelling, sensory impairment of the plantar aspect of the toes and forefoot, presence of blisters (mainly hemorrhagic "red").
- ***Radiographic assessment***. Conventional calcaneal radiographs include:

– Lateral calcaneal view, usually showing the following findings in cases of displaced posterior facet fractures:
  Decrease of the calcaneal height,
  Depression of the posterior facet ("horizontal" or "vertical" compression),
  Perturbation of the obtuse angle formed between the anterior and the posterior calcaneal facets (Gissane angle: increased with the horizontal depression, and decreased with the vertical depression of the posterior facet).
– Axial (Harris or Böhler) view for assessment of (Fig. 42.11),
  The width of the calcaneus (usually increased),
  Varus–valgus deformity of the posterior tuberosity,
  The sustentaculum tali fragment,
  The subtalar joint displacement.

- ***CT scan is irreplaceable*** for:
  – Precise analysis of the fracture pattern,
  – Better assessment of the displacement,
  – Surgical indication and planning,
  – Disclosure of any associated injuries (e.g., fibular tendons dislocation) (Fig. 42.12).

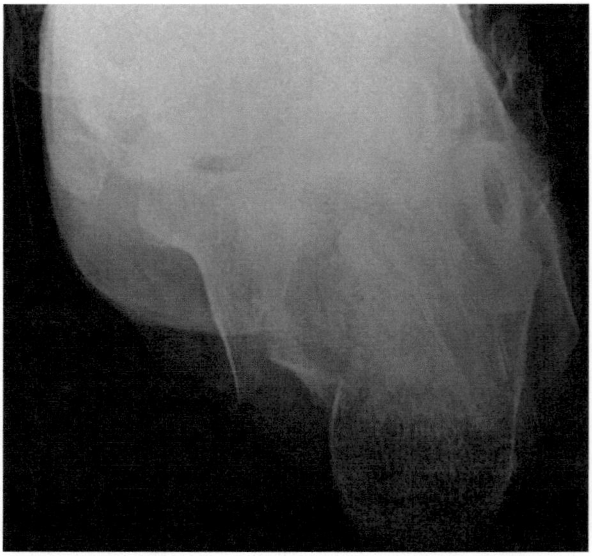

Fig. 42.11 Retro-tibial axial calcaneal radiographic view (Harris or Böhler)

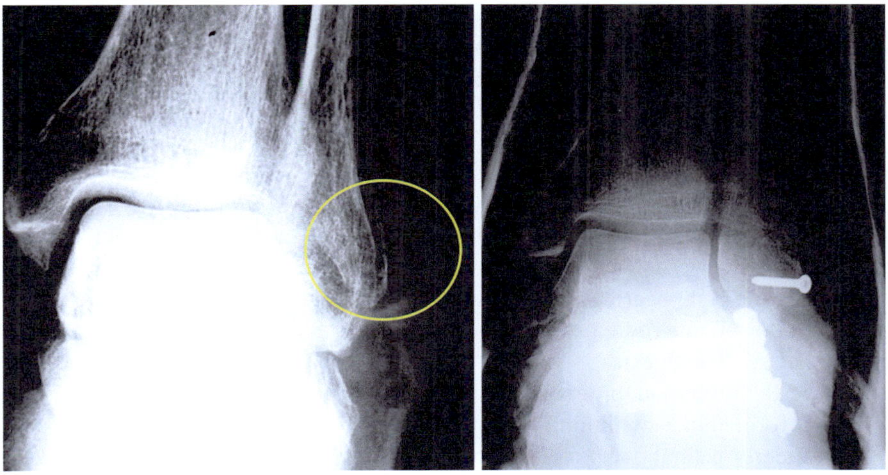

Fig. 42.12 Fracture of the calcaneus associated with a dislocation of the fibular tendons (observe the bony chip on the lateral malleolus)

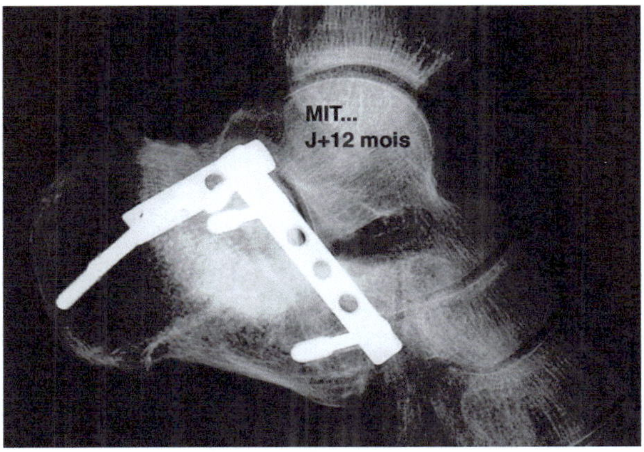

Fig. 42.13 Calcaneus lateral radiograph after open reduction and internal fixation using two plates and screws (with restitution of the subtalar congruence)

42.2.3 Management

- **Displaced fractures are usually treated surgically**
  - Presence of blisters and significant swelling should delay the surgical procedure (risk of skin necrosis and infection),
  - It is highly recommended to wait until the swelling resolves and the wrinkle sign appears (usually 10–14 days).
  - Surgical treatment is performed in the absence of contraindications (peripheral artery disease, elderly patient, heavy smoker, alcohol abuse, etc.).
  - It usually consists of reduction and internal fixation with restitution of the articular subtalar joint congruence (Fig. 42.13).

  - If an orthopedic surgeon is not available for early surgical treatment: apply the RICE protocol (Rest, Ice, Compressive dressing impregnated with alcohol and glycerin, and Elevation) in order to avoid or to reduce the risk of blisters while awaiting for surgery.
  - *Red Flag*: do not put the foot in elevated position for patients with peripheral artery disease.
- **Undisplaced fractures are usually treated conservatively**
  - For young patients who are able to walk using crutches: functional treatment as following:

    No weight bearing for 8–12 weeks,

    Use of anti-edema compression socks or elastic bandage,

    Use of analgesics,

    Rehabilitation program for progressive weight bearing and ROM performed in a swimming pool.
- For elderly patients who are not able to walk without weight bearing, a below-knee cast is applied with the following characteristics:
  - Window made in the cast, at the plantar aspect of the heel,
  - Rigid walking heel applied to the cast just anterior to window, along the longitudinal axis of the tibia,
  - Weight bearing as tolerated, with walking assistance device.

42.3 Fractures of the Tarsal Navicular Bone (Refer Also to Chap. 41)

42.3.1 Patho-Anatomy

- Fractures of the tarsal navicular are usually located to the body of the bone.
  - They usually present as a simple vertical fracture (Fig. 42.14).
  - Complex fracture pattern may occur (comminuted, fragmentary).
  - Some fractures may present an "enucleation" of the navicular fragment from the "talo-naviculo-cuneiform space" (Fig. 42.15).
- The fracture line may affect the medial tuberosity of the navicular bone.
  - It usually involves an avulsion of the posterior tibialis tendon insertion.
  - It may be misinterpreted as an accessory bone (os navicularis or os tibiale externum).
- A particular fracture type is represented by the "stress fracture," usually undiagnosed with conventional radiographs (refer to Chap. 41).

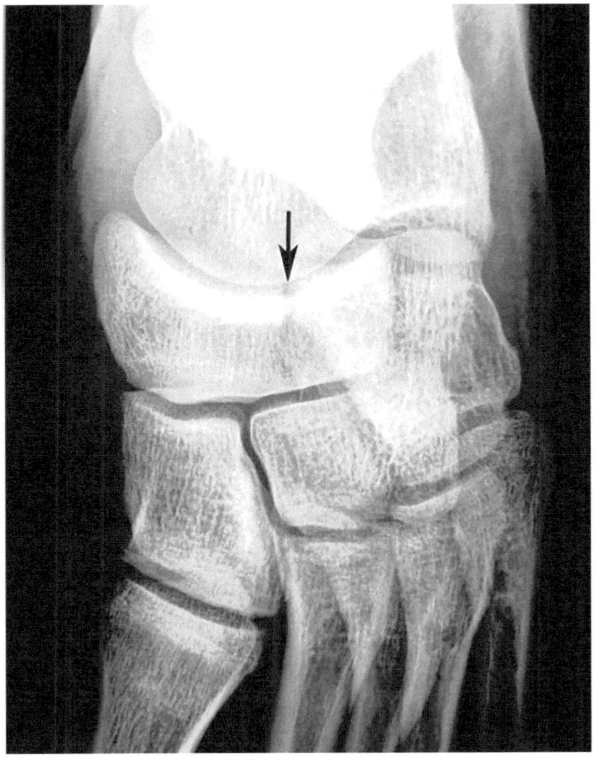

Fig. 42.14 AP foot X-ray showing a sagittal fracture of the tarsal navicular bone

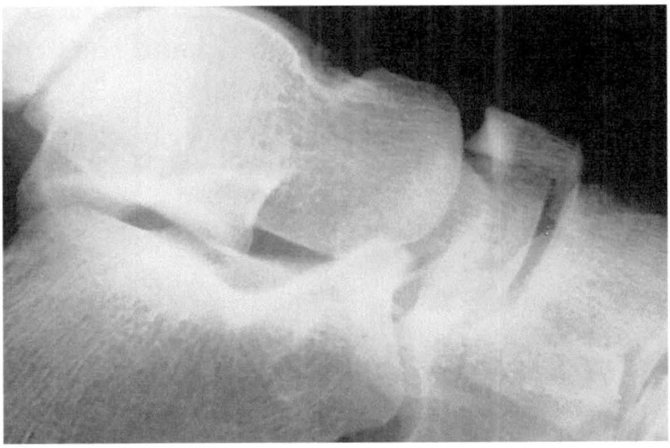

Fig. 42.15 Lateral foot X-ray showing an "enucleation" of the fractured navicular fragment out of the "talo-naviculo-cuneiform space"

42.3.2 Clinical Presentation

- The diagnosis is suspected when the patient presents with swelling and localized pain at the site of the navicular bone (dorso-medial aspect of the midfoot). The pain is increased with weight bearing.
- The clinical presentation may be subtle with mild edema and pain.

42.3.3 Radiographic Diagnosis

- The radiographic assessment includes AP, lateral, and internal and external oblique views of the midfoot.
- *CT scan* is mandatory in any doubtful cases.

42.3.4 Management

- **Displaced fractures are treated surgically**.
  - Early open reduction and internal fixation.
  - If the surgical treatment has to be delayed (unavailable surgeon for example) either a RICE protocol or a cast immobilization (anti-edema) is applied while awaiting for surgery.
- **Undisplaced fractures are treated conservatively**.
  - Below-knee non-weight bearing cast is applied for 8 weeks,
  - Rehabilitation after cast removal.

42.4 Fractures of the Cuboid and the Cuneiform Bones

- The pain is localized at,
  - The medial and dorso-medial aspect of the midfoot for cuneiform bones fractures,
  - The lateral aspect of the midfoot for cuboid bone fractures.
- Fractures of these bones may represent a part of a more complex fracture pattern (e.g., multiple associated fractures or fracture–dislocations of the foot).
- The primary radiographic assessment includes AP, lateral, and oblique (internal and external) views (Fig. 42.16).
- *CT scan* is a must, especially in case of any doubt.
- Treatment.
  - Undisplaced fractures: usually conservative treatment with below-knee cast for 6–8 weeks followed by rehabilitation after cast removal.
  - Displaced fractures: open reduction and internal fixation.

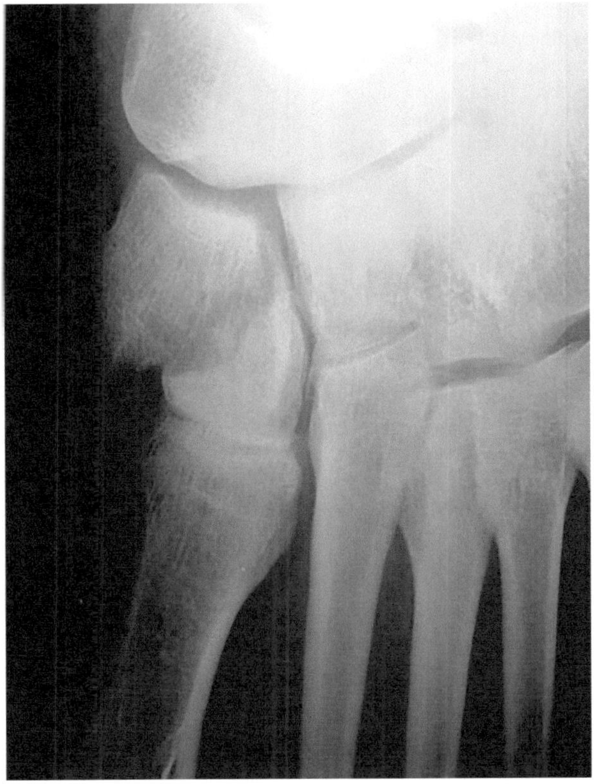

Fig. 42.16 AP foot radiograph revealing a displaced fracture of the first cuneiform bone

42.5 Fractures of the Metatarsal Bones

42.5.1 Patho-Anatomy

1. The fracture line may be located in the base, the shaft, or the neck of the metatarsal (Fig. 42.17).
2. One or more metatarsals can be affected at the same time.
3. Fractures of the metatarsal shaft may be, transverse, oblique, spiral, wedge, or comminuted.
4. **Fractures of the base of the first and fifth metatarsals have some particularities**.
   (a) ***Fractures of the base of the first metatarsal bone***
   - May be extra or intra-articular,
   - In the event of intra-articular fracture, it may induce *dorsal sub-luxation* of the base of the metatarsal with plantar flexion of the bone, leading to plantar impingement and prominence of the metatarsal head with secondary metatarsalgia if not properly reduced.

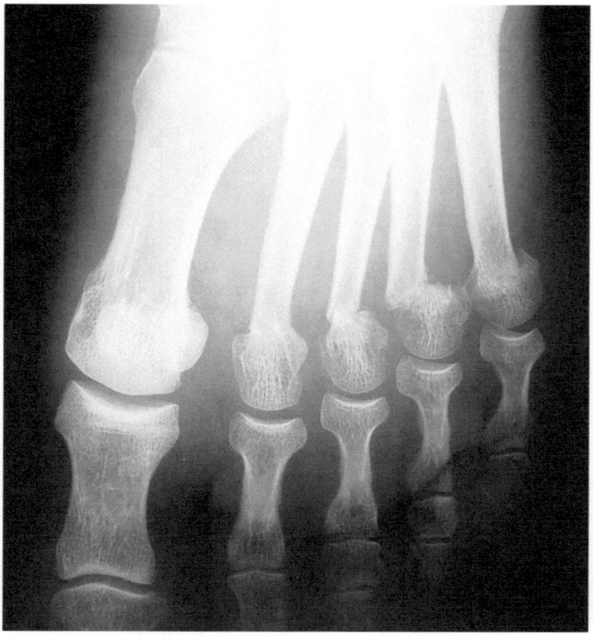

Fig. 42.17 AP foot radiograph showing fractures of the neck of the second, third, fourth, and fifth metatarsal bones

- *CT scan* is very helpful for adequate analysis of the fracture pattern and displacement.

(b) ***Fractures of the base of the fifth metatarsal bone***

- The radiographic evaluation includes AP, lateral, and oblique views of the foot.
  - The presence of an "os vesalianum" may be mistaken for a fracture of the metatarsal base.
  - The line that separates the "os vesalianum" from the metatarsal base is typically parallel to the long axis of the metatarsal.
  - The line of a true fracture of the base of the fifth metatarsal is usually oblique or perpendicular to the long axis of the metatarsal.
- They usually correspond to fracture-avulsion of the peroneus brevis tendon.
- They are commonly classified in three types based on the location of the fracture:
  - Type 1: fracture of the tip of the styloid process of the fifth metatarsal (corresponds to fracture-avulsion secondary to contraction of the peroneus brevis tendon),
  - Type 2: fracture located at the base of the styloid process (metaphyso-diaphyseal junction).
  - Type 3: fracture of the proximal metatarsal diaphysis (Jones fracture).

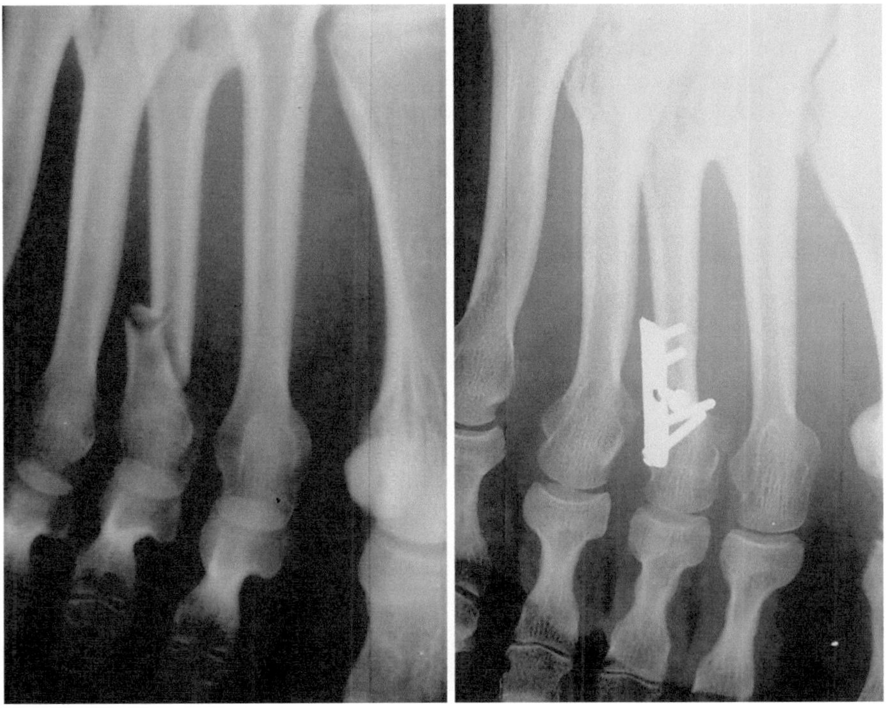

Fig. 42.18 Pre- and post-operative AP forefoot radiographs showing a fracture of the third metatarsal bone (before and after fixation with plate and screws)

42.5.2 Management

- ***Perfect reduction of metatarsal fractures is mandatory*** to restore the length, the angulation, and the orientation of the metatarsals and to reestablish the normal alignment of the metatarsal heads. Failure to achieve these requirements may lead to metatarsalgia with chronic pain and long-term functional disability.
- ***Displaced fractures require surgical treatment*** (Fig. 42.18).
  - Adequate radiographs are necessary to reveal any displacement that may require surgical treatment.
  - Open reduction and stable internal fixation is performed to restore the metatarsal heads alignment.
  - Cast immobilization after surgical fixation is not necessary.
  - Residual displacement may lead to chronic metatarsalgia, a disabling condition of difficult treatment.
- ***Undisplaced fractures require conservative treatment***
  - Fractures of the styloid process of the fifth metatarsal are treated using either a strapping or a removable brace for 6 weeks. The fracture line may remain visible on the radiographs for 6 months.

- Fractures of the other metatarsals are treated using either:
  Below-knee cast,
  Special shoes that shift the weight bearing area to the heel, keeping the forefoot in non-weight bearing during walking and standing position.
  The time required for bone healing is 6–8 weeks.

42.6 Fractures of the Phalanges

- ***Fractures of the* phalanges *of the lesser toes***
  - Undisplaced fractures are usually managed conservatively with functional treatment (temporary syndactylization by strapping the fractured toe to the adjacent intact toes using adhesive elastic tape for 4 weeks).
  - Displaced fractures are reduced using local anesthesia (interdigital nerve block), followed by syndactylization as previously.
- **Displaced fractures of the first phalanx of the big toe** are preferably treated surgically (reduction with internal fixation).

Foot and Ankle Dislocations

43

43.1 Dislocation of the Tibiotalar Joint

- Isolated tibiotalar joint dislocation is a rare condition (Fig. 43.1).
- It is often associated with malleolar fracture (one malleolus, e.g., posterior malleolus, or more).
- The dislocation should be relocated in emergency, preferably under general anesthesia, to prevent soft tissue and neuro-vascular complications. The reduction consists of applying a traction-relocation maneuver following the opposite direction of the dislocation.
- A post-reduction radiographic control is a must.
- A temporary below-knee cast is applied while awaiting for the final treatment (radiographs are repeated after immobilization to check the reduction).
- A specialized orthopedic opinion is warranted, especially in the case of associated malleolar fracture.

D. Saragaglia, A. Hassan Chamseddine, *Traumatology for the Emergency Doctor*, https://doi.org/10.1007/978-3-031-63196-2_43

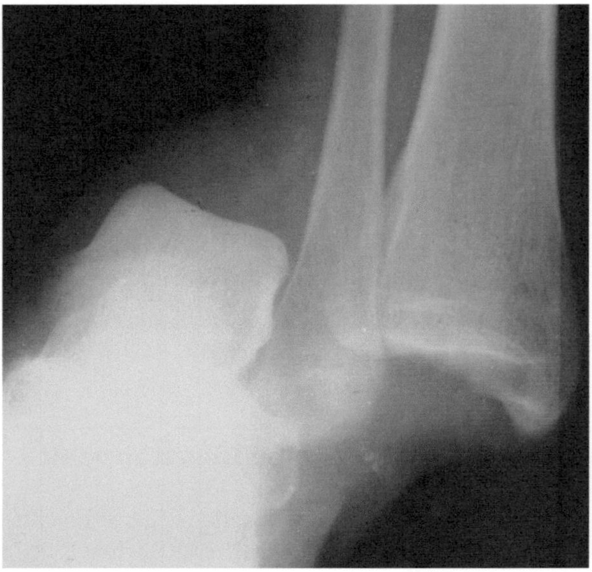

Fig. 43.1 AP ankle radiograph revealing a pure tibiotalar dislocation

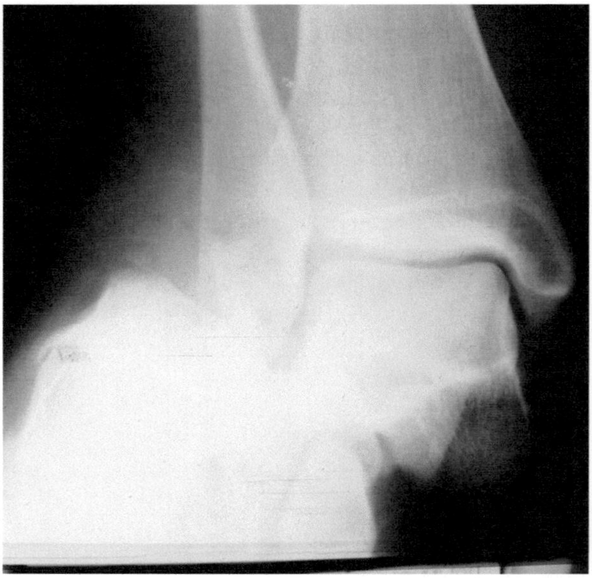

Fig. 43.2 AP right ankle radiograph revealing a subtalar lateral dislocation

43.2 Subtalar Dislocation

- It is often associated with a *talonavicular dislocation*.
- It may be associated with a fracture of the talar bone.
- The dislocation is *either medial or lateral* (Fig. 43.2).

- Management.
  - Relocation of the dislocation in emergency, preferably under general anesthesia.
  - Post-reduction below-knee cast immobilization for 4 weeks.
  - An irreducible dislocation should elevate the possibility of soft tissue incarceration, namely the posterior tibialis tendon: surgical open reduction is indicated in this case.
  - In case of associated fracture of the talar neck: open reduction and internal fixation of the talus is recommended.

43.3 Midtarsal Dislocation (Chopart Joint Line Dislocation)

- Mid-tarsal dislocation is rarely an isolated injury.
- It is commonly associated to a subtalar dislocation or a fracture of the navicular or cuboid bone (Fig. 43.3).
- A closed reduction and below-knee immobilization under anesthesia should be performed in emergency.
- A secondary early internal fixation (using temporary pinning) is often required for:
  - Stabilization of the dislocation (as the reduction is often unstable),
  - Reduction and fixation of associated displaced fracture (navicular and cuboid bones).

Fig. 43.3 AP foot radiograph showing a midtarsal dislocation with a fracture of the cuboid bone

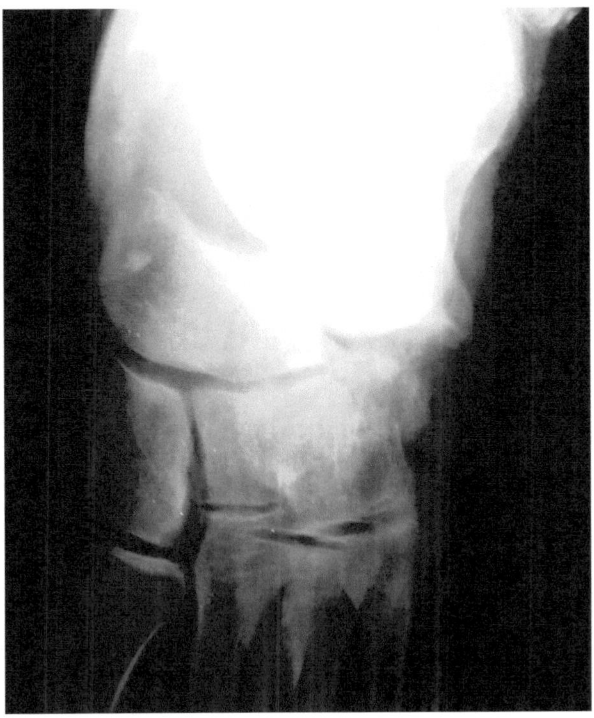

43.4 Tarsometatarsal Dislocations and Fracture–Dislocations (Lisfranc Joint Line Dislocations)

- Tarsometatarsal dislocation is either,
  - *A complete homolateral dislocation*: all metatarsals are dislocated (1st to 5th) in the same direction (usually dorso-lateral),
  - A Partial Lisfranc dislocation,

    Medial column dislocation: medial dislocation of the first ray (first metatarsal),

    Lateral column dislocation: lateral dislocation of the lateral column (2nd to 5th metatarsals) (Fig. 43.4).
  - *A complete divergent dislocation* (medial dislocation of the medial column with lateral dislocation of the lateral column).
- Associated fractures are common:
  - Fracture of the base of the second metatarsal (most common),
  - Fracture of the base of the other metatarsals,
  - Fracture of the cuneiform bones.

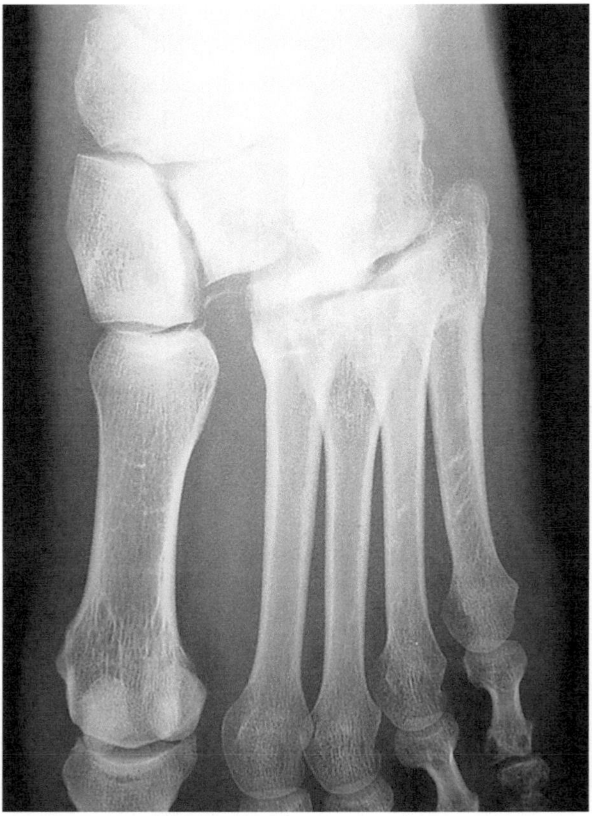

Fig. 43.4 AP foot radiograph showing a tarsometatarsal dislocation, the so-called Lisfranc dislocation, resulting in a lateral dislocation of the whole lateral column of the foot (from the second to the fifth metatarsal)

- Treatment is surgical.
  - Open reduction with internal fixation is required (using multiple pinning or mini-plates),
  - Post-reduction below knee immobilization for 6–8 weeks.

43.5 Metatarsophalangeal and Interphalangeal Dislocations

- They are relocated using manual traction maneuvers under local anesthesia.
- Temporary syndactylization is recommended for 3–4 weeks (strapping of the affected toe to the adjacent intact toes using adhesive elastic tape).
- Open reduction and temporary pinning is indicated in rare circumstances when the dislocation is irreducible (because of the interposition of the flexor, extensor tendon, or capsule).

44 Tendino-Muscular Injuries of the Lower Limb

44.1 Thigh

- Most tendino-muscular injuries of the thigh region affect the muscle bellies and rarely require surgical management (refer to Chap. 12, "Acute Muscular Injuries").
- Injuries that may require surgical treatment mainly correspond to avulsion injuries, such as avulsions of,
  - The proximal insertion of the hamstrings tendon on the ischial tuberosity,
  - The distal insertion of the rectus femoris (distal junction with the vastus intermedius) (Fig. 44.1).
- The diagnosis is frequently missed during emergencies and is often only made at a late stage, which subsequently leads to more difficult treatment.
- Efforts should be directed toward making an early diagnosis (which is correlated with more satisfactory outcomes). This is generally achieved with,
  - Well-oriented clinical assessment.

    The presence of two points of pain and tenderness is a usual finding: one in the muscle belly and the other at the zone of insertion of the muscle (*"bipolar" pain*).

    In some cases, the retraction of the muscles is obvious (proximal for the rectus femoris and distal for the hamstrings tendon),

    Significant functional disability.
  - *Ultrasound* assessment should explore the entire course of the muscle from the proximal to the distal insertion.
  - *MRI examination* is highly sensitive and specific.
- Early surgical treatment is indicated for athletes (before the occurrence of retraction and fibrosis). Non-operative treatment, which may include the RICE protocol, can be considered for non-athletes.

D. Saragaglia, A. Hassan Chamseddine, *Traumatology for the Emergency Doctor*, https://doi.org/10.1007/978-3-031-63196-2_44

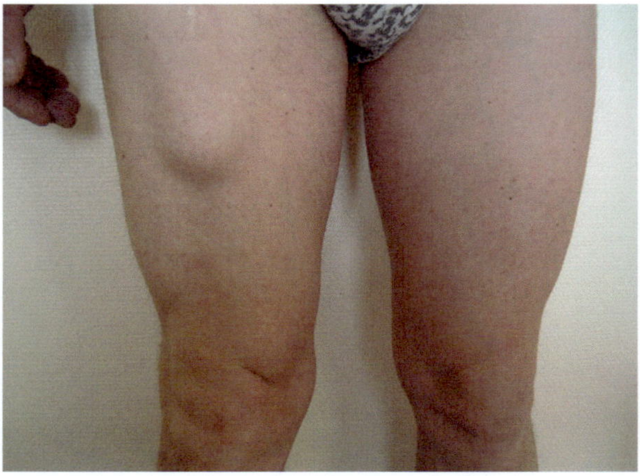

Fig. 44.1 Photo of the anterior aspect of the thigh of a patient with a late presentation of an avulsion of the distal insertion of the rectus femoris

44.2 Knee

- Tendino-muscular injuries of the knee usually correspond to either,
  - **Rupture of the patellar tendon**

    Avulsion at the proximal insertion, from the inferior pole of the patella (with or without bony fragment),

    Mid-substance tear,

    Avulsion at the distal insertion, from the anterior tibial tubercle (with or without bony fragment).
  - **Rupture or avulsion of the quadriceps tendon** at the proximal border of the patella (with or without bony fragment).
- **The clinical history** should look for any associated risk factors (especially for quadriceps tendon rupture): diabetes mellitus, systemic rheumatoid disease (rheumatoid arthritis, lupus, etc.), chronic renal disease and renal failure, previous local steroid injections, etc.
- **The clinical diagnosis** is often evident:
  - History of severe quadriceps contraction during jumping or landing effort,
  - Audible popping with pain at the time of accident,
  - Swelling,
  - Functional disability, with knee instability (giving way during walking),
  - Patient *unable to perform active knee extension* (straight leg raise form the bed).
  - *Painful palpable gap* at the superior or inferior pole of the patella (according to the site of rupture).

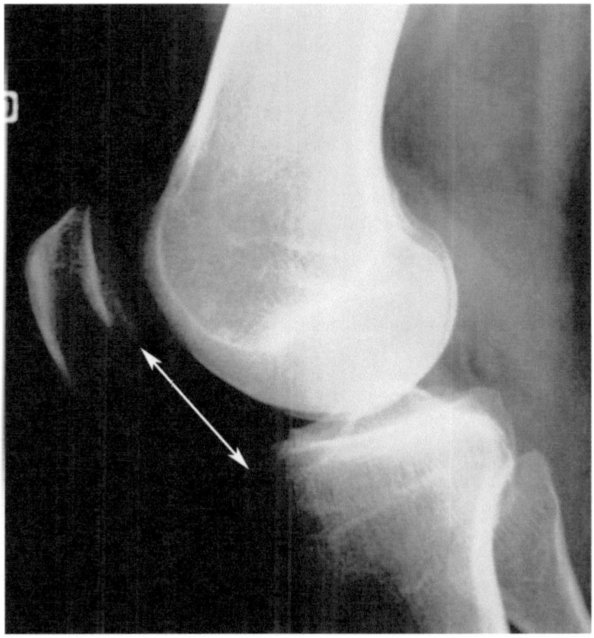

Fig. 44.2 Lateral knee radiograph showing a normal patellar height

   - Bilateral rupture of the quadriceps tendon may occur in patients with associated systemic diseases.
- **The radiographic assessment uses comparative radiographic AP and lateral knee views, and commonly shows**:
   - Patella in "high" position (patella alta) on the lateral view (compared to the opposite side): indicative of a complete rupture of the patellar tendon (Figs. 44.2 and 44.3).
   - Patella in "low" position (patella baja) with *anterior tilt* of the proximal pole of the patella (Figs. 44.4 and 44.5), suggestive of a complete rupture of the quadriceps tendon.
- **Ultrasound and MRI** are not really beneficial for the diagnosis, except for:
   - Diagnosis of partial rupture,
   - Identification of the exact site of rupture (mid-substance, size of the distal or proximal stump, retraction).
   - Presence of intra-tendinous degenerative changes (sign of chronic process).
- **Treatment** involves surgical intervention in almost all the cases.

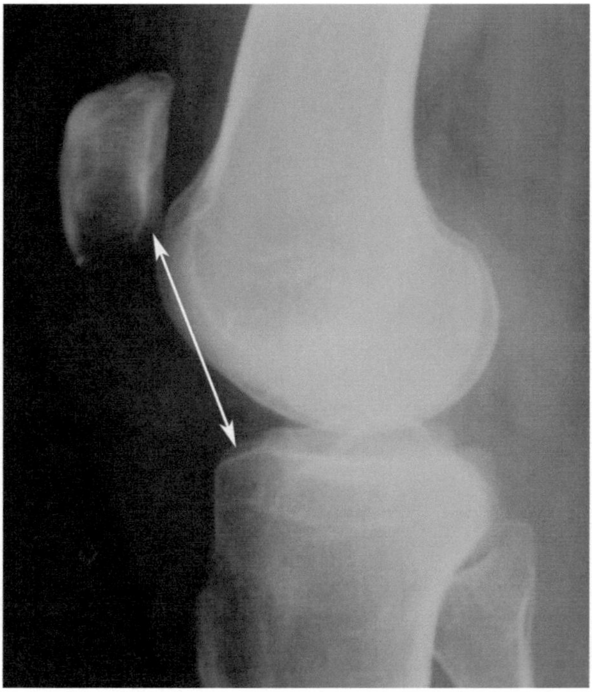

Fig. 44.3 Lateral knee radiograph showing a patella alta, indicative of rupture of the patellar tendon (patella in high position compared to Fig. 44.2. However, for a better analytic comparison, the two radiographs should be performed with the same degree of knee flexion position)

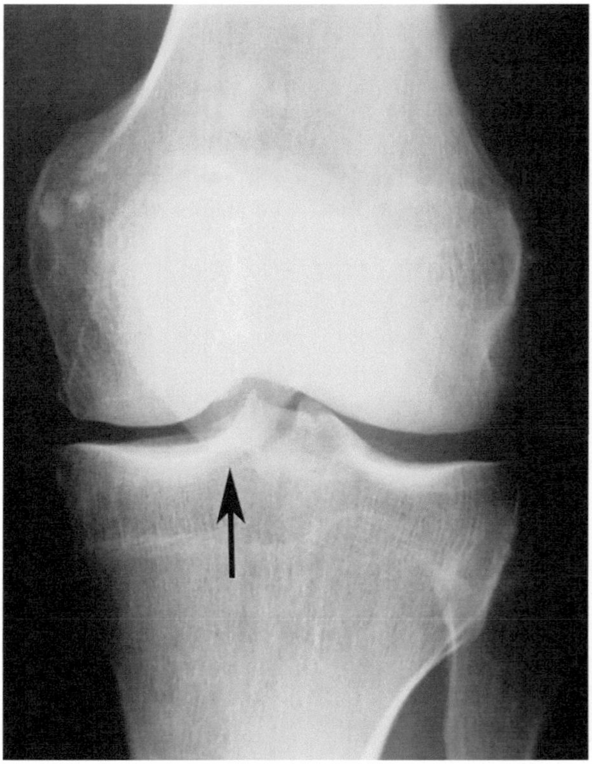

Fig. 44.4 AP knee radiograph in extension position showing the distal pole (tip) of the patella in lower position than normal (distal to the femoro-tibial joint line), indicative of rupture of the quadriceps tendon

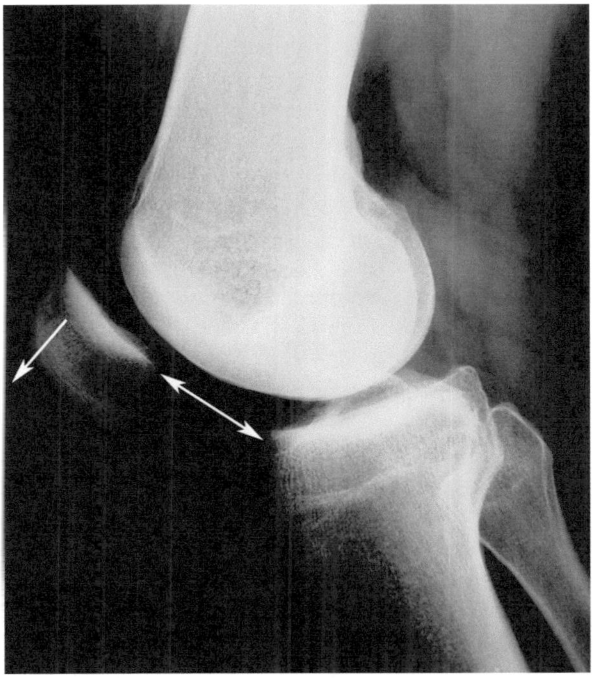

Fig. 44.5 Lateral knee radiograph of the same patient as shown in Fig. 44.4 showing patella baja (patella in lower position than normal) with an anterior tilt of the proximal pole of the patella, indicative of a rupture of the quadriceps tendon

44.3 Leg

44.3.1 Tennis Leg

- It involves injury of the distal insertion of the medial gastrocnemius muscle.
- It may be associated with rupture of the plantaris tendon.
- Different degrees of severity are identified based on the extent of the rupture, whether it is partial or complete.
- **Diagnosis**
  - Severe sudden pain of the calf with sensation of "popping" or "snapping" during the accident,
  - Immediate moderate functional disability following the accident.
  - The injury usually occurs during a sudden movement that involves knee extension with forced dorsal flexion of the ankle.
  - Physical exam.

    Focal tenderness at the distal part of the medial gastrocnemius,
    Swelling,
    Palpable gap at the site of rupture (when the patient presents early),
    Proximal retraction of the medial gastrocnemius (if complete rupture).
  - *Ultrasound* is generally disappointing despite the findings of,

    Hematoma or fluid collection around the distal medial gastrocnemius,
    Tear of the fibers of the distal medial gastrocnemius.

  - ***MRI*** is more performing (more sensitive and specific), especially if it is bilateral and comparative, and made without and with contraction of the triceps surae.
- **Treatment**
  - For partial tear: conservative treatment using below-knee weight bearing cast immobilization for 4–6 weeks in order to avoid recurrent rupture.
  - For complete tear with proximal retraction of the muscle: surgical treatment is recommended.
  - Red Flag: observe for compartment syndrome (rare) in case of severe swelling that may require fasciotomy.

44.3.2 Achilles Tendon (Calcaneal Tendon)

- Achilles tendon rupture generally occurs during sports activities.
- Usually secondary to sudden antagonist dorsi-flexion of the ankle during contraction of the triceps surae.
- **Diagnosis**
  - Clinical presentation.

    Severe sudden pain at the posterior aspect of the ankle or the heel, with *sensation of "popping"* or "snapping" during the accident,

    Immediate moderate functional disability following the accident: the patient is able to walk with limping and partial weight bearing.
  - ***Physical exam is fundamental*** (patient in prone position) and made in comparison to the opposite side:

    Palpable gap at the posterior aspect of the ankle or the heel (distal part of the Achilles tendon),

    The foot is in spontaneous increased dorsi-flexion position at rest, which is observed in both knee extension and flexion, resulting in the *loss of the physiological equinus* resting position of the foot,

    Weakness (or deficit) of active plantar flexion of the ankle against resistance by the hand of the examiner,

    Increased passive dorsi-flexion of the ankle at 90° knee flexion,

    Positive provocative Thompson test: absence of plantar flexion of the foot when the calf is squeezed by the hand of the examiner.

    Inability to perform tip toe walking exercise.
  - Ultrasound may be misleading, as it frequently concludes to the erroneous diagnosis of partial rupture.
  - MRI is indicated in case of confusing or ambiguous physical exam.
- **Treatment** is usually surgical, unless presence of contraindications (elderly, peripheral artery disease, comorbidities, etc.).

Part IV

Limbs Trauma in Pediatric Patients

45 Particularities of Pediatric Fractures

Management of traumatic injuries in pediatric patients adheres to special considerations related to the unique characteristics of the musculoskeletal system at this age:

- The potential of residual growth in the immature pediatric skeleton.
- The spontaneous ability to progressively correct certain angular deformities without any therapeutic intervention.
- The risk of progressive deformation or increased residual deformities due to specific injuries (such as those of the growth plate or physis) which may result in epiphysiodesis (partial or complete premature fusion of the growth plate), leading to permanent limb deformity (angular deviation and shortening).

45.1 Fractures

45.1.1 Torus or Buckle Fractures (Fig. 45.1)

- Correspond to a particular fracture type in baby and infant.
- Commonly affect the metaphyseal areas of long bones.
- Typical radiographic aspect: compression of one cortex with intact opposite cortex.
- Most frequent localization: distal radius.
- May be overlooked in emergency setting because of,
  - Inadequate or bad quality radiographic views,
  - Lack of oblique views.
- Healing time 3–4 weeks.

45.1.2 Greenstick Fractures (Fig. 45.2)

- Correspond to a particular type of diaphyseal fractures in young children.

D. Saragaglia, A. Hassan Chamseddine, *Traumatology for the Emergency Doctor*, https://doi.org/10.1007/978-3-031-63196-2_45

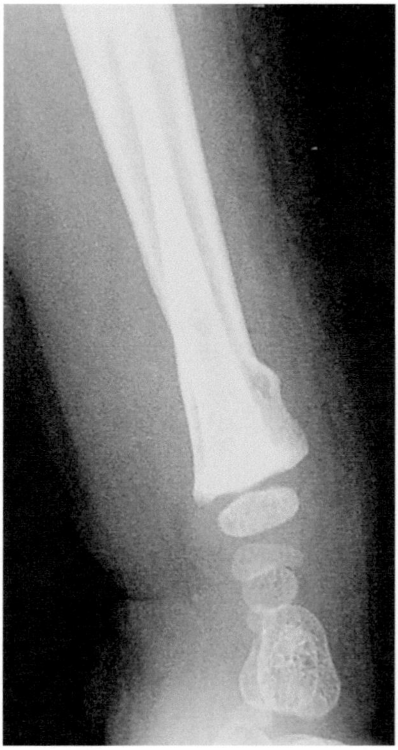

Fig. 45.1 Lateral wrist radiograph showing a torus or a buckle fracture of the distal radius

- Most common site: the forearm.
- Secondary to a bending force that causes an incomplete fracture, leading to a radiographic "bowing" appearance of the affected bone with,
  - a complete fracture of the convex side of the diaphysis,
  - and a plastic bending deformity without fracture–rupture of the concave side, with the periosteum remaining intact.
- Treatment typically involves closed reduction: the maneuver of reduction should induce a complete fracture *by breaking the bent concave side* to prevent the recurrence of the plastic deformity.

45.1.3 Diaphyseal Long Bone Bowing (Fig. 45.3)

- Corresponds to a plastic deformity without interruption of bone continuity.
- Most common site: the forearm (where one bone may be bowed while the other one fractured).
- Always consider the possibility of associated injuries, such as:
  - *a plastic bowing of the ulna* with an associated dislocation of the radial head at the elbow (Monteggia lesion),

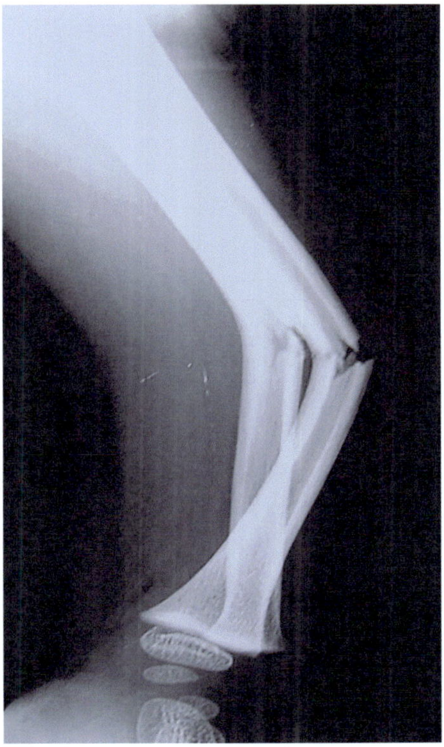

Fig. 45.2 Forearm radiograph showing a greenstick fracture of both bones (radius and ulna)

- *or a plastic bowing of the radius* with an associated dislocation of the ulnar head at the wrist (Galeazzi lesion).

45.2 Fractures Involving the Growth Plate (Salter-Harris Fractures)

They are categorized into five types based on the relationship of the fracture line to the growth plate or physis, according to the *Salter-Harris classification* (Fig. 45.4).

- **Type I**
  - Represents a transverse fracture line through the growth plate.
  - Results in pure epiphyseal displacement or separation, without extending into the metaphysis or the epiphysis.
  - Carries a low risk of growth disturbance.
  - There is a risk of avascular necrosis for the slipped proximal femoral epiphysis and the slipped radial head epiphysis.
- **Type II**
  - Is the most frequent type.
  - Results in a fracture line that runs through the growth plate and the metaphysis.

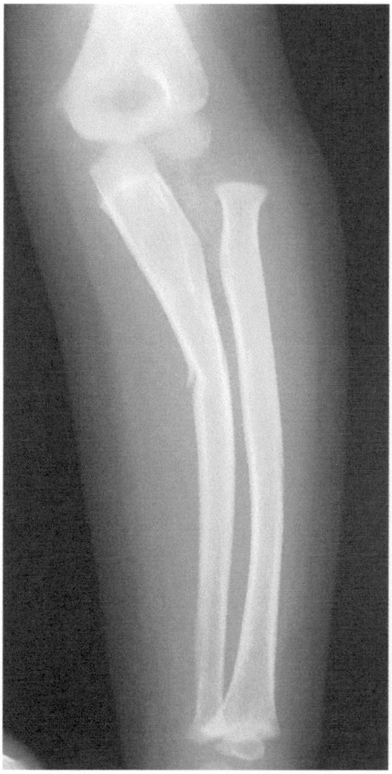

Fig. 45.3 Forearm radiograph showing a plastic bowing of the ulna associated with a dislocation of the radial head at the elbow (Monteggia lesion)

  - The epiphysis remains uninvolved.
  - Carries a prognosis similar to that of type I, with generally good outcomes expected.
- **Type III**
  - Corresponds to an epiphyseal fracture with partial displacement, involving both the growth plate and the epiphysis.
  - The metaphysis remains unaffected.
  - It carries a risk of post-traumatic epiphysiodesis, which can lead to future growth disturbances, especially if the reduction is imperfect and residual displacement persists.
- **Type IV**
  - Corresponds to a fracture that involves all three structures: the fracture line traverses the metaphysis, the growth plate, and the epiphysis.
  - It carries a risk of epiphysiodesis and potential future growth disturbance.
- **Type V**
  - It corresponds to compression of the growth plate.
  - It results in a reduction of the physeal line space, which can be difficult to visualize on X-rays.
  - The X-rays may appear normal.

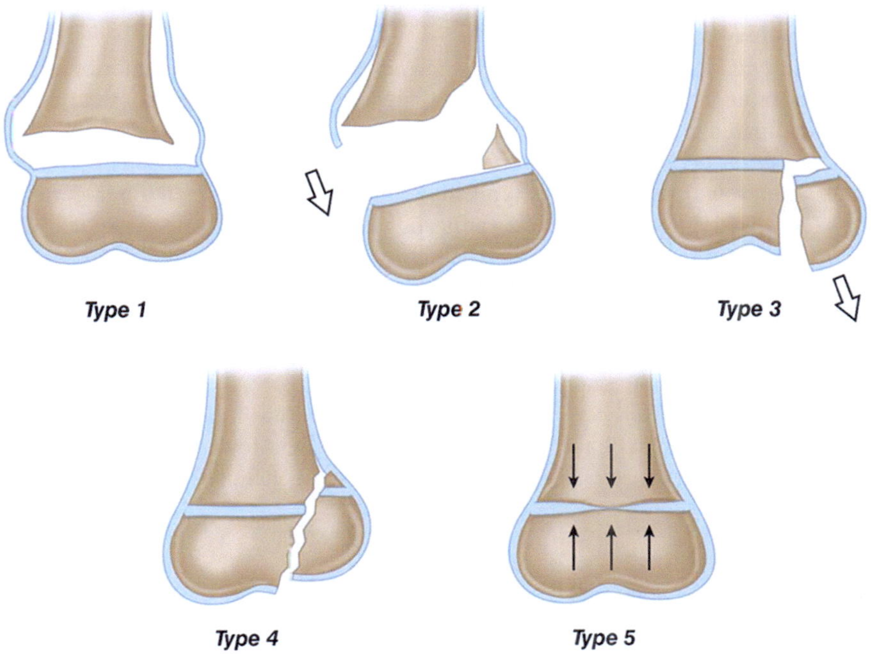

Fig. 45.4 Illustration of the Salter-Harris classification for fractures involving the growth

- The compression of the growth plate may be associated with one of the previous fracture types.
- It carries a high risk of epiphysiodesis with consequent future growth disturbance.

Regular radiographic monitoring is recommended until the end of growth (bone maturity) for all types of Salter-Harris fractures.

It is essential to inform the parents about the potential risk of growth disturbances. Should growth disturbances occur, therapeutic intervention may be necessary to minimize their functional impact.

45.3 Characteristics and Distinctive Features of Evolution

- **Delayed union and nonunion** are exceptional in pediatric patients.
- **The capacity for bone remodeling** and the spontaneous progressive correction of residual deformities, known as malunion, is a significant characteristic of pediatric fractures:
  - *Frontal angulations* with varus or valgus malunion are prone to spontaneous progressive realignment. The capacity of correction is generally inversely

proportional to the child's age, meaning younger children have a greater potential for natural correction.

- *Sagittal angulations* with malunion in *flessum or recurvatum* (anterior or posterior angulation respectively) tend to undergo slower spontaneous correction compared to frontal angulations.
- *Rotation malunions* (malrotation) are not subject to spontaneous correction with growth, meaning they typically require surgical intervention to correct.
- For distal humerus fractures: varus and valgus malunions are associated with a poorer prognosis and less satisfactory outcomes compared to malunions with residual sagittal angulation (flexion or extension).
- Malunion secondary to Salter-Harris type fractures may lead to more severe axial deformities, which tend to have more significant consequences for the lower limb than the upper limb.
- *Limb length discrepancy* may occur in the medium to long term and has a more severe functional impact when it affects the lower limbs. Diaphyseal fractures can cause over growth of the affected bone, particularly in younger patients.

Pediatric Injuries 46

In pediatric patients, the same fractures as in adults can be found. We will only focus on the most common fractures and other lesions (sprains, dislocations, etc.).

46.1 Upper Limb

46.1.1 Clavicle

- Orthopedic treatment typically involves the use of a "figure of 8" bandage in almost all cases.
- Bone healing occurs within 3–4 weeks.
- Hypertrophic (exuberant) bone callus may occur and may worry the parents.
- Remodeling and vanishing of the exuberant callus progressively occurs with growth.

46.1.2 Shoulder

- **Shoulder dislocation**
  - Occurs only in adolescent.
  - Treatment is same as in adult (see Shoulder dislocations).
- **Fractures of the proximal humerus**
  - Most commonly correspond to Salter-Harris type II fractures (Fig. 46.1).
  - For undisplaced or moderately displaced fractures (up to 30°–45° angulation), orthopedic treatment typically involves a sling and swathe (shoulder brace or immobilizer) for 3–4 weeks, followed by self-rehabilitation.
  - For significantly displaced fractures,

    Closed reduction under general anesthesia may be performed, followed by the same immobilization and rehabilitation protocol as for less severe fractures,

D. Saragaglia, A. Hassan Chamseddine, *Traumatology for the Emergency Doctor*, https://doi.org/10.1007/978-3-031-63196-2_46

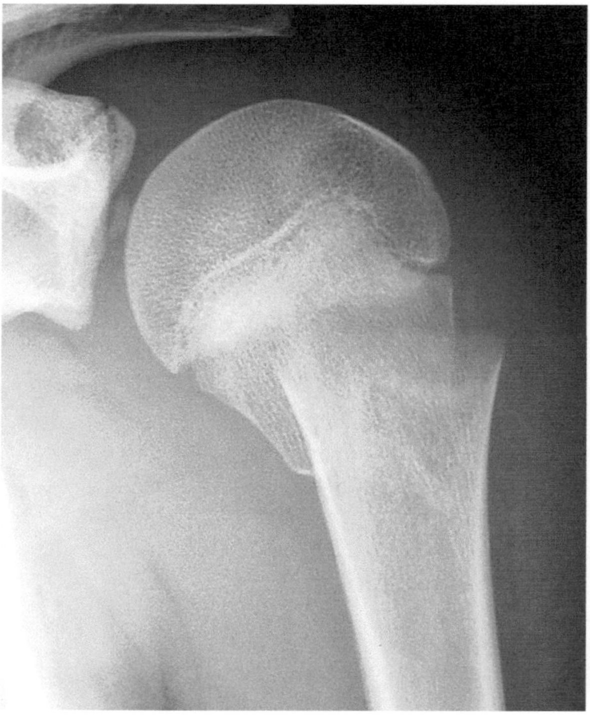

Fig. 46.1 AP shoulder X-ray showing a fracture of the proximal humerus, Salter-Harris type 2

Open reduction may be necessary for irreducible fractures, often due to soft tissue interposition such as the long head of the biceps.

46.1.3 Humeral Shaft Fractures

- They typically do not cause complications.
- It is important to always check for associated radial nerve palsy.
- Orthopedic treatment is commonly applied, using either sling and swathe immobilization or a hanging cast.
- Surgical treatment should generally be reserved for exceptional cases, even if performed percutaneously.
- Residual malalignment is usually well tolerated and spontaneous progressive correction with growth, so surgical correction should not be necessary.

46.1.4 Elbow

- **Supra-condylar fractures**
  - Are very common in children.
  - They are categorized into flexion and extension type fractures.

– It is important to always carefully check for any associated neuro-vascular injuries, particularly in displaced fractures.
– *Extension type fractures* are the most common, and can be categorized into four types:

  Type I

    Undisplaced fractures.

    Treatment is conservative using immobilization with either an above elbow cast or the Blount method (at 120° elbow flexion) for 4 weeks.

  Type II

    Minimal displacement,

    Displacement only in the sagittal plane, with anterior opening of the fracture line, visible on lateral elbow view,

    Intact posterior cortex and periosteal hinge.

    Treatment is the same as for type I.

  Type III (Fig. 46.2)

    Displaced fracture with preservation of interfragmentary contact,

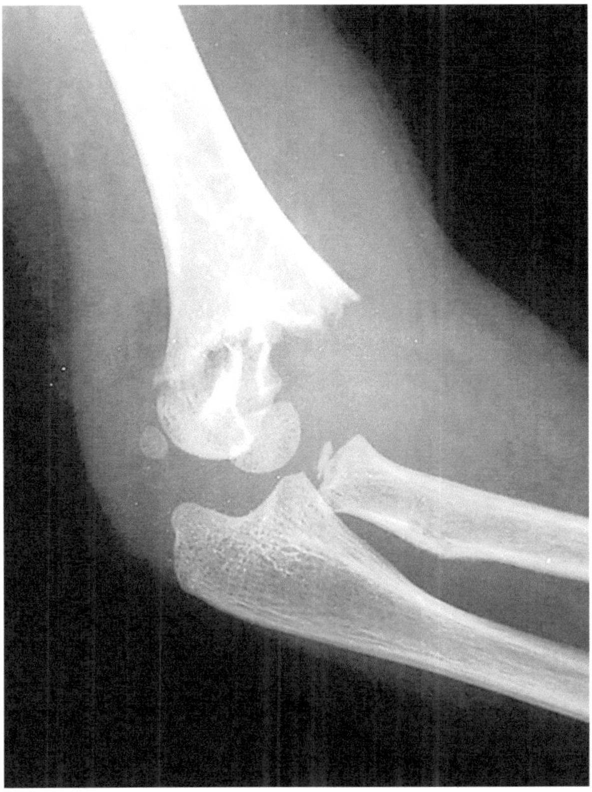

Fig. 46.2 Elbow X-ray showing a grade 3 supra-condylar fracture of the distal humerus (extension type)

Treatment involves either closed reduction and immobilization under general anesthesia or closed reduction with percutaneous pinning. Open reduction is exceptional and only if irreducible.

Type IV (Fig. 46.3)

Major displacement with loss of interfragmentary contact,

It is important to carefully assess for associated neuro-vascular lesions,

Represents a *surgical emergency*: urgent specialized orthopedic consultation is required for urgent reduction and fixation which may involve either closed reduction and percutaneous pinning or open reduction with pinning if irreducible by closed maneuvers.

- **Fracture of the lateral condyle** (Fig. 46.4a, b)
  - The fracture line involves the articular cartilage, making it an articular fracture.
  - It often requires surgical reduction and fixation.
  - If not diagnosed and treated appropriately, it may progress to nonunion.
- **Elbow dislocation and fracture of the medial epicondyle**
  - *An apparent "isolated" fracture* of the medial epicondyle (Fig. 46.5a, b) is often associated with an elbow dislocation that has spontaneously reduced. A displaced fracture typically requires surgical reduction and stabilization to prevent nonunion, as the medial epicondyle is subject to continuous traction by the origin of the flexor tendons.
  - *Elbow dislocations* are uncommon in pediatric patients but are frequently associated with fractures of the medial epicondyle. It is crucial to check for intra-articular incarceration of the medial epicondyle both at presentation and

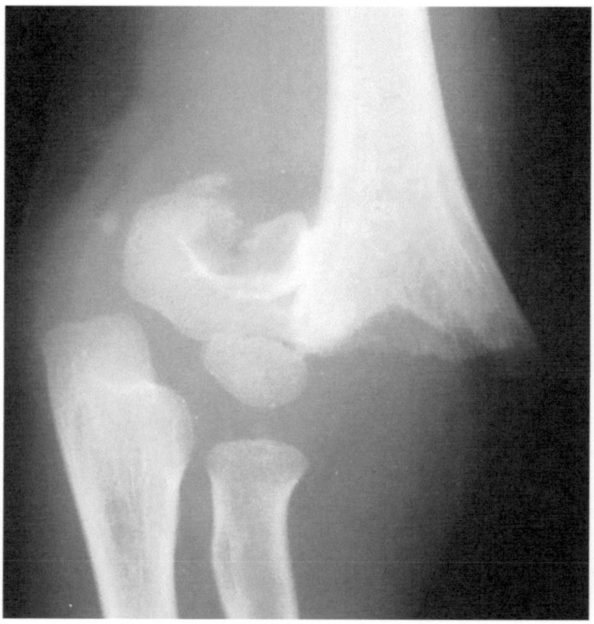

Fig. 46.3 Elbow radiograph showing a grade 4 supra-condylar fracture of the distal humerus (extension type)

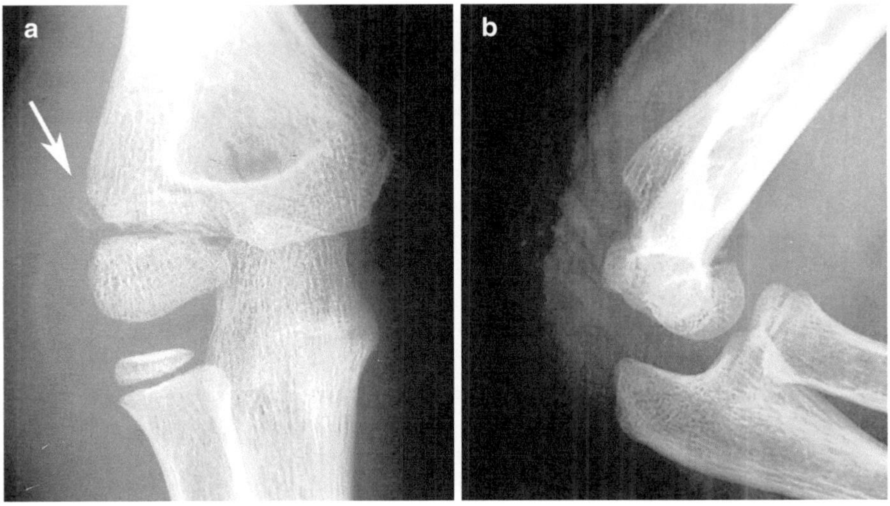

Fig. 46.4 (**a**) AP elbow radiograph showing a fracture of the lateral condyle of the distal humerus. (**b**) Lateral radiograph of the same elbow as shown in (**a**) with a fracture of the lateral condyle of the distal humerus

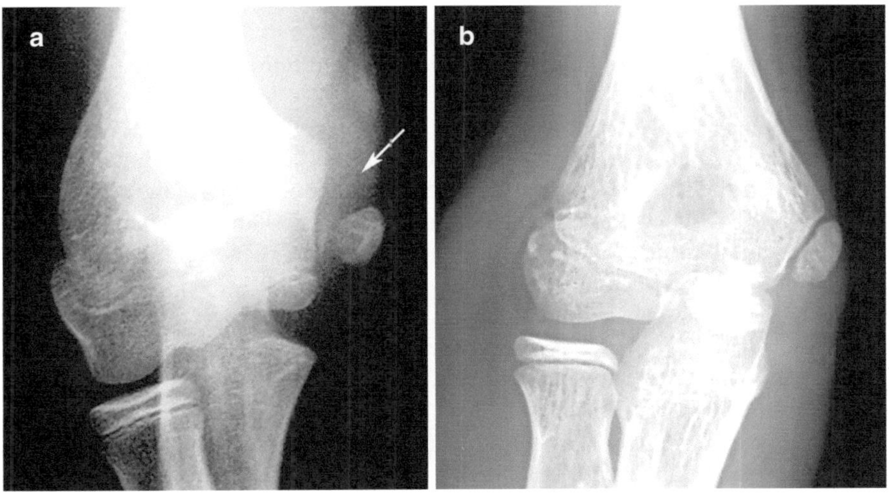

Fig. 46.5 (**a**) AP elbow radiograph showing a displaced fracture of the medial epicondyle of the distal humerus (observe the widening of the humeral-ulnar joint line). (**b**) AP elbow radiograph showing a normal image of the medial epicondyle of the distal humerus

after reduction. An Irreducible dislocation should prompt consideration of the diagnosis of incarceration.

- Treatment

The ER physician should be capable of reducing an elbow dislocation, especially if an orthopedic surgeon is not immediately available. Post-reduction radiographs are crucial to verify the reduction, assess the congruence of the joint, and detect any potential incarceration of the medial epicondyle.

If the dislocation is "simple," without associated fractures, an above elbow cast is applied for 3 weeks, followed by self-rehabilitation.

If the dislocation is associated with a fracture of the medial epicondyle, a specialized orthopedic consultation is necessary.

- **Nursemaid's elbow**
  - It is the most common elbow injury in children between the ages of 1 and 4 years.
  - It involves the subluxation of the annular ligament and radial head, typically due to traction applied on the hand or forearm along the axis of the upper limb.
  - The clinical diagnosis is usually straightforward:

    The child often refuses to use their hand and holds their upper limb in an antalgic position with the elbow extended at the side of the body and the forearm in pronation.

    Physical examination reveals pain and tenderness at the lateral aspect of the elbow.
  - Elbow radiographs are typically not necessary as they usually do not contribute to the diagnosis.
  - An Elbow ultrasound may be beneficial to confirm the diagnosis in cases of uncertainty.
  - Treatment involves closed reduction where the physician puts the forearm in extreme supination along with forced elbow flexion, and simultaneously applies direct pressure on the lateral aspect of the elbow (over the radial head). A palpable and audible click often indicates successful reduction. Following reduction, the child is immediately able to use their hand again.
- **Radial head and neck fractures**
  - They are relatively common.
  - They typically involve fracture-compression of the radial neck with tilt and angulation of the radial head (Fig. 46.6).
  - Treatment options include:

    For mild and to moderate radial head tilt (up to 30°): immobilization with an above elbow cast for 3 weeks, followed by self-rehabilitation.

    For significant radial head tilt (>30–40°), a specialized orthopedic consultation is recommended for percutaneous reduction and fixation.
- **Fracture of the olecranon process**
  - Undisplaced fractures are typically treated with an above elbow cast for 4–6 weeks.
  - Displaced fractures (>2–3 mm displacement): a specialized orthopedic consultation is recommended to evaluate the need for potential surgical treatment.

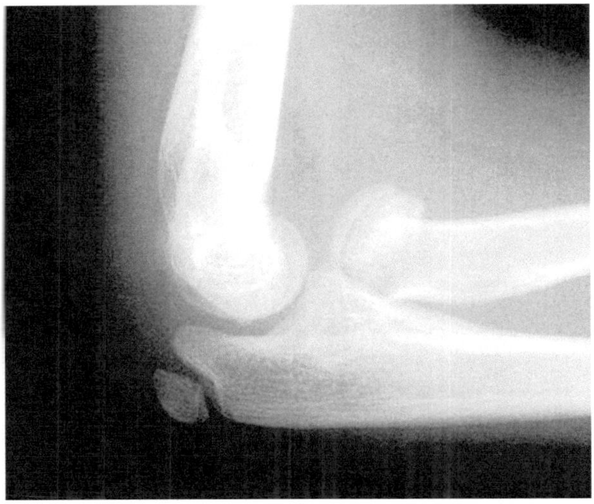

Fig. 46.6 Lateral elbow X-ray showing a displaced fracture of the neck of the radius

46.1.5 Forearm Fractures

1. **Both bone forearm fractures** (Fig. 46.7)
   (a) Common fractures in children.
   (b) They require proper reduction to restore full pronation-supination range of motion.
   (c) Greenstick and bowing fractures are frequently seen.
   (d) *For children < under 10 years*
   - Orthopedic treatment is generally the first choice unless there is significant displacement or unstable reduction which may indicate the need for surgical treatment.
   - Plastic deformation (bowing), greenstick fractures, and displaced fractures often necessitate closed reduction under general anesthesia. This is followed by immobilization with an above elbow cast for a minimum of 2 months, then a protective forearm cast for 1 month.
   - The healing process of these fractures is "slow," and there is a known risk of re-fracture after cast removal.

   (e) For children > over 10 years
   - The same guidelines apply as for younger children.
   - Surgical treatment tends to be more commonly indicated for displaced fractures.
2. **Fracture of one bone**
   (a) Treatment follows similar principles as fractures involving both bones of the forearm.
   - Orthopedic treatment is more commonly pursued for children under 10 years old.

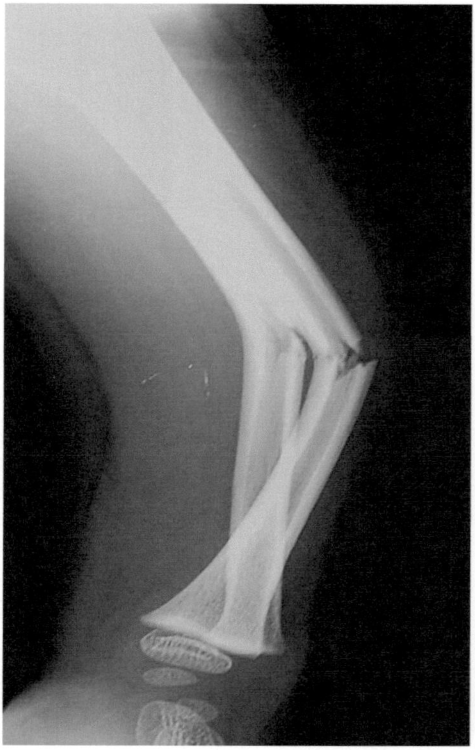

Fig. 46.7 Radiographic view of a fracture of both forearm bones (radius and ulna)

- Surgical intervention is more frequently indicated for patients over 10 years old.
- Achieving perfect reduction and restoring the radial curvature is essential for proper healing.

(b) *Red flags*

- Isolated ulna fracture: always consider the possibility of a Monteggia lesion, which is an associated dislocation of the radial head at the elbow. Appropriate elbow X-rays are necessary to rule out this injury (Fig. 46.8).
- Apparent isolated radial head dislocation: Be vigilant for plastic deformation of the ulna that may accompany the dislocation.
- Isolated radius fracture: always check for a Galeazzi lesion, which involves an associated dislocation of the ulnar head at the wrist. Wrist X-rays are required to confirm this injury.
- Injuries with these red flags should be evaluated by a specialized orthopedic surgeon due to the potential need for surgical treatment.

3. **Distal metaphyseal fractures**

(a) They are specific to children.
(b) They can affect one or both bones of the forearm.
(c) They encompass a variety of types, ranging from buckle fractures to completely displaced fractures (Fig. 46.9).

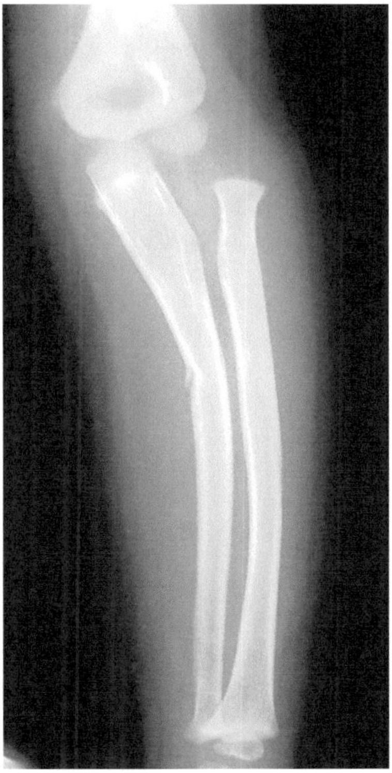

Fig. 46.8 Monteggia lesion resulting in a plastic deformity (bowing) of the ulna with radial head dislocation

(d) Treatment.
   - For undisplaced fractures: treatment typically involves an above elbow cast for 4–6 weeks.
   - For moderately displaced fractures: these may require a closed reduction under general anesthesia with an above elbow cast immobilization for 6 weeks.
   - For completely displaced fractures: emergency reduction with surgical stabilization of the fracture site are indicated if there is significant instability that could lead to secondary displacement.

4. **Salter-Harris fractures of the distal radius**
   (a) The type II is the most common, followed by type I.
   (b) Dorsal displacement occurs more frequently than volar displacement.
   (c) The fracture can be isolated (affecting only the radius) or associated with a fracture of the distal ulna.
   (d) Displacement can range from undisplaced to completely displaced, depending on the severity of the trauma (Fig. 46.10).
   (e) Type V fractures may be overlooked due to the normal appearance of radiographs, as they involve compression of the growth plate.
   (f) Treatment

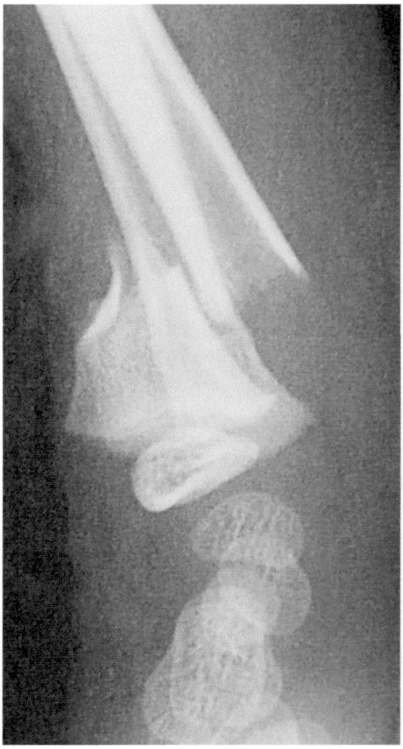

Fig. 46.9 Lateral wrist X-ray showing a displaced fracture of the distal metaphysis of the radius

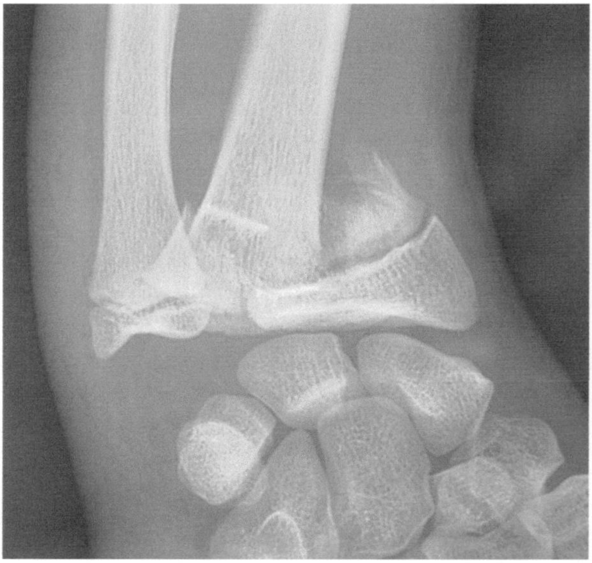

Fig. 46.10 AP wrist radiograph showing a Salter-Harris type 2 fracture of the distal radius

- For undisplaced fractures: cast immobilization for 4–6 weeks is recommended with radiographic control at 1 week despite the low risk of secondary displacement.
- For displaced fractures:
  - Closed reduction under general anesthesia is necessary.
  - Post-reduction below elbow cast immobilization should be performed in volar flexion of the wrist (for initial dorsal displacement) for 4 weeks.
  - These fractures heal quickly, making correction of secondary displacement by closed maneuvers nearly impossible after 10–14 days.

46.1.6 Wrist and Hand

The guidelines and rules for managing adult wrist and hand trauma are applicable. For detailed information, refer to the chapter "Trauma of wrist and hand."

Salter-Harris fractures of metacarpals and phalanges are not uncommon in pediatric cases.

46.2 Lower Limb

46.2.1 Pelvis and Hip

- Bone avulsions are relatively common during sports activities in adolescents, particularly at the antero-superior iliac spine, antero-inferior iliac spine, and ischial tuberosity. Treatment of these avulsions is similar to that in adult (refer to the chapter "Traumatic injuries to the pelvic ring").
- Fractures of the acetabulum and hip dislocations are rare.
- These injuries often require a specialized orthopedic consultation for potential surgical treatment.

46.2.2 Femur

- **Femoral neck fracture** (Fig. 46.11a, b)
  - Femoral neck fractures and acute slipped capital femoral epiphysis are rare.
  - They often require a specialized orthopedic consultation for urgent surgical treatment, as they involve a risk of avascular necrosis of the femoral head.
- **Femoral shaft fractures**
  - They are relatively common.
  - They need to be managed by an orthopedic team.
- **Distal femur Salter-Harris types' fractures** (Fig. 46.12)
  - They are relatively common.
  - They require to be managed by an orthopedic team.

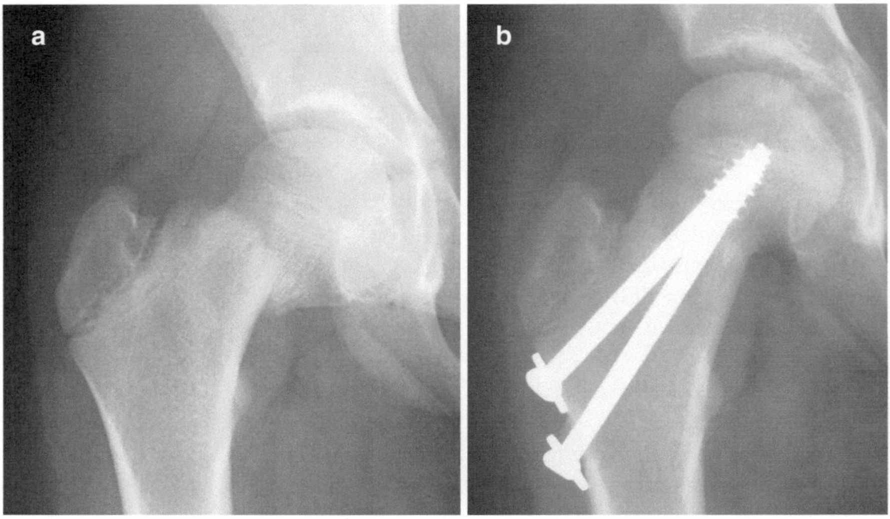

Fig. 46.11 (**a**) AP hip radiograph showing a displaced femoral neck fracture (intra-capsular fracture). (**b**) AP radiograph of the same hip depicted in (**a**) at 2-months follow-up after reduction and internal fixation with two cancellous screws

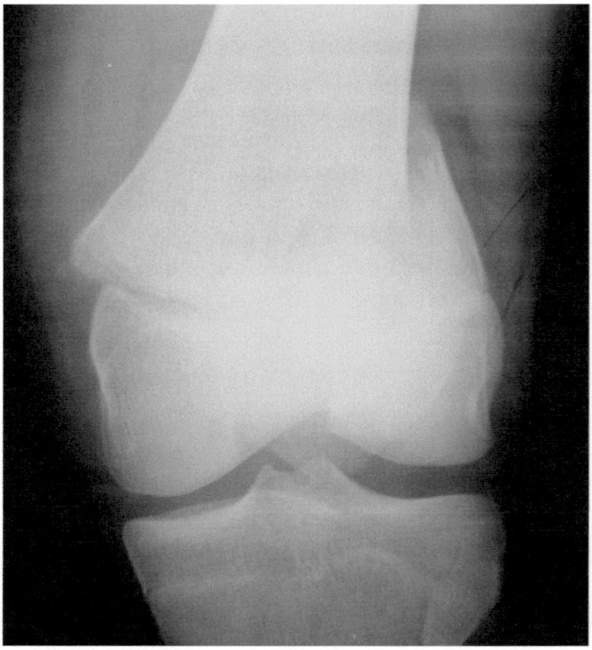

Fig. 46.12 AP knee X-ray showing a Salter-Harris type 2 fracture of the distal femur resulting in a moderate displacement

– They involve a risk of premature fusion of the growth plate that may result in growth disturbances, such as limb length discrepancy, and frontal or sagittal malalignment.

46.2.3 Knee

- **Avulsion of the tibial spines** is the most frequent injury of the pediatric knee.
  – For undisplaced avulsion: above-knee cast immobilization is required for 4 weeks.
  – For displaced avulsion: a specialized orthopedic consultation is required for potential surgical treatment.
- **Rupture of the anterior cruciate ligament (ACL):**
  – Is becoming more frequent than before.
  – Surgical treatment may be required based on individual cases.
  – The decision for surgical repair is weighted by the status of the growth plate and its remaining potential for growth and the possibility of associated menisci injuries.
  – Conservative treatment is applied while awaiting for the final surgical treatment (around the time of growth maturity). It prohibits sports activities that involve major risk of instability (football, basketball, etc.).

46.2.4 Leg

1. **Proximal tibia epiphyseal fractures (Salter-Harris types)** (Fig. 46.13a, b).
   (a) They are rare.
   (b) They frequently result in growth disturbances and long-term malalignment of the proximal tibia.

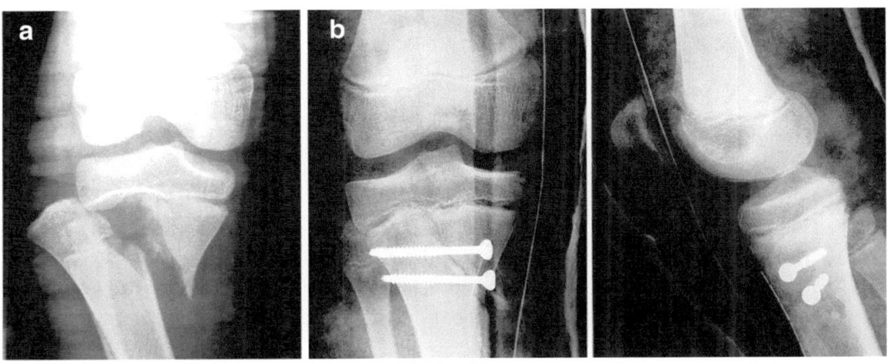

Fig. 46.13 (**a**) AP knee X-ray showing a Salter-Harris type 2 fracture of the proximal tibia resulting in a significant displacement. (**b**) AP and lateral X-rays of the same fracture as shown in (**a**) after open reduction and internal fixation with two screws

   (c) They require a specialized orthopedic consultation in all cases to determine the best treatment option.
   (d) For displaced fractures: urgent reduction and stabilization are necessary.
2. **Tibial shaft fractures**
   (a) Tibial shaft fractures may be isolated (Fig. 46.14) or be associated with a fracture of the fibula.
   (b) Closed reduction of displaced isolated tibial fractures is often difficult to achieve.
   (c) Isolated tibial fractures treated with closed reduction and cast immobilization may present a secondary displacement with varus malalignment. They consequently require close observation using weekly radiographic control for early recognition and correction.
   (d) *Red Flag*: Displaced fractures require immediate clinical evaluation and secondary close observation during treatment, as they may induce compartment syndrome.
   (e) In babies and young child: "hairline" fracture is common and may be missed on the initial radiographs. A fine clinical examination along with an analysis of the mechanism often helps making the diagnosis. Early periosteal reaction (meaning callus formation) confirms the initial diagnosis of fracture after 10–14 days of immobilization.

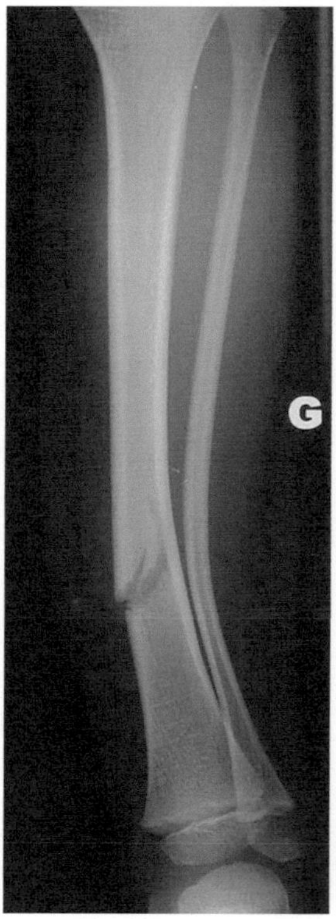

Fig. 46.14 AP leg X-ray showing an isolated fracture of the tibia associated with a plastic deformity (bowing) of the fibula

(f) Treatment
- *For undisplaced and minimally displaced fractures*: orthopedic treatment is indicated.
  - Long leg cast immobilization (ankle and knee included) for an initial period of 6 weeks.
  - Same type of cast for 4 weeks in young child with "hairline" fracture (sub-periosteal fracture).
  - Below-knee walking cast for 4 additional weeks after removal of the initial long leg cast.
  - Weekly radiographic control (for the first 3 weeks) for early detection and correction of any secondary displacement.
- *For displaced fractures*: a specialized orthopedic consultation and management for reduction and immobilization under general anesthesia (long leg cast, or fixation using percutaneous intra-medullary elastic nails).

3. **Distal metaphyseal tibial fractures** (Fig. 46.15)
   (a) They often correspond to a compression-fracture of the anterior metaphyseal cortex with posterior angulation.
   (b) A closed reduction followed by a conventional immobilization is often inadequate, as these fractures require an immobilization with the ankle and foot in plantar flexion and equinus position.

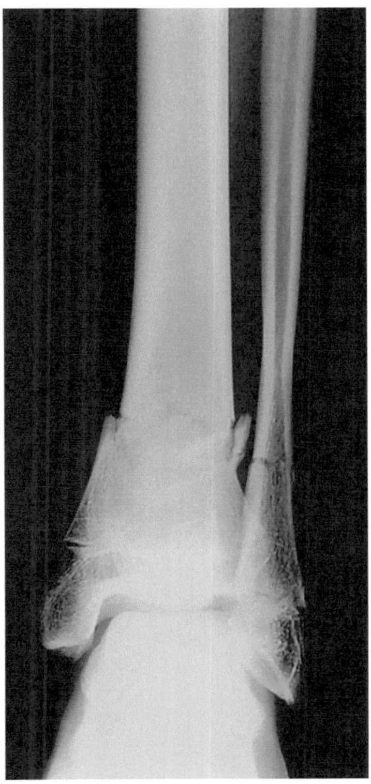

Fig. 46.15 AP distal leg radiograph showing associated fractures of the distal metaphyses of the tibia and fibula

   (c) They usually have a good prognosis.
4. **Distal tibial epiphyseal fractures (Salter-Harris types)** (Fig. 46.16)
   (a) They often occur between the ages of 10 and 15 years.
   (b) All types of Salter-Harris may occur.
   (c) The most common types are I and II.
   (d) Fracture of Chaput or Tillaux tubercle is a specific fracture pattern that often occurs in the adolescents, near to skeletal maturity (13–15 years). It corresponds to a Salter-Harris type III fracture of the distal tibial epiphysis (involving the antero-lateral tubercle) with an avulsion of the antero-inferior tibio-fibular ligament.
   (e) The triplane fracture is a specific pattern that associates together three fracture lines: a sagittal trans-epiphyseal line, a horizontal trans-physeal line, and a frontal trans-metaphyseal line (Fig. 46.17a, b).
   (f) A specialized orthopedic consultation is required (risk of premature growth plate fusion resulting in progressive ankle deviation or deformity).

46.2.5 Ankle

1. **Ankle sprains**

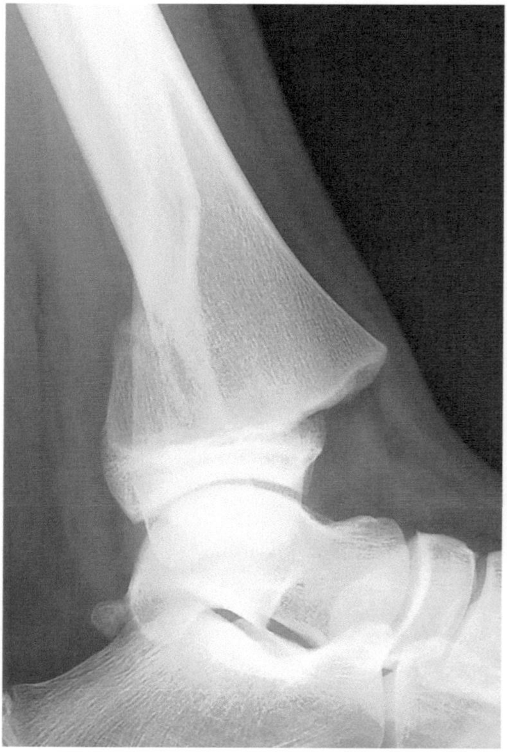

Fig. 46.16 Lateral ankle radiograph showing a Salter-Harris type 2 fracture of the distal tibia

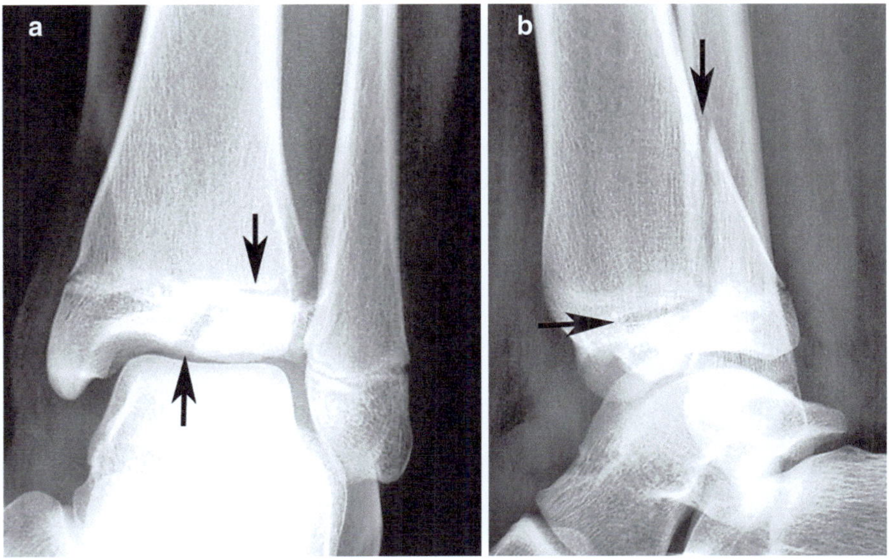

Fig. 46.17 (**a**) AP ankle radiograph of a distal tibial "triplane" fracture. (**b**) Lateral ankle radiograph of a distal tibial "triplane" fracture

(a) They are rare in young children, before the age of 12 years.
  - They often correspond to a fracture of the lateral malleolus (Salter-Harris type) that is rarely seen on the radiographs.
  - The diagnosis is usually based on the clinical presentation: lateral ankle pain and tenderness, with functional disability and normal radiographs.
  - The treatment is a below-knee cast immobilization for 3 weeks.

(b) In adolescent patients,
  - Ankle sprain is more common than in young children.
  - Radiographic Stress views are not essential for the diagnosis.
  - Same management as for adult patients.

2. **Bi-malleolar fractures**
   (a) They are rare.
   (b) They require a specialized orthopedic management and care.
3. **Lateral malleolus fractures**
   (a) They are not rare.
   (b) They commonly involve a fracture of the tip of the malleolus.
   (c) The treatment is a below-knee cast immobilization for 6 weeks.

46.2.6 Foot

- In young children: fractures of the metatarsals and phalanges are common and are treated conservatively.
- In adolescent: fractures of the bones of the foot are similar to fractures in adult and should receive the same management and care.

Part V

Head and Spine Trauma

47 Management of Head Trauma

The first and most important action for the ER physician dealing with a patient admitted for head trauma is to define the degree of severity of the injury:

- **Is it a mild trauma with no further progression or consequences?**
- **Or is it a severe injury requiring a specialized consultation and care?**

A primary careful systematic physical examination is fundamental for the initial decision making: a simple close clinical observation is usually required for a mild head trauma, while reanimation measures are applied for a severe one.

Scalp wounds have been discussed in Chap. 7. However, the hemorrhagic character of these wounds is often pejorative for the condition of a patient with a severe head trauma. This condition may consequently require an urgent control of the bleeding.

47.1 After Admission of a Patient with Head Trauma, The ER Physician Should Answer Four Questions

- Are there any signs of brain damage?
- Is the head injury open (penetrating injury)?
- Are there any associated multiple traumatic injuries (polytrauma patients)?
- Was there any brain injury prior to the current trauma?

47.1.1 Are There Any Signs of Brain Damage?

- The occurrence of any *loss of consciousness* necessitates a full investigation into its timing and duration: was it initial, concomitant with the trauma, or after the trauma? Was it brief or prolonged (lasting more than 20 min)?

D. Saragaglia, A. Hassan Chamseddine, *Traumatology for the Emergency Doctor*, https://doi.org/10.1007/978-3-031-63196-2_47

- Is there any post-traumatic *memory disturbance or amnesia* (memory deficit) manifested as either "retrograde" or "anterograde" amnesia?
- *Are there any focal signs, such as:*
  - Motor deficit on one side of the body, in form of hemiparesis or hemiplegia,
  - Cranial nerves deficit: abnormality in pupillary size (Miosis, mydriasis), pupillary light reflex, and accommodation reflex, oculomotor nerve paralysis, or weakness or loss of movement in facial muscles.
- Glasgow Coma Scale (GCS)
  - It is a clinical scale used to measure and observe the level of consciousness in patients (above 2 years of age) with acute brain injury through serial and repetitive assessments.
  - The scale evaluates three components: eye opening, motor response, and verbal response.
  - The score or note given by the examiner for each tested component is based on the best response provided by the patient at a given time:

Glasgow coma scale (GCS)

Eyes (4)	Opening response	Spontaneous	4
		To verbal command	3
		To pain	2
		No opening	1
Best motor response (6)	To verbal command	Obeys command	6
	To pain	Localizing	5
		Withdrawal from pain stimuli	4
		Abnormal flexion to pain	3
		Abnormal extension to pain	2
		No motor response	1
Best verbal response (5)		Orientated	5
		Confused and disorientated	4
		Inappropriate words	3
		Incomprehensible sounds	2
		No verbal response	1
	Total		**15**

- Calculation of the Glasgow Coma Scale: The final score is made by the combined scores of the three components together (total ranging from 3 to 15) and the score of each tested component separately at the time of assessment (example: patient with Eyes = 2, Verbal = 3 and Motor = 4 is given a total score of 9 and designated as "GCS 9 = E2, V3, M4").

47.1.2 Is the Head Injury Open (Penetrating Injury)?

- A penetrating head injury involves a breach of the dura mater.

– A fracture of the base of the skull may clinically manifest in the form of cerebrospinal fluid or blood drainage from the nose (rhinorrhea) or the ear (otorrhea).

47.1.3 Are There Any Associated Multiple Traumatic Injuries (Polytrauma Patient)

The patient should be carefully assessed for any associated injuries:

- Internal and/or external hemorrhage, which has a pejorative prognosis for a patient with head trauma, should be compensated.
- Intra-thoracic and intra-abdominal injuries.
- Limbs, spine, and pelvis fractures.
- Cervical spine injury with systematic X-rays and a CT scan in case of doubt.

47.1.4 Was There Any Brain Injury Prior to the Current Trauma?

- Pre-existing or previous brain damage has a pejorative prognosis effect on brain function.
- It is important to investigate and take a detailed past history for:
  - Drug overdose,
  - Alcoholism,
  - Epilepsy,
  - Previous head trauma,
  - Psychiatric conditions.

47.2 Subsequent to the Above Assessment and Investigation, the ER Physician Should Be Able to Distinguish the Following

- **Severe head trauma**
  - Glasgow Coma Score ≤7,
  - Loss of consciousness for more than 6 h,
  - Amnesia lasting for more than 24 h,
  - Presence or absence of focal signs,
  - Presence or absence of associated traumatic injuries (polytrauma).

Patients with severe head trauma should benefit from an urgent **brain CT scan** and be transferred under the care of a specialized neurosurgical reanimation team.

- **Moderate head trauma:** Glasgow Coma Score 9–12.

The patient should be admitted for observation to a facility with specialized reanimation and neurosurgical teams.

- **Minor head trauma**
  - Glasgow Coma Score >12,
  - Absence of focal signs,
  - Initial loss of consciousness lasting for less than 20 min,
  - Amnesia lasting for less than 24 h.

Patients with minor head trauma should be admitted for *skull radiographs and observation*. If a fracture is present, or if the patient experiences clinical aggravation with symptoms of intracranial hypertension (such as somnolence, fatigue, headaches, nausea and vomiting, tinnitus, loss of peripheral vision, etc.), then an *urgent CT scan* and specialized neurosurgical consultation should be requested.

- **Minor head trauma with focal signs**

Patients with minor head trauma and focal signs should undergo an *urgent CT scan* and receive a specialized neurosurgical consultation.

- **Open or penetrating head trauma**

Patients with open head trauma should be transferred to the care of a specialized neurosurgical team, regardless of the degree of severity indicated by the GCS.

47.3 Particular Presentations of Severe Head Trauma

47.3.1 Extradural (or Epidural) Hematoma

- It is considered a vital neurosurgical emergency.
- It corresponds to a collection of blood between the inner table of the skull and the outer aspect of the dura mater.
- It is usually caused by a fracture of the skull that unduces injury to the middle meningeal artery.
- It is characterized by the presence of a **free interval of consciousness** between the accident and the occurrence or aggravation of the neurologic symptoms.
- The free interval of consciousness may follow an initial brief episode of loss of consciousness due to the accident. This is followed by clinical aggravation of neurologic symptoms and impairment of consciousness and vigilance, usually associated with disturbances of the pupillary reflexes.
- In pediatric patients, severe headaches and brain edema on the initial CT scan (which should be requested even for minimal doubt) are alarming. These symptoms necessitate close observation by a specialized neurosurgical team,

regardless of the clinical neurologic assessment, even if the neurologic examination is normal.

47.3.2 Acute Subdural Hematoma

- It corresponds to a collection of blood between the inner aspect of the dura mater and the outer aspect of the arachnoid mater within the brain's meningeal layers.
- It is usually caused by rupture of the bridging veins located in the subdural space.
- It is commonly associated with injury to the brain cortex. It therefore has a severe prognosis.
- It is clinically manifested by an immediate and severe disturbance of vigilance and level of consciousness. An initial free interval of consciousness is rare.
- Requires urgent attention from a specialized neurosurgical team.

In Summary

- ER physicians often face many different types of head and brain injuries, a few of them require specialized neurosurgical care.
- Special attention is necessary to avoid misdiagnosing or underestimating head injuries susceptible to *secondary aggravation,* such as extradural hematomas.
- Some clinical presentations are misleading, and any misjudgment by the ER physician may lead to medical error with serious medico-legal burden.
- A detailed history and careful systematic clinical examination, along *with appropriate radiographic and CT assessments*, are crucial for minimizing the risk of diagnostic errors.

48 Spine Trauma

Signs and symptoms of spine injury may be limited to localized pain and muscle contracture. Confirmation of a vertebral injury is based on radiographic assessment.

48.1 Radiographs of Normal Cervical Spine

48.1.1 Standard Views

1. **Anteroposterior view** (Fig. 48.1)
   (a) The spinous processes must be aligned in the midline.
   (b) The spaces between the spinous processes are even.
   (c) The uncinated processes and lateral masses must be aligned on both sides (right and left).
   (d) The shadows of the larynx and trachea are aligned in the midline.
2. **Lateral view** (Fig. 48.2)
   (a) Is the most informative and useful for diagnosing cervical spine traumatic injuries.
   (b) Consists of a strict lateral projection of the cervical spine without rotation.
   (c) Must include the C7-T1 junction.
   (d) The normal radiographic landmarks correspond to:
      - A harmonious lordosis of the entire cervical spine, characterized by three smoothly aligned curves:
        – The anterior border of the vertebral bodies,
        – The posterior border of the vertebral bodies,
        – The spino-laminar line (at the base of the spinous processes).
      - The predental space should measure ≤3 mm in adult and ≤5 mm in children, (defined as the space between the posterior border of the anterior ring of C1 and the anterior margin of the odontoid process of C2).
      - Regular and even intervertebral disc spaces.
      - Regular inter-spinous spaces.

D. Saragaglia, A. Hassan Chamseddine, *Traumatology for the Emergency Doctor*, https://doi.org/10.1007/978-3-031-63196-2_48

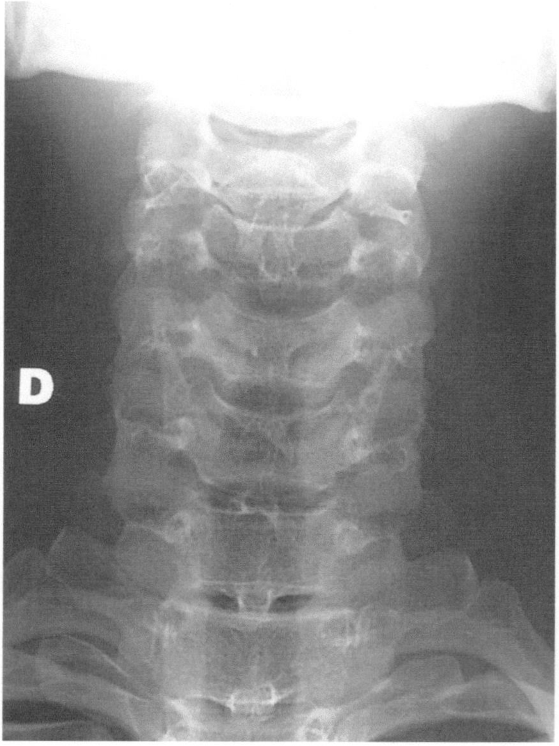

Fig. 48.1 AP cervical spine radiograph showing a "normal" image

- Articular facets that are well visualized and perfectly superimposed.
- The shadow of the pre-vertebral soft tissues must be as follows:
  - C1–C4 $\leq$7 mm,
  - Below C4 $\leq$22 mm (less than the width of the vertebral body at this level).

3. **Odontoid view (open mouth view)**
   (a) The distance between the vertical edge of the odontoid process and the edge of lateral mass should be equal on both sides,
   (b) The borders of C1 and C2 should be aligned.
4. **Oblique views (right and left)** (Fig. 48.3)
   (a) Regular alignment of the vertebral bodies,
   (b) Regular and harmonious aspect of the intervertebral foraminae.

48.1.2 CT Scan

- Is mandatory when radiographic images are doubtful.
- Should involve a complete assessment of the soft tissues and bony structures.
- Should include coronal, axial, and sagittal views, with 3-D reconstruction.

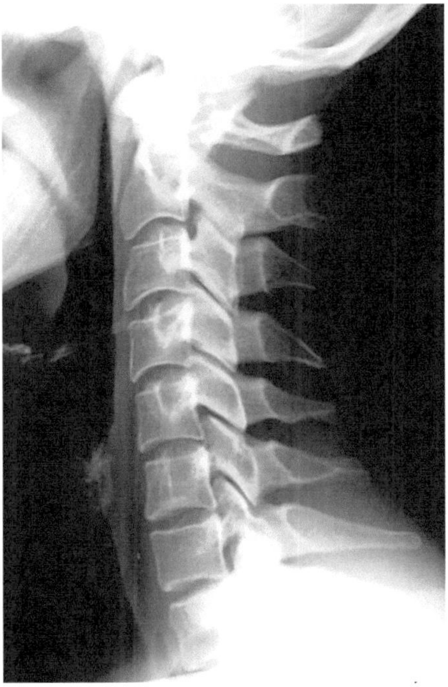

Fig. 48.2 Lateral cervical spine radiograph showing a "normal" image

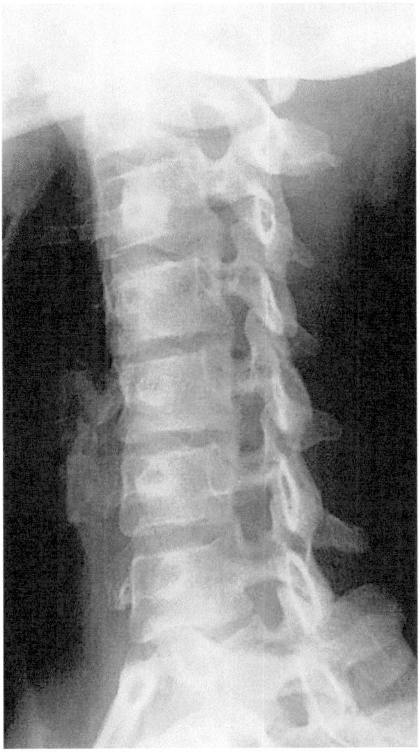

Fig. 48.3 Oblique cervical spine radiograph showing a "normal" image

48.2 Radiographs of Normal Thoraco-Lumbar Spine

48.2.1 Standard Views

- **Anteroposterior view** (Fig. 48.4)
  - Straight vertical alignment of the vertebral bodies and spinous processes with no evidence of translation.
  - Regular spaces between the spinous processes.
  - A regular increase in the height of the vertebral bodies from proximal to distal.
  - Vertical alignment of the pedicles, with regular interpedicular spaces and no evidence of rotation.
  - Integrity of the transverse processes in the lumbar spine.
- **Lateral view** (Fig. 48.5)
  - Presence of the normal physiological thoracic kyphosis and lumbar lordosis.
  - Harmonious alignment of the vertebral bodies with smooth curves along the anterior and posterior borders.
  - Regular rectangular shape of the vertebral bodies.
  - Integrity of the posterior vertebral wall for each vertebra.
  - Regular inter-spinous spaces.

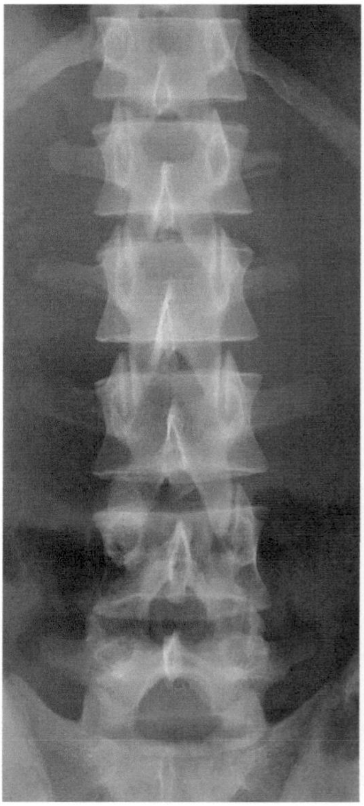

Fig. 48.4 AP lumbar spine radiograph showing a "normal" image

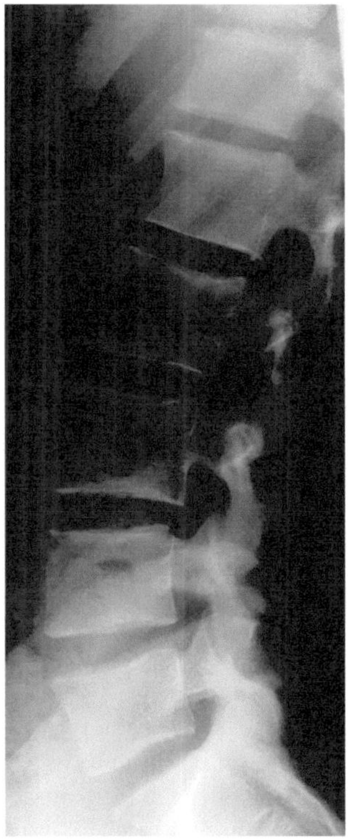

Fig. 48.5 Lateral lumbar spine radiograph showing a "normal" image

- Integrity of the intervertebral disc spaces, with a regular mild increase from L1–L2 through L4–L5, and a minimally narrower L5–S1 compared to L4–L5.

48.2.2 CT Scan

- Is mandatory when radiographic images are doubtful.
- Should involve a complete assessment of the soft tissues and bony structures.
- Should include coronal, axial, and sagittal views, with 3-D reconstruction.

48.3 Patho-Anatomic Types of Spine Injuries

Three patho-anatomic types of injuries are recognized: disco-ligamentous, disco-corporeal, and mixed injuries.

48.3.1 Disco-Ligamentous Injuries

- They are secondary to horizontal shear trauma.
- They include *sprains, dislocations, and fracture–dislocations*.
- They cause rupture of the intervertebral ligaments and disc between two adjacent vertebrae, with or without bony avulsion.
- They result in "horizontal" acute and *chronic instability*.
- They usually fail to achieve spontaneous healing.
- They occur more commonly in the cervical spine (75%) and are rare in the lumbar spine (6%).

48.3.2 Disco-Corporeal Injuries

- They are secondary to axial compression trauma.
- They involve vertebral body crushing by the intervertebral disc, which penetrates the superior end-plate of the adjacent inferior vertebra, resulting in a variable degree of vertebral bursting.
- They result in "vertical" instability with impairment of the vertebral posture and balance.
- They include anterior marginal fractures, corporeal compression fractures, and comminuted fractures ("burst fractures").
- They occur more commonly in the lumbar spine (76%) and are rare in the cervical spine.

48.3.3 Mixed Injuries

- They combine the two previous modes of injuries and instabilities.
- They correspond to the *"tear drop fracture"* in the cervical spine and *the Chance fracture* in the lumbar spine.
- The thoracic spine is a common site of "mixed injuries" due to its reduced mobility compared to the cervical and lumbar spines.

48.4 Neurologic Examination of a Patient with Spine Trauma

It should be simple and systematic to evaluate the level of the spinal cord injury and determine whether it is complete. It includes:

- Clinical confirmation of spinal cord injury, excluding any cranial nerve deficits and intracranial lesions,
- Functional assessment of the muscles of the upper and lower limbs, on their innervation by the brachial plexus (C5-T1) and lumbo-sacral plexus (L2-S1), respectively,

- Assessment of the objective cutaneous sensation of the trunk and limbs using various tests to localize the site and level of the neurologic injury. The results of the assessment are then reported on a body map form,
- Assessment of the osteotendinous reflexes (i.e., Biceps: C5, C6; Brachio-radialis: C6; Triceps: C7; Patellar: L4; Achilles tendon: S1).
- Examination of the perineal area for evaluation of,
  - Cutaneous sensation,
  - Anal reflex, which is tested by introducing a gloved finger into the anus and asking the patient to squeeze it.
- **Determination of the ASIA scale** (American Spinal Injury Association) based on the physical examination for evaluation of the grade of neurologic impairment as follows:
  - *Complete spinal cord injury*: Absence of sensory and motor functions and reflexes for the injured metameric level, resulting in either paraplegia or tetraplegia. Note: any patient with paralysis of the lower limbs and loss of interosseous muscles function of the hands is considered **"tetraplegic."**
  - *Incomplete spinal cord injury:* Persistence of one or more conscious and/or voluntary neurologic functions below the level of injury, such as preservation of sensory function in a specific cutaneous territory or the perineal area, or voluntary contraction of a particular muscle group.
  - *Cauda equina syndrome,* secondary to spinal injury below the L2 level is characterized by severe low back pain radiating to the lower limbs, saddle anesthesia or paresthesia (in the perineum, external genitalia, and peri-anal area), and urinary bladder and fecal incontinence or loss of control.

Following the history and physical examination, the diagnosis of spinal cord injury is confirmed by **MRI**, depending on accessibility.

48.5 Pitfalls of Cervical Spine Trauma

48.5.1 Upper Cervical Spine: C1–C2

- **Jefferson fracture** (Fig. 48.6a, b)
  - It involves a fracture of both the anterior and posterior arches of the C1 vertebra also known as the "Atlas."
  - It usually results from an axial load mechanism, such as diving headfirst into shallow water in a marine environment or swimming pool.
  - AP radiographs of the cervical spine show abnormal widening of the space between lateral masses of C1.
  - CT scan axial cuts show the fracture line and its location and reveal any possible displacement.
  - The typical treatment is conservative, involving immobilization with a hard collar.

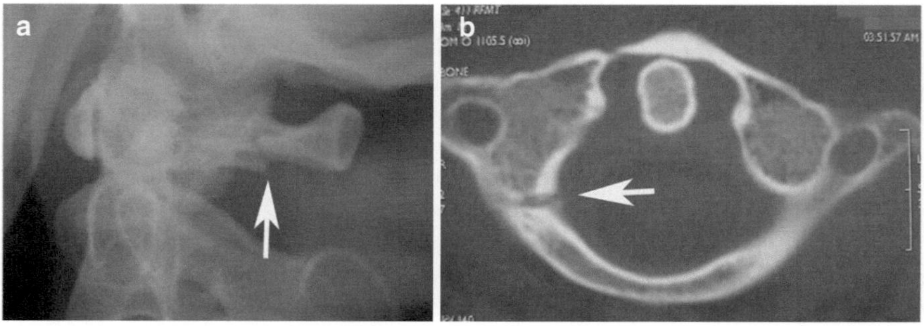

Fig. 48.6 (**a**) Lateral X-ray of an upper cervical spine showing a Jefferson fracture of the C1 vertebra. (**b**) Axial cut CT scan showing a Jefferson fracture of the C1 vertebra

- **Fractures of the odontoid process of C2** (Fig. 48.7)
  - They involve a fracture of the "Dens," also known as the Odontoid process of the C2 vertebra, which is also called the "Axis".
  - They can result from various mechanisms, such as sudden forward and backward movements, hyperflexion, or hyperextension of the neck.
  - They are usually visualized on the AP "open mouth" radiographic view.
  - *CT scans with 3D reconstruction* have supplanted plain radiographs for diagnosis and fracture pattern identification.
  - Three types of fractures are usually described:

    Type I fractures involve the tip of the odontoid process; they are usually stable and typically require only simple immobilization.

    Type II fractures involve the base of the odontoid process; they are the most common type, usually unstable with a high incidence of nonunion, and often require surgical treatment for stabilization.

    Type III fractures extend into the body of the C2 vertebra and may be stable or unstable.
- **"Bi-pedicular" fractures of C2** (Fig. 48.8)
  - They involve fractures of the isthmus of the C2 vertebra, commonly known as "*Hangman's fracture.*"
  - The most common mechanism is a violent hyperextension with concomitant distraction of the neck, such as during judicial hanging.
  - Other mechanisms include:

    Sudden aggressive hyperextension of the neck during abrupt deceleration, where the face or the chin of the victim powerfully strikes an object while the neck remains extended, such as in a frontal vehicle collision during a road traffic accident.

    Diving accidents, among others.
  - As the fracture involves the two pedicles of the C2 vertebra, it tends to enlarge the spinal canal dimensions at that level, usually without signs of neurologic impairment.

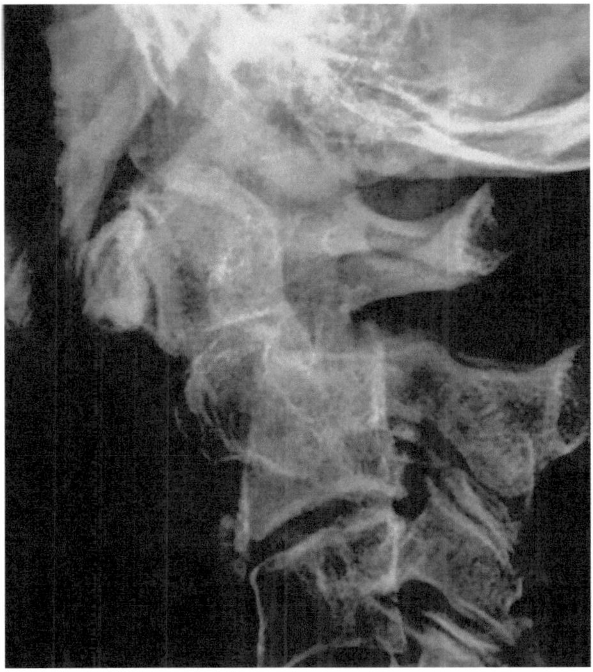

Fig. 48.7 Lateral X-ray of an upper cervical spine showing a displaced fracture of the odontoid process

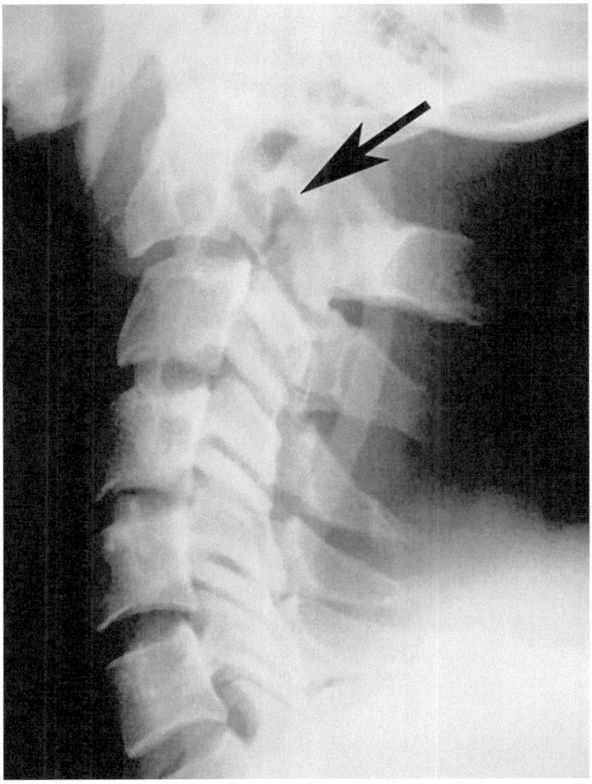

Fig. 48.8 Lateral cervical spine X-ray showing a "bi-pedicular" fracture of the C2 vertebra

- Treatment options are:

  Conservative, using hard collar immobilization, when the C2–C3 intervertebral disc is intact.

  Surgical, involving C2–C3 arthrodesis, when the C2–C3 disc is disrupted, as indicated by the disturbance of the C2–C3 disc space on lateral radiographs.

48.5.2 Lower Cervical Spine: C3–C7

1. **Disco-ligamentous injuries** (75%)
   (a) *Neck Sprains*
   - Refer to an injury of the intervertebral stabilizer ligamentous system of the cervical spine.
   - May induce acute or chronic cervical spine instability with variable degrees of severity.
   - Radiographic assessment is key to diagnosis.
     - Simple radiographs show anterior flexion of the cervical segment, proximal to the level of injury (Fig. 48.9).
     - *Dynamic radiographs in flexion-extension,* performed after a few days of treatment with painkillers, NSAID's, and muscle relaxants, reveal localized intervertebral instability with anterior flexion of the proximal cervical segment.
     - *Note*: each person has one intervertebral disc space that is more mobile than the others, and this varies with age.

   (b) *Dislocations and fractures of the cervical facets*

   They represent a spectrum of injuries that includes:
   - *Unilateral facet dislocation* (Fig. 48.10)
     - The radiographic presentation may be ambiguous, and the diagnosis can be missed on the lateral view radiograph.
     - It is better visualized on the oblique views.
     - It involves encroachment of the inferior facet of the superior vertebra into the foramen on one side, commonly resulting in neck pain with unilateral radiculopathy.
   - *Bilateral facet dislocation*
     - Radiographic diagnosis is obvious on the lateral view, showing vertebral dislocation, or displacement of more than 50% of the vertebral width.
     - It commonly results in significant injury to the spinal cord.
   - *Facet fractures*
     - They can be unilateral or bilateral.
     - Involvement of the superior facet of the inferior vertebra is more common.

   (c) *Treatment of these injuries is typically surgical, involving arthrodesis of the affected intervertebral disc space after reduction of the displacement.*

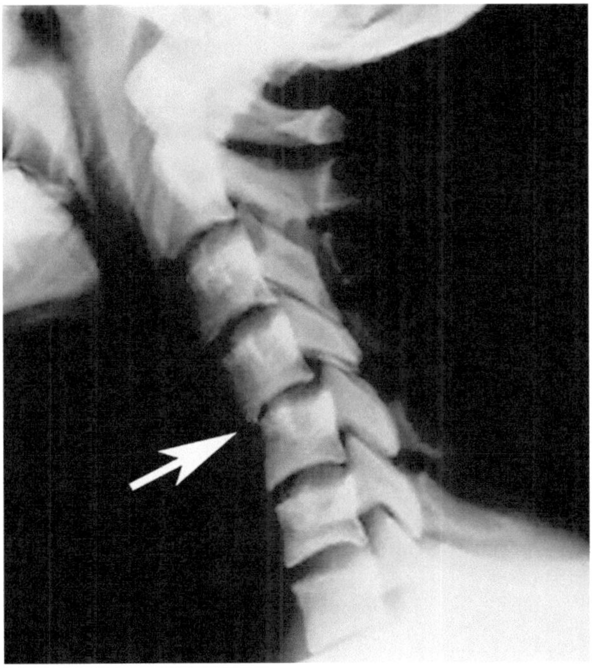

Fig. 48.9 Cervical spine simple lateral X-ray showing an anterior flexion of the cervical segment proximal to C4–C5 level, indicative of C4–C5 disco-ligamentous severe sprain injury

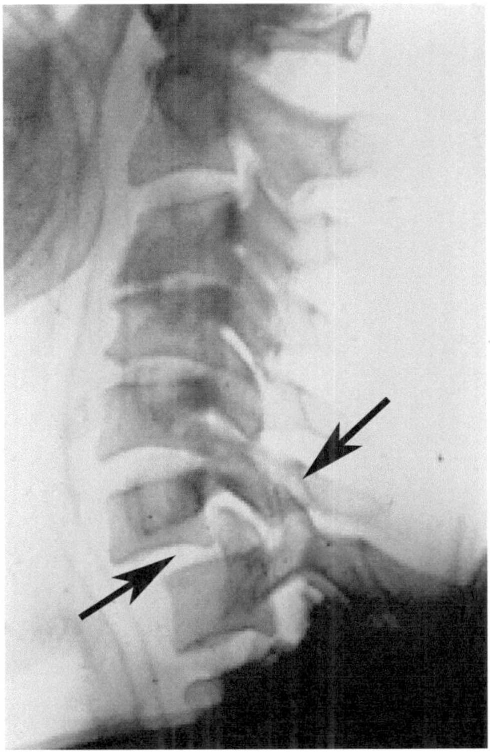

Fig. 48.10 Lateral cervical spine X-ray showing a C6–C7 unilateral facet dislocation

2. **Disco-corporeal injuries** (5%)
   (a) They may manifest in the form of compression fractures or burst-type fractures.
   (b) The diagnosis is evident on simple radiographs, showing widening of the interpedicular distance on the AP view and retropulsion of vertebral bony fragment into the spinal canal on the lateral view.
   (c) The CT scan provides a satisfactory estimation of the vertebral injury and any bony impingement on the spinal cord.
   (d) The treatment commonly involves surgery, such as corpectomy (excision of the fractured vertebra), along with bone grafting and arthrodesis of the affected level.
3. **Mixed injuries** (20%)
   (a) Are associated with the "*tear drop fracture,*" which is almost always located at the C5 vertebra (Fig. 48.11).
   (b) The "tear drop fracture" is an unstable fracture that commonly causes spinal cord injury.
   (c) This fracture pattern puts the cervical spine in a flexion position, which poses a threat to the spinal cord.

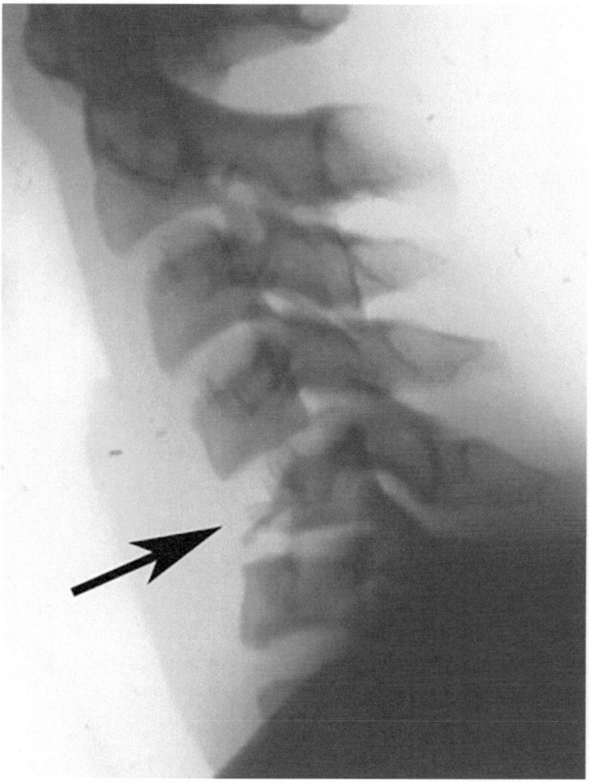

Fig. 48.11 Lateral cervical spine X-ray showing a C5 "tear drop fracture"

(d) It involves fracture-avulsion of the antero-inferior corner of the vertebral body, along with an associated tear of the superior and/or inferior intervertebral disc.
(e) The mechanism of injury is usually diving headfirst into shallow water, such as in a marine environment or swimming pool, or a fall onto the apex of the head.
(f) Treatment is surgical, involving arthrodesis with or without corpectomy of the affected vertebra (C5).

The majority of the aforementioned injuries are unstable and pose a threat to the spinal cord. The use of *hard collar immobilization in a neutral neck position* is crucial from the first moment of collection-evacuation. It remains essential during transport, physical evaluation, and radiographic assessment of injured patients. Reduction maneuvers are allowed only in a specialized medico-surgical unit, under strict neurologic observation, and in the immediate pre-operative period.

4. A special note is warranted for patients with pre-existing degenerative cervical spine conditions.
   (a) Commonly these are elderly patients over 60–65 years,
   (b) Known to have severe cervical spine spondylosis (arthrosis/arthritis) with borderline spinal canal dimensions and spinal cord impingement, yet without neurological clinical expression,
   (c) Minimal trauma, such as a simple fall, may decompensate the previously precarious neurological situation, resulting in the occurrence of tetraparesis (quadriparesis) or tetraplegia (quadriplegia),
   (d) Transfer to the care of a specialized team is mandatory.

48.6 Pitfalls of Thoracic Spine Trauma

The thoracic spine has minimal range of mobility as compared to the cervical and lumbar spines. It can be subject to different types of injury:

48.6.1 Compression or Wedge Fractures

- They are induced by a flexion mechanism or axial compression trauma.
- They are usually stable.
- They involve minimal or moderate compression (loss of height) of the anterior border of the vertebra.
- The posterior vertebral arch remains intact, and the spinal canal is not compromised.
- Treatment is usually conservative, involving the use of a thoraco-lumbar brace and a rehabilitation program to strengthen the paravertebral muscles.

48.6.2 Mixed Injuries

- They combine significant vertebral compression in one or more vertebrae with fractures of the posterior arch, which contribute to progressive instability, worsening the kyphotic displacement over a few weeks.
- These injuries require a *CT scan* and, in most cases, a specialist's consultation to perform posterior osteosynthesis on several levels.

The following remarks should be noted:

- Injuries to the spinal cord in the thoracic region are often severe, typically resulting in permanent complete paraplegia,
- The cervico-thoracic junction and the upper thoracic spine are not well visualized on standard plain radiographs due to image superposition with the shoulder girdles. Therefore, a *CT scan* is highly recommended for exploring these areas.

48.7 Pitfalls of Lumbar Spine Trauma

The lumbar spine is a mobile and load bearing segment. The thoraco-lumbar junction is a fulcrum zone of mobility (between the fixed thoracic spine and the mobile lumbar spine); it is therefore often involved in spinal injuries, especially T12–L1–L2.

48.7.1 Disco-Corporeal Injuries

They correspond to the most frequent injuries (76%). The severity of lesion of a given vertebra regularly follows the energy of the trauma received by the vertebra according to a reproducible scheme.

- **Anterior marginal fractures**
  - Are regularly benign.
  - The vertebral static posture remains unmodified.
  - Treatment is usually conservative (functional).
- **Anterior compression fractures** without involvement of the posterior vertebral wall (Fig. 48.12a, b)
  - The spinal canal remains intact.
  - Treatment is either conservative or surgical according to the amount of compression or loss of the anterior vertebral wall height (local vertebral and regional angulations), the patient's age and physical condition and activities.
- **Burst fractures**
  - The entire vertebral body is crushed.
  - The injury pattern typically includes fracture of the posterior arch, and displaced postero-superior *bony fragment into the spinal canal* with possible spinal cord injury.

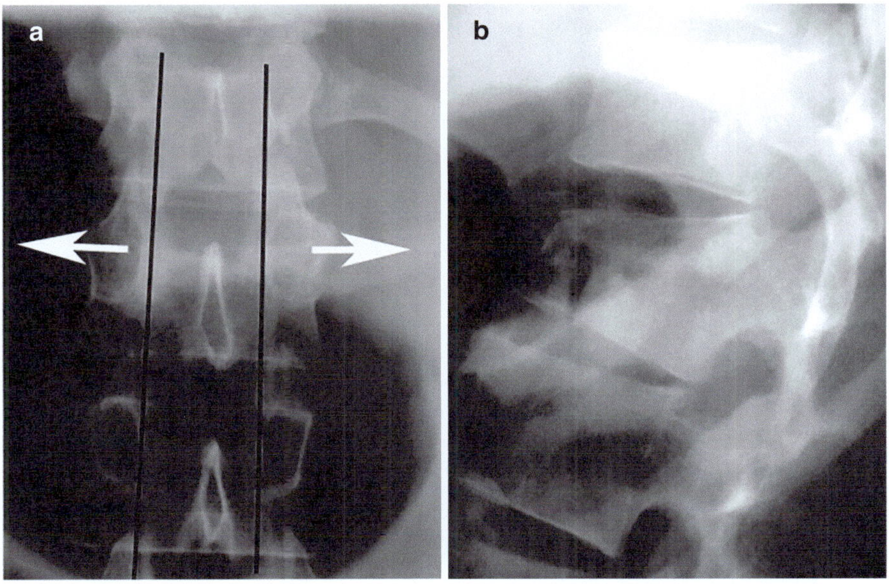

Fig. 48.12 (**a**) AP spot T12-L2 spine X-ray showing a widened interpedicular space of the L1 vertebra. (**b**) Lateral spot T12-L2 spine X-ray of the same patient as shown in (**a**) showing a cuneiform anterior compression-fracture with preservation of the posterior wall of the L1 vertebra

- CT scan assessment is mandatory.
- Surgical treatment is often indicated (decompression with internal fixation).

48.7.2 Disco-Ligamentous Injuries

- Are rare (6%).
- May manifest in the form of intervertebral dislocation, a very painful and unstable injury with an important neurological threat (Fig. 48.13).
- Treatment is surgical (reduction with internal fixation).

48.7.3 Mixed Injuries

- Represented by the **Chance fracture** (18%).
- The injury pattern includes vertebral body fracture-compression with horizontal fracture of the posterior arch involving fracture of the spinous process, facet joints (or articular processes) and pedicles. It corresponds to a posterior transverse "opening" of the affected vertebra (Fig. 48.14).
- Treatment is surgical (reduction with internal fixation).

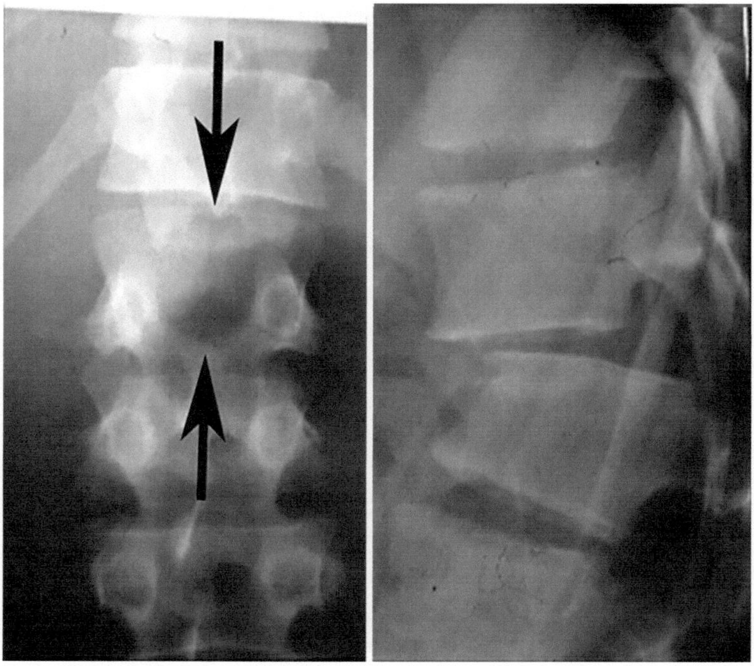

Fig. 48.13 AP and lateral X-rays showing a lumbar dislocation (T12-L1). Note the widening of the T12-L1 inter-spinous space on the AP view

Fig. 48.14 CT scan reconstruction of a chance fracture

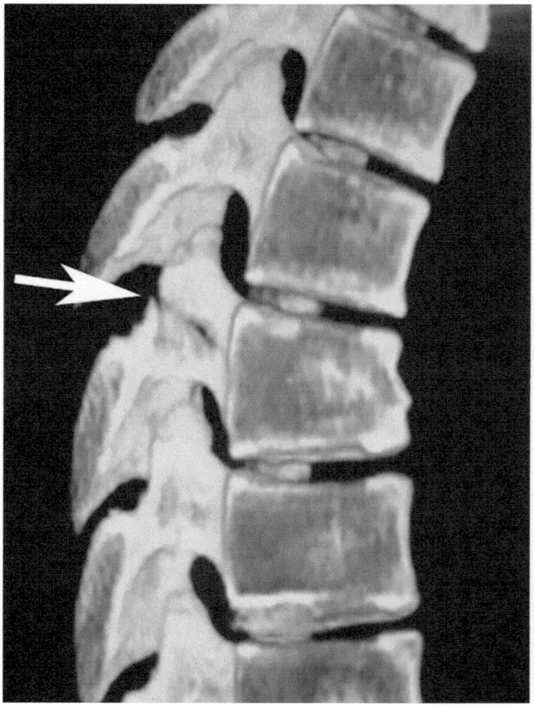

48.8 Fractures of the Sacrum and Coccyx

48.8.1 Isolated Fractures of the Sacrum

- Are usually secondary to posterior direct trauma.
- May occur in osteoporotic elderly patients (insufficiency fracture).
- Can occur in young patients after a fall from a height onto their buttocks.
- The fracture line is horizontal and typically runs through the third or fourth sacral foramina.
- Radiographic diagnosis can be easily obscured by the presence of intestinal gas.
- *A CT scan* is a must for an adequate diagnosis, and in case of doubt.
- Conservative treatment,
  - Is indicated for undisplaced fractures and for minimally displaced fractures (<1 cm) without neurologic impairment.
  - It involves bed rest for 3 weeks followed by partial weight bearing as tolerated.
- Surgical treatment is indicated for:
  - displaced fractures after failure to reduce anterior displacement of the distal fragment with closed external maneuvers,
  - displaced fractures with soft tissue compromise,
  - fractures associated with a neurologic deficit.

48.8.2 Fractures of the Coccyx

- Are rare.
- Difficult radiographic diagnosis (to differentiate from a "hook-shaped coccyx").
- Diagnosis is based on history (fall in a seated position), physical examination (pain, bruise, swelling), and tenderness on rectal examination.
- Treatment
  - Conservative treatment is almost always indicated,
    - Use of a "donut" cushion to reduce pressure in a seated position,
    - Use of high-fiber foods and/or "laxatives" to prevent constipation,
    - Use of painkillers with or without NSAIDs.
  - Surgical treatment is rarely indicated,
    - For severe and/or persistent coccydynia (even after fracture healing),
    - Consists of coccygectomy (excision of the coccyx).

MIX
Papier aus verantwortungsvollen Quellen
Paper from responsible sources
FSC® C105338

If you have any concerns about our products,
you can contact us on
ProductSafety@springernature.com

In case Publisher is established outside the EU,
the EU authorized representative is:
Springer Nature Customer Service Center GmbH
Europaplatz 3, 69115 Heidelberg, Germany

Printed by Libri Plureos GmbH
in Hamburg, Germany